PSYCHOLOGICAL ASPECTS OF A FIRST PREGNANCY AND EARLY POSTNATAL ADAPTATION

Psychological Aspects
of a First Pregnancy
and Early Postnatal Adaptation

Editors:

Pauline M. Shereshefsky, M.S.S.W.

Leon J. Yarrow, Ph.D.

Raven Press, Publishers ▪ New York

Made in the United States of America

International Standard Book Number 0-911216-65-0
Library of Congress Catalog Card Number 73-87877

Preparation and publication of the present volume was made possible by the National Institute of Child Health and Human Development (Contract No. NIH-72-C-259).

Foreword

This monograph has long been needed by those in obstetrics, pediatrics, nursing, psychiatry, and social sciences who deal continuously with the problems associated with pregnancy, family dynamics, and, ultimately, infant and parent well-being. Its emphasis is upon the behavioral rather than the biological facets of pregnancy. This is most encouraging, for research relevant to infant morbidity and mortality had previously emphasized the physiological and pathological aspects of pregnancy outcome, neonatal adaptation, and infant well-being. The impact of behavioral aspects has been neglected.

The study sought to draw expertise from multiple medical and paramedical specialties, with close collaboration with the obstetrical management of the pregnant women, their husbands, and their offspring. Of great significance is the obscure barrier between patient and obstetrician about "extramedical concerns" that requires skillful and emphatic communication with the patient. The effects of these concerns on the ultimate outcome of the pregnancy were significant.

This study has laid to rest some previous dogma related to psychiatric pathology during pregnancy; it has, however, raised questions of how intrapsychic conflicts, disharmonies of marriage, and previous maternal-mother relations can be adjusted during nine months to optimize the outcome of pregnancy and infant performance.

The results presented here leave open alternate interpretations; however, the data are there—exhaustively collected, critically analyzed, and highly significant. The fact that this volume confines itself to "normal" primigravidas from a middle-class urban population should not detract from the significance or motivation for reexamination of the traditional aspects of ante- and postpartum care. It should, in fact, stimulate further inquiry or questions concerned with the psychodynamics of pregnancy and maternal infant relationships.

The results of this study are especially provocative in their implications for the care of pregnant women. Just as there are populations at risk by reason of physiological vulnerabilities, there are women at risk because of psychosocial problems. Much needs to be done to develop techniques to identify, early in pregnancy, women with psychosocial hazards and to develop appropriate services to ameliorate these hazards.

Eileen G. Hasselmeyer, Ph.D., R.N.
Director,
Perinatal Biology and Infant Mortality Branch
National Institute of Child Health and
    Human Development
National Institutes of Health

Research Staff
and Collaborators

The planning of the research design for this study and carrying out its various phases has been done by a multidisciplinary team that included the following:

PROJECT AFFILIATION   **CURRENT AFFILIATIONS**

Thomas M. Arnett, M.D.
Medical Program Administrator,
Group Health Assn., Inc.
Co-Director of Project
(1964-1968)

Consultant in Health Maintenance
   Organization Programs

Jesse F. Casey, M.D.
Principal Investigator
(March, 1963 to June, 1964)
Consulting Psychiatrist

Consultant in Psychiatry,
Mental Health Programs

Elaine Gerson, Ph.D.
Psychologist
Infant Observer

Clinical Psychologist, Private Practice

Robert D. Gillman, M.D.
Consulting Psychiatrist

Psychoanalyst,
Private Practice with Adults and Chil-
   dren;
Supervising and Training Analyst,
   Baltimore-District of Columbia
   Institute for Psychoanalysis

Rhoda S. Goodwin, M.A.
Psychologist
Infant Observer

Research Psychologist,
Psycholinguistics Department,
Mass. Institute of Technology

Nancy Kalina
Administrative Assistant

Business Executive

Henry H. Lichtenberg, M.D. (deceased)
Formerly Chief of Pediatrics,

Group Health Assn., Inc.
Pediatrician on Project
 Research Staff

Beatrice Liebenberg, A.C.S.W.   Psychiatric Social Worker, Private
Psychiatric Social Worker   Practice;
                                  Faculty, Group Therapy Training Pro-
                                     gram, Washington School of Psychiatry;
                                  Part-time Faculty, Smith College
                                     School for Social Work

Robert F. Lockman, Ph.D.   Measurement Psychologist, Center for
Consulting Statistician   Naval Analyses;
                                Instructor in Psychology,
                                   Montgomery College, Maryland

John Lukasik, M.D.   Private Practice, Obstetrics and Gyne-
Obstetrician   cology

Harold Plotsky, M.D.   Psychoanalyst in Private Practice;
Principal Investigator   Psychiatric Consultant, Episcopal
(June, 1964 to December, 1966)   Center for Children;
Consulting Psychiatrist   Instructor, Washington Psychoanalytic
                                Institute

Josiah Sacks, M.D.   Private Practice, Obstetrics and Gyne-
Obstetrician   cology;
                          Clinical Instructor, George Washington
                             University Hospital Medical School

Sara Saltzman, M.A.   Clinical Psychologist, Private Practice;
Clinical Psychologist   Instructor, Washington School of Psy-
                             chiatry;
                          Guest Lecturer, Washington
                             Psychoanalytic Institute

Melvin Sandmeyer, M.D.   Private Practice, Obstetrics and Gyne-
Obstetrician   cology;
                          Assistant Clinical Professor, Obstetrics
                             and Gynecology, George Washington
                             University Medical School

Toby Schneidman   Psychological Consultant, Mobile
Psychologist   Health Unit Project, Children's Hospital
Infant Observer   of Washington, D.C.

Benjamin A. Shaver, M.D.   Pediatrician, Group Health Assn., Inc.
Pediatrician on Project
 Research Staff

Pauline M. Shereshefsky, M.S.S.W.
Principal Investigator
(December, 1966 to July, 1968)
Psychiatric Social Worker

Psychiatric Social Worker, Private Practice

Louise Stone Schwartz, M.S.W.
Psychiatric Social Worker

Psychiatric Social Worker, Private Practice;
Psychiatric Social Work, Counseling, Annunciation School, Washington, D.C.;
Faculty, Washington School of Psychiatry

Leon J. Yarrow, Ph.D.
Research Consultant

Chief, Social and Behavioral Sciences Branch, NICHD

Since completion of the project, further analyses of selected aspects of the data were undertaken by Research Associates in the Social and Behavioral Sciences Branch, NICHD; their studies are included in this volume. They are:

Walter A. Brown, M.D.

Assistant Professor of Psychiatry, Yale University School of Medicine

Gordon W. Keating, M.D.

Fellow in Child Psychiatry, University of Washington School of Medicine

Tracey Manning, M.A.

In process of completing her doctoral dissertation, Psychology Department, Catholic University of America

Acknowledgments

Financial support for the research reported here was through an extramural grant from the National Institute of Mental Health (NIMH Project No. 5-R01 MH 14733-05) for the first years of operation of the study. As the project progressed, a wealth of data became available bearing on the more theoretical aspects of the study, namely the psychological factors in pregnancy and early postnatal adaptation. Funds provided under contract from the National Institute of Child Health and Human Development made possible the analyses of these data and the preparation of a number of separate reports covering analyses which otherwise would not have been undertaken (NICHD Contract No. PH43-68-642). Through its extramural grant program, the Perinatal and Infant Mortality Branch of NICHD has also made possible the preparation and publication of the present volume (Contract No. NIH-72-C-259).

The research presented here was initially planned with the late Henry H. Lichtenberg, M.D., then Medical Program Administrator and Chief of Pediatrics, Group Health Association, and subsequently (until his death in 1966) pediatrician member of the research team. His vision of the preventive potential in medical group practice played a crucial role in enabling the project plan to become a reality.

We are deeply indebted to the patients who accepted participation in the project. In providing data generously and sharing feelings and deeply personal experiences, they, especially, enabled the project plan to become a reality.

The initial stimulus for undertaking a study on the psychology of pregnancy was provided by the work of Gerald Caplan, M.D., Chairman of the Laboratory of Community Psychiatry at Harvard University; his studies of pregnant women were initiated in Jerusalem, Israel, as early as 1950.

For their imaginative insight and dedication to broad mental health objectives, which were important determinants in the decisions leading to sponsorship of this undertaking, we are greatly indebted to Caroline Chandler, M.D., E. James Lieberman, M.D. (both formerly of the

Center for Studies of Child and Family Health, NIMH), and Eileen G. Hasselmeyer, Ph.D., Chief of Perinatal and Infant Mortality Branch, NICHD.

Dr. Dorothy S. Huntington, now Coordinator of Preschool Programs, Community Mental Health Center, Peninsula Hospital and Medical Center, in California, has shared her knowledge of the field most generously, advising us in the early stages of planning the research and reviewing this final result with empathetic understanding of limitations and fine, discriminating perception of goals and issues.

We acknowledge with gratitude the specialized consultation made available from other investigators in related research areas, especially Howard A. Moss, Ph.D., and Robert G. Ryder, Ph.D., of the Child Research Branch, NIMH; and the group of psychoanalysts of the Washington School of Psychiatry who were simultaneously conducting a study on the emotional aspects of pregnancy: Edith V. Weigert, M.D., Naomi K. Wenner, M.D., Mabel B. Cohen, M.D., John M. Fearing, M.D., Robert G. Kvarnes, M.D., and Edward M. Ohaneson, M.D.

Within Group Health Association, the project made considerable demands on the medical and nursing staffs of the Obstetrics and Pediatrics Department of GHA for their active help in the research program; special thanks is extended to them for their fine cooperation.

We take this opportunity to express appreciation for the significant contribution made by each member of the research team.

Mrs. Nancy Kalina, Administrative Assistant, had the interest and capacity to learn the language of each discipline in the multidisciplinary research team in order to perform tasks specific to the needs of each member of the team. In the preparation of this volume, we are especially indebted to her and Mrs. Christine Sutton for their painstaking work and alert attention to detail.

Some years before he became associated with the National Institute of Child Health and Human Development, Dr. Leon Yarrow accepted an invitation from GHA to design the research plan for the project, and was subsequently prevailed upon to provide overall consultation to the staff. We are grateful that NICHD freed his time sufficiently to enable him to share the editorship for this volume as well. More than any other single person, he has provided leadership, knowledge, and continuity of theoretical approach.

Thomas M. Arnett, M.D.
Medical Program Administrator, GHA, 1961-1972, and Co-Director of Project, 1964-1968

Pauline M. Shereshefsky
Principal Investigator, 1966-1968

Preface

There could hardly be a more auspicious moment for the appearance of this monograph. Both its contents and the process by which it came to be are now at the forefront of attention in the fields of human service and social science. That the project from which it grew was conceived a decade ago is a tribute to the vision of its founders.

This is a good example of applied research, involving fine clinicians willing to be accountable in detail, and fine researchers willing to bend their instruments to measure the awesome and commonplace reality of first pregnancy. The project is also a model of cooperation between health and mental health professionals. Obstetricians, pediatricians, and mental health workers all have a place in the lives of young primigravidous couples, but rarely have they been so well integrated. Thirdly, this is a model of a preventive service: theoretically sound, sensibly carried out, carefully evaluated.

The results are by no means free of problems, and much in the interpretation will depend upon the reader. The investigators would be the first to say it could be done better. But, as a result of their monumental efforts, we see that it can be done. The study comes at a time when obstetricians and pediatricians are reappraising their roles. Birth rates are down, some hospital wards are shrinking or closing, and there is time now—there always was great need—to pay attention to the emotional and counseling needs of young families.

In the decade since this project began, a revolutionary change in family formation has come about. Whereas most first pregnancies in the United States were then accidental in terms of timing, by now it appears that the majority are the result of deliberate intent—as was the case in the study population. Vital as family planning is in protecting and promoting health and mental health, there is more to be done. This project illustrates the range of resources needed to promote a level of parenthood and child development commensurate with human potential, adequate not only to survive but to master an uncertain future.

E. James Lieberman, M.D.
Mental Health Project Director
American Public Health Association

Contents

Psychological Aspects of a First Pregnancy
and Early Postnatal Adaptation.
Raven Press, New York © 1974

Chapter I
Premises and Assumptions

Pauline M. Shereshefsky

INTRODUCTION

Myth, cultural patterns, and idiosyncratic personal experience all converge in determining the individual meaning of the new experience of a first pregnancy. Anthropologists have noted the central importance that culture accords to the birth experience: "All known societies pattern the behavior of human beings involved in the process of reproduction" (Mead and Newton, 1967, p. 147). Psychoanalytic thought, at an early stage in its development, saw the meaning of childbirth as a reliving for the woman of the experience of her own birth (Rank, 1929).

The study reported in this volume deals with the psychological aspects of pregnancy and early mother-infant adaptation. During a period in which the biomedical sciences have steadily contributed a substantial body of literature on the physiology of the pregnant woman, and perhaps even more on the fetus and the infant, relatively little systematic research has been directed to an understanding of the psychodynamics of the pregnant woman and its relation to her interaction with the infant in the early postnatal period. The project described in this report was developed to enhance understanding of the psychodynamics of pregnancy and contribute to a recognition of the psychological factors in pregnancy maintenance, pregnancy outcome, and maternal-infant adaptation.

The project was conducted from 1963 to 1968 at the Group Health Association, Inc. of Washington, D.C., a medical consumer cooperative which provides obstetrical care as part of its comprehensive medical services. It was established as a demonstration project in preventive mental hygiene measures, on the premise that the mother's psychological state is one of the crucial early influences affecting infant development. An important assumption of the research was that a first pregnancy, as a major experience affecting the growth pattern of the maturing woman, is generally accompanied by some degree of stress which can be reduced by an adequately supportive emotional environment. It was hypothesized that such a supportive emotional environment could be achieved through a social work counseling service as an adjunct to the obstetrical services. A research design was built into the project to explore the psychodynamics associated with individual differences in adjustment to the pregnancy experience and early mother-infant adaptation, and to permit some evaluation of the effects of social work counseling on the course of pregnancy and on maternal adaptation.

The conclusions of earlier investigators on which this study was based centered on issues of psychodynamics and intervention, which will be set forth briefly. Data from medical and sociological studies pointing to differences in the incidence of reproductive casualty among different class groups had bearing on the selection of the sample from a middle-class group.[1]

PSYCHODYNAMICS

Several investigators (Sontag, 1944; Caplan, 1957, 1959, 1961; Bibring et al., 1961) have concluded that the mother's psychological state during pregnancy may significantly affect the fetus *in utero* and may also affect the mother's later relationship with her infant. In an exhaustive review of the research literature on psychological factors in pregnancy, Grimm, referring especially to Sontag (1944), states, "In studies conducted over a number of years...it has been demonstrated that emotional disturbances and severe fatigue in the mother during the last stage of pregnancy were associated with an increase in activity of the fetus *in utero* and disturbances such as irritability, gastrointestinal disorders, higher than average heart rate, vasomotor irritability, or changes in respiratory pattern in the newborn" (Grimm, 1967, p. 35).

In earlier studies, the fact of psychological stress was almost universally reported as accompanying a first pregnancy. Caplan (1959) sees the pregnancy period as a "biologically determined psychological crisis. During pregnancy both the intrapersonal forces in the pregnant woman and the interpersonal forces in her family are in a state of disequilibrium." In later writing, when "crisis" was more sharply defined in his conceptual framework, Caplan modified his view of pregnancy as a crisis, placing emphasis on the whole period of pregnancy as one of increased susceptibility to crises. He still sees pregnancy as a period of "altered behaviour,...of disequilibrium compared with the normal state of the family;...a period of emotional upset in the woman, and often in her husband and her other children" (Caplan, 1961, p. 65).

Bibring also conceives of pregnancy as a period of crisis and disequilibrium. She postulates that, like puberty and the menopause, pregnancy is associated with significant somatic and psychological changes. She states, "The crisis of pregnancy is basically a normal occurrence and indeed even an essential part of growth, which must precede and prepare maturational integration" (Bibring et al., 1961, p. 22). During this period, unsettled or partially resolved conflicts from earlier developmental stages are revived. The resolution of these conflicts is of tremendous significance for the mastery of the subsequent developmental stage, .i.e., motherhood.

PSYCHOLOGICAL INTERVENTION

Several investigators recognize the readiness of pregnant women to participate in programs of psychological study and to make effective use of psychotherapy at this time (Caplan, 1961; Bibring et al., 1961; Wenner and Cohen, 1968; Grimm, 1969). Based on his view of pregnancy as a period of disequilibrium, Caplan postulates the value of therapeutic intervention as a preventive measure. During a period of disequilibrium, he hypothesizes, the individual is more susceptible to influence than in periods of stable functioning, so that even minimal therapeutic intervention at such a period may be significantly effective.

There have been few attempts to provide special services geared to the needs of the normal, married pregnant woman and her family, and fewer still to study the effectiveness of the services made available in this circumstance. Notable exceptions are the studies of Caplan (1954; also reported by Cyr and Wattenberg, 1957); the Gordons (Gordon and Gordon, 1959, 1960); the more recent researches, including Wenner and Cohen (1968), Chertok (1969), Deutscher (1970), Larsen (1970); and those of Mann (1959) and Mann and Grimm (1962). The last two investigators were dealing with women with a defined problem in connection with pregnancy—habitual abortion with no known organic basis. This group of women has been found to be responsive to psychotherapy, to an impressive extent, in carrying to term when in psychotherapeutic treatment during the pregnancy; Grimm (1967) reports that two separate research teams, in one of which she was involved, found comparable results in extended work on this problem.

SCOPE OF STUDY

This research was established on the basis of the premises presented above: the significance of a first pregnancy in the personal development of the woman and its relation to the functioning of the infant, the psychologically stressful impact of pregnancy for the primigravida especially, and the greater accessibility of women to psychological intervention during pregnancy.

Some 60 families collaborated in this study. They represent a sample of young, middle-class American families living in an urban setting. Each family was involved in the project for a period of one year, from three months prenatally during the course of their first pregnancy until six months postnatally. To permit evaluation of the effectiveness of counseling, half of these families were randomly assigned to a counseled group and were engaged in a program of casework counseling during the pregnancy; the other half were similarly assigned to a control group and participated on a non-counseling basis. For all families, adaptations were evaluated periodically during the six months' postnatal period.

CRITERIA FOR SELECTION OF FAMILIES

The project sample was planned to consist of normal married couples undergoing a first pregnancy. The women were selected from primigravidae accepted for obstetrical care by GHA who met the following criteria:

The pregnant woman was living with her husband.

She had had no previous pregnancy experience.

No children were living in the family, whether by previous marriage of husband, adoption, etc.

Pregnancy was diagnosed within the first trimester.

The pregnant woman was not currently undergoing psychotherapy.

Neither husband nor wife was suffering from a marked physical handicap or deformity.

There was no wide gap between cultural backgrounds of husband and wife.

A few additional criteria derived from actual experience were added after the project was begun:

Age limits of 18 to 28 years inclusive for the pregnant woman. A minimum educational requirement, i.e., the equivalent of a four-year high school education for the woman.

A requirement of at least normal intelligence.

Both practical and theoretical considerations determined the socio-economic group included in this project. On the practical side was the reality of a sponsoring agency and setting, the Group Health Association, Inc. of Washington, D.C.[2] The availability of a middle-class group coming to one center for obstetrical care made it possible to set up the criteria developed for a population representative of normal, middle-class, young married couples undergoing a first pregnancy.

The theoretical considerations bearing on the nature of the group selected are of significance in any approach to a study of the maternity cycle. Two considerations are presented, in brief, below.

Social Class and Its Impact in Pregnancy

The higher incidence of reproductive disturbance among lower-class as compared with middle- and upper-class groups is well documented from studies in many countries. The sociologist Illsley (1967, p. 82), reviewing a comprehensive body of data, concludes that "stillbirth, neonatal death, congenital malformations of the central nervous system, birth weight, gestation period, and difficulty in labor are all influenced by the socio-economic status of the parents." Discussing this finding, Richardson (1967, p. ix) warns, "The findings...do not mean that social class causes differences in reproductive risk but, rather, point the way to further research on such factors as poor nutrition, stunting of physical growth, poor hygiene, prevalence of infectious disease, large numbers of pregnancies, and close spacing of children, which may contribute to reproductive disturbances." The data strongly suggest that the childbearing group in our lower classes constitutes a "population at risk," with need for a wide array of social-medical services which are not in fact available in modern societies.

The anthropological approach represented by Mead and Newton suggests as well that it is not the lower-class group alone that may be affected by lacks in emotional support and in ancillary services during pregnancy. Writing of cultural patterns surrounding childbearing in primitive and modern societies, they point out that, through the ages, human societies have patterned their practices around childbearing so as to assure material and emotional supports to the pregnant woman. They state specifically that "traditional forms of providing economic and practical help to childbearing women and infants appear to be less common in modern American society than elsewhere" (Mead and Newton, 1967, p. 195).

The impact of commonly held cultural attitudes of relative indifference towards the pregnant woman in modern American society and the lack of the kinds of material and emotional supports which other societies have deemed essential for childbearing obviously have major significance for an understanding of the psychodynamics of pregnancy. These broad issues constitute a separate area of inquiry, and especially of cross-cultural study, beyond the scope of this undertaking.

Selection of a Psychologically Normal Sample

It seemed desirable to study psychodynamics in a setting in which the focus on the pregnancy itself would not be distorted or blurred as it might be if the sample were to include only "problem" cases (an alternative that was considered in the light of the additional interest in therapeutic intervention). To emphasize the pregnancy as the center of interest, therefore, and not to risk intensification of stress by problems already in the situation at the time of the pregnancy, the decision was made to select an essentially normal group.

BRIEF DESCRIPTION OF PROJECT POPULATION

The detailed description of socio-economic characteristics presented in the next chapter indicates that the sample consisted of young people: the mean age for the women is 23 years, five months, for the men 27 years, one month. They were predominantly Protestant; Jews and Catholics each represented over one-fifth of the sample. Seventy-nine per cent were white, and 21 per cent were Negro.

Consistent with the criteria listed above, the project participants emerge as fairly homogeneous in socio-economic terms: the men predominantly college-educated and in professional occupations; the women with a minimum of a high school education and many engaged in professional and semi-professional work when the pregnancy occurred. They were socially upward mobile. Few had been exposed to psychologically oriented professionals, except for the usual under-graduate courses in psychology, and, under the selection criteria, none was currently involved in psychotherapy nor had any been earlier engaged, to any appreciable extent, in a program of psychotherapy. Like other studies dealing with normal populations, the sample represented the relatively broad spectrum of emotional adjustment.

CONCEPTUALIZATION OF THE VARIABLES

Some six sets of variables were conceptualized as basic to an understanding, of the psychology of a first pregnancy and its relationships to maternal adaptation and infant behavior in the first half year of life. Four sets of variables were specific to the prenatal period: life history; current personality of the woman; current life situation, especially the marriage and external stresses; and the pregnancy experience itself. Two sets of variables were specific to the postnatal period: maternal adaptation and infant functioning.

The first set of variables, *life history,* was directed to determining influences from the woman's childhood that might be expected to be operative in the development of a sense of identity and especially in her current adaptation. We hypothesized that the single, most vital influence would be found in the woman's early relationships with her mother. Psychoanalysts who have studied the intrapsychic life of women have seen the mother-daughter relationship as crucial in the young woman's adaptations to pregnancy and maternity (Deutsch, Vol. II, 1945; Benedek, 1952; Bibring et al., 1961; Caplan, 1961).

A number of variables were concerned with the woman's own experience in being mothered. Other childhood and premarital experiences seen as contributing to the development of a sense of identity included: identification with a parent or both parents, school and work adjustments, peer relationships, and interest in children and experience with them (during the woman's own childhood and adolescence). This last item was included on the basis of an earlier study indicating its predictive value with respect to maternity (Levy, 1958).

The second set of variables, *the personality of the woman,* was studied early in the pregnancy and again a year later at the end of the period for project participation, since we were interested from the beginning in seeing to what extent pregnancy and maternity were associated with personality changes in the woman. Personality variables have been used frequently in studies of pregnancy: to determine whether the later emotional adjustment during pregnancy can be predicted; to establish the relationship of specific personality characteristics to specific pregnancy risks and complications such as habitual abortion (Mann, 1959; Grimm, 1962), prolonged labor (Cramond, 1954), and toxemia (Coppen, 1958); or, as in one long-term investigation, to study women with immature personality with special reference to their response over time to motherhood (Pavenstedt, 1961, 1965). A substantial body of studies, including those referred to here, have been reviewed and summarized by Grimm, who concludes, "In all studies on the subject, personality variables measured fairly early in pregnancy have been found to relate to a woman's emotional adjustment and the occurrences of physiological symptoms, within the normal range later in pregnancy" (Grimm, 1967, p. 33).

The variables comprising the personality study included 28 items which were concerned with assessment of the woman's predominant defenses, characteristic way of expressing feeling, sense of her own identity, achievement of an adult role, qualities designed to indicate feminine identification, and, generally, her adaptive behavior (how adequate her defenses were in dealing with her needs). In addition, a diagnostic psychiatric classification was made (a number of classifications were differentiated within the range of the "normal" and a few classifications were developed for those who could be expected not to fall within the range of normalcy by psychiatric definition), and an intelligence test was administered.

Current life situation, the third broad set of variables, was directed to two aspects of the woman's current situation that were seen as likely to affect her attitude toward her pregnancy and mothering role: marital adaptation, with special reference to the impact of the husband, and external stresses not specific to pregnancy. The husband's impact on adaptation to the maternity cycle was conceptualized as one of the major areas for investigation, more on the basis of clinical experience than of research findings. Later reports by Wenner and Cohen (1968) and Deutscher (1970) affirm the validity of this approach. With the general objective of evaluating the amount of support on which the woman might be able to draw, the variables for evaluating the husband's impact and family adaptation included: dependency behavior of the husband, empathy, affection, sexual adjustment, ease of decision making as a couple, emotional reaction to the pregnancy, and fostering of self-confidence in the wife as a mother. These were largely adapted from a significant work in progress at NIMH on early marriage relationships (Goodrich et al., 1968; Ryder, 1970). Other variables, suggested by the study in progress at the Washington School of Psychiatry (Wenner and Cohen, 1968), related to congruence of the pregnancy with the couple's current way of life and with their long-term plans.

A number of investigators have pointed to the special stresses inherent in pregnancy, particularly for primiparae, and several studies have indicated that external events aggravate the stresses associated with the pregnancy experience and may contribute to certain pregnancy complications (Gordon and Gordon, 1960; Hetzel et al., 1961; Larsen, 1966). Assessment was concerned with such factors as: financial difficulties, illness of husband or wife, illness or death in the extended family, job dissatisfaction, and religious differences. We hypothesized that, if the psychology of pregnancy is to be understood in realistic terms, it is important to concern ourselves not only with psychodynamic processes but also with the external events that impinge on the pregnant woman.

The fourth and last set of variables specific to the prenatal period was related to the *pregnancy experience* itself. From the outset it was recognized that the physiological aspects of the pregnancy must constantly be kept in view, and to this end the woman's psychological reactions to the medical course of the pregnancy were observed and recorded by the obstetrician for each visit. The variables that were evaluated by the psychiatric research team included: predominant mood, expectations and hopes with respect to the sex of the child, intensity or lack of anxiety and fears characteristic of pregnancy (such as those relating to body image, physical fears for herself, concern over the unborn child, feelings of inadequacy to undertake infant care), dependency pattern in relation to husband and others, narcissism, sense of physical well-being (or the reverse), capacity to see herself in the role of mother and confidence about assuming that role, current adjustment to husband and mother, and evidence of any movement of the couple toward identification as a family (with some disengagement from their families of origin).

Labor and delivery were seen as part of the pregnancy experience. It was assumed that much of the adaptive energies of the woman throughout pregnancy would be directed to labor and delivery and it was therefore appropriate to include evaluations of this experience among the set of variables designed to assess the psychological adaptations during the entire pregnancy experience. The variables specific to labor and delivery were directed to an overall medical assessment as well as an assessment of the emotional aspects, so that the woman's subjective reaction could be compared with data from medical evaluations. The obstetrician's observations were thus of major importance, and the variables he reported included: false labor, normal delivery or not, whether on time, overdue or premature, stage of admission to hospital, complications, anxiety, use of anesthetics and their timing, reaction to pain, response to baby, and mood. Physiological developments and changes over time, and changing psychological reactions during the course of the pregnancy, indicated the need for assessment of the pregnancy situation at more than one time period.

Included among the variables centered on the pregnancy experience were a few items on the response of the couple to counseling. The counseling service was assessed in terms of its effectiveness in reducing the degree of emotional disturbance associated with the stress of pregnancy, in helping to promote satisfactory husband-wife relationships, and in helping to facilitate the assumption of satisfactory parental roles. It was assumed that effectiveness of the counseling could be evaluated in terms of a comparison of the two groups with respect to the outcome criteria for the project—an assumption that was found to be oversimplified when unanticipated complexities tended to obscure the effects of counseling.

In the postnatal period, of the two sets of variables encompassing the six months' postpartum evaluation, those dealing with *maternal adaptation* were developed in relation to: the mother's interaction with her infant, her satisfaction in her new role as mother, and the level of satisfying interaction within the family. With respect to the mother-infant interaction, we drew primarily on Yarrow's heuristic conceptualization of the mother's role in early infancy (Yarrow, 1963; Yarrow and Goodwin, 1965; also Brody, 1956, 1965). Drawing on his categories of maternal care in mother-infant interaction, we were concerned with the mother's role in helping the infant satisfy his needs and bring about reduction in tension under conditions which were sensitively related to his capacities and individual characteristics. We were also interested in determining how and to what extent the mother provided needed stimulation to him, as well as in ascertaining her underlying feelings for him in terms of emotional involvement, individualization of the infant, and overall acceptance or "the extent to which the mother is able to accept the child as he is" (Yarrow and Goodwin, 1965, p. 476). Over and beyond her interaction with the infant, we saw maternal adaptation as involved in the woman's readjustment in intrapsychic terms—anxieties, reactions and gratifications in response to the new practical and emotional demands, and her prevailing mood since the birth of the infant—and we were concerned with the husband-wife relationship as both adjusted to their new roles in relation to the infant and to each other.

The last set of variables, *infant characteristics,* was directed to an assessment of the final outcome criterion, the infant's functioning.[3] Even more than the variables for maternal adaptation, this set of variables was selected from those conceptualized and developed by Yarrow in his studies on development of focused relationships in infancy and analyses of the effective environment of the infant (Yarrow, 1963, 1967, 1968, 1972). It was planned that the infant would be studied in his natural setting at home (Moss, 1967). The variables for assessment of the functioning and characteristics of the infant covered: intellectual and motor functions, including activity level and state of tension; affective behavior, including characteristic mood and expression of negative feeling (in the nature of his crying); social responsiveness; and coping characteristics, which involved such qualities as adaptability, irritability, vulnerability to stress, and goal-directedness. Additional data were obtained by the pediatrician during pediatric examinations, including the infant's weight, feeding behavior and adjustment to routines, physical and neurological status, and observations of mother-infant interaction.

NATURE OF THIS VOLUME

The project was a multidisciplinary undertaking; the research team included persons trained in medicine, psychiatry, clinical and research psychology, psychiatric casework, and statistical methodology. The contributions of the entire research team are represented and incorporated in this volume. Sections or chapters written by individual members of the team will be identified accordingly; the separate chapters center around the following major problems of the study as a whole.

1. Study of variables in the woman's life history, personality, and current life situation (marital adaptation and external stresses) that are related to the psychological adaptation to pregnancy, labor, and delivery.
2. Investigation of the personality variables of the woman and her psychological adjustment during pregnancy as they are related to pregnancy outcomes, with special reference to postpartum psychiatric disorders.
3. Analyses of the predictability of adaptation to the maternal role from several sets of variables: life history, current personality, marital situation, external stresses, and psychological adaptation to the pregnancy experience.
4. Analyses of the relationship between selected aspects of infant adaptation and the variables of maternal personality, adaptation to the maternal role, and postnatal marital adjustment.
5. Comparison of counseled and non-counseled groups on selected variables.

In a last summary chapter, the premises, assumptions, and hypotheses that have been set forth here will be reexamined in the perspective of the intimate knowledge obtained in studying sixty women in depth during their first pregnancy, observing the impact of the pregnancy on them and their husbands, and evaluating adaptations of the new family unit in the first six months.

---

[1]In general, the term "middle class," as used with special reference to this study population, is analogous to class status defined by the Hollingshead and Redlich studies, which differentiate five classes ranging from Class I, as the most advantaged, through Class V, as the least advantaged (socially, economically, and educationally). On the basis of their groupings, our project population falls in Classes II and III (Hollingshead and Redlich, 1958, pp. 85-104).

[2]The Group Health Association is a medical consumer organization which provides comprehensive prepaid medical care; as of June, 1968, when the official report of the study was completed, it served some 70,000 participants in the Greater Washington area. See Appendix A for further description of the Group Health Association, Inc.

[3]The earlier research design did not include any intensive study of the infant. When the subtlety and complexity of evaluating mother-infant interaction was more fully recognized in

the process of developing research methods and tools, it became clear that a separate study of the infant would be needed. It was then that a psychologist with specialized training and experience in studying infant behavior was added to the research team to supplement the physical examinations and the observations of the pediatrician, already a member of the research staff. It was also found desirable to extend the postpartum period of study of each family from three to six months.

REFERENCES

Benedek, T. (1952) *Psycho-Sexual Functions in Women.* New York: The Ronald Press.

Bibring, G.L., Dwyer, T.F., Huntington, D., and Valenstein, A.F. (1961) A Study of the Psychological Processes in Pregnancy and of the Earliest Mother-Child Relationship. I. Some Propositions and Comments. *The Psychoanalytic Study of the Child,* Vol. XVI. New York: International Universities Press.

Brody, S. (1956) *Patterns of Mothering.* New York: International Universities Press.

Brody, S. (1965) Mental Health Interventions—Infant Development Research Project. In: *Report of Proceedings, Conference on Mental Health in Pregnancy.* Child Mental Health Section, NIMH, Bethesda, Md. (Unpublished).

Caplan, G. (1954) Preparation for Healthy Parenthood, *Children,* 1:171-175.

Caplan, G. (1957) Psychological Aspects of Maternity Care. *American Journal of Public Health,* 47:25-31.

Caplan, G. (1959) Concepts of Mental Health and Consultation. Washington, D.C.: Children's Bureau, Publication No. 373.

Caplan, G. (1961) *An Approach to Community Mental Health.* New York: Grune and Stratton.

Chertok, L. (1969) *Motherhood and Personality. Psychosomatic Aspects of Childbirth.* Philadelphia: J.P. Lippincott.

Coppen, A.J. (1958) Psychosomatic Aspects of Pre-eclamptic Toxaemia. *Journal of Psychosomatic Research,* 2:241-265.

Cramond, W.A. (1954) Psychological Aspects of Uterine Dysfunction, *Lancet,* 2:1241-1245.

Cyr, F.E., and Wattenberg, S.H. (1957) Social Work in a Preventive Program of Maternal and Child Health, *Social Work,* 3:32-39.

Deutsch, H. (1945) *The Psychology of Women: Motherhood,* Vol II. New York: Grune and Stratton.

Deutscher, M. (1970) Brief Family Therapy in the Course of First Pregnancy: A Clinical Note. *Contemporary Psychoanalysis,* 7:21-35.

Goodrich, W., Ryder, R.G., and Rausch, H.L. (1968) Patterns of Newlywed Marriage. *Journal of Marriage and the Family,* 30:383-391.

Gordon, R.E., and Gordon, K. (1959) Social Factors in the Prediction and Treatment of Emotional Disorders of Pregnancy. *American Journal of Obstetrics and Gynecology,* 77:1074-1083.

Gordon, R.E., and Gordon, K. (1960) Social Factors in Prevention of Postpartum Emotional Problems. *Obstetrics and Gynecology,* 15:433-437.

Grimm, E.R. (1962) Psychological Investigation of Habitual Abortion. *Psychosomatic Medicine,* 24:369-378.

Grimm, E.R. (1967) Psychological and Social Factors in Pregnancy, Delivery and Outcome. In: *Childbearing—Its Social and Psychological Aspects,* edited by S.A. Richardson and A.F. Guttmacher. Baltimore: Williams and Wilkins Co.

Grimm, E.R. (1960) Women's Attitudes and Reactions to Childbearing. In : *Modern Woman,* edited by G.D. Goldman and D.S. Milman. Springfield, Ill.: Charles C. Thomas.

Hetzel, B.S., Bruer, B., and Poideven, L.O.S. (1961) A Survey of the Relation Between Certain Common Antenatal Complications in Primiparae and Stressful Life Situations during Pregnancy. *Journal of Psychosomatic Research,* 5:175-182.

Hollingshead, A.B., and Redlich, F.C. (1958) *Social Class and Mental Illness; A Community Study.* New York: John Wiley and Sons.

Illsley, R. (1967) The Sociological Study of Reproduction and Its Outcome. In: *Childbearing—Its Social and Psychological Aspects,* edited by S.A. Richardson and A.F. Guttmacher. Baltimore: Williams and Wilkins Co.

Larsen, V.L. et al, (1966) Attitudes and Stresses Affecting Perinatal Adjustment. Mental Health Research Institute, Ft. Steilacoom, Washington. Report to NIMH.

Larsen, V.L. (1970) Social Stresses of First Time Parents. Unpublished paper, presented at American Orthopsychiatric Assn. Annual Meeting, March 1970.

Levy, D.M. (1958) *Behavioral Analysis.* Springfield, Ill.: Charles C. Thomas.

Mann, E.C. (1959) Habitual Abortion: A Report in Two Parts on 160 Patients. *American Journal of Obstetrics and Gynecology,* 77:706-718.

Mann, E.C., and Grimm, E.R. (1962) Habitual Abortion. In: *Psychosomatic Obstetrics, Gynecology, and Endocrinology,* edited by W.S. Kroger. Springfield, Ill.: Charles C. Thomas.

Mead, M., and Newton, N. (1967) Cultural Patterning of Perinatal Behavior. In: *Childbearing— Its Social and Psychological Aspects,* edited by S.A. Richardson and A.F. Guttmacher. Baltimore: Williams and Wilkins Co.

Moss, H.A. (1967) Sex, Age and State as Determinants of Mother-Infant Interaction. *Merrill-Palmer Quarterly* 13:19-36.

Pavenstedt, E. (1961) A Study of Immature Mothers and Their Children. In: *Prevention of Mental Disorders in Children,* edited by G. Caplan. New York: Basic Books.

Pavenstedt, E. (1965) A Comparison of the Child-Rearing Environment of Upper-Lower and Very Low-Lower Class Families. *American Journal of Orthopsychiatry,* 35:89-98.

Rank, O. (1929) *The Trauma of Birth.* London: Kegan Paul.

Richardson, S.A. and Guttmacher, A.F. (eds.) (1967) *Childbearing—Its Social and Psychological Aspects.* Baltimore: Williams and Wilkins Co.

Ryder, R.G. (1970) A Topography of Early Marriage. *Family Process,* 9:385-402.

Sontag, L.W. (1944) War and the Fetal Maternal Relationship. *Marriage and Family Living,* 6:1-5.

Wenner, N.K., and Cohen, M.B. (eds.) (1968) Emotional Aspects of Pregnancy. Final Report of Washington School of Psychiatry Project. Washington, D.C.

Yarrow, L.J. (1963) Research in Dimensions of Early Maternal Care. *Merrill-Palmer Quarterly,* 9:101-114.

Yarrow, L.J., and Goodwin, M.R. (1965) Some Conceptual Issues in the Study of Mother-Infant Interaction. *American Journal of Orthopsychiatry,* 35:473-481.

Yarrow, L.J. (1967) The Development of Focused Relationships during Infancy. In: *Exceptional Infant, The Normal Infant,* Vol. I, edited by J. Helmuth. Seattle, Washington: Special Child Publications.

Yarrow, L.J. (1968) Conceptualizing the Early Environment. In: *Early Child Care,* edited by L. Dittmann. New York: Atherton Press.

Yarrow, L.J. Rubenstein, J.L., Pedersen, F.A., and Jankowski, J.J. (1972) Dimensions of Early Stimulation and Their Differential Effects on Infant Development. *Merrill-Palmer Quarterly,* 18:205-218.

*Psychological Aspects of a First Pregnancy
and Early Postnatal Adaptation.*
Raven Press, New York © 1974

Chapter II
Research Design and Methodology

Robert F. Lockman

INTRODUCTION

The preceding chapter presented the two major foci of inquiry in this study, outlined the research design in brief, and set forth the criteria for selection of the project sample. Concepts and hypotheses which led to the development of the variables used in the study were presented, and, finally, five major problems were outlined as central to the study as a whole.

This chapter describes the research design in more detail and outlines the methods used in data collection and data analysis, including rater agreement and data reduction. It also contains a description of the final set of factors that represent the main body of quantitative data and a full description of social characteristics of the project population.

DESIGN OF THE STUDY

The research was designed to (1) explore psychological aspects in adjustment of women to a first pregnancy and early mother-infant adaptations, and (2) evaluate the effects of social work counseling on the course of pregnancy and early maternal adaptation.

For the first purpose, relationships among all sets of variables were calculated for all 57 subjects. For the second purpose, tests of significance of differences between counseled and control groups were involved, using a two-randomized-groups design. This design was necessitated by the fact that potential subjects did not, of course, become pregnant at the same time. These two purposes are not incompatible, since variables affected by counseling on which the two groups differ significantly can be standardized within groups to permit estimates of relationship for the total sample.

To make use of parametric statistics, the goal was 30 subjects in each group. A larger sample would have been desirable; however, the initial study of the woman's personality and current situation, including her family adaptation, and assessments at several intervals over a twelve-month period was a costly undertaking.

DATA COLLECTION

Procedures

In the time span chosen for study, the first trimester of pregnancy to six months postpartum, assessment of the physiological and psychological changes in the woman and changes in the social circumstances of each family required repeated measurements over time. To follow the procedures in detail, a Procedural Data Collection Chart is presented in Table 1. It outlines the data collection steps for the total sample, indicates which of the several professional disciplines is involved in the given procedure, and lists those procedures in the prenatal period that were specific to the counseled group only.

Prenatal Period of Study. Initially advised of the project by the obstetrician who conducted the medical examination and confirmed the diagnosis of pregnancy, each woman who was interested in exploring the possibility of participating was scheduled for a screening interview with a social worker of the project team. The project administrative assistant, using a series of random numbers, assigned the woman to either the counseled or control group. Prior to the screening interview, the administrative assistant informed the social worker of the group assignment for the particular woman. No other member of the project staff was informed of the group assignment. Each woman was given an interpretation of the purpose and nature of the project and was told what would be required if she decided to participate: the control group members were told of the research orientation, and the counseled group members were told, in addition, of the counseling orientation. The number of interviews involved was also explained.

TABLE 1. *Procedural data collection chart*

Pregnancy period	Delivery and neonatal period	Postnatal period

Three or four months (counseled and control groups)
Casework interviews with woman—2
Psychiatric interviews with woman—2
Psychological evaluation
  Rorschach Examination
  Thematic Apperception Test
  Figure Drawing Test
  Rotter Sentence Completion Test
  Wechsler Adult Intelligence Scale
Casework interview with husband—1
 	
Three to seven months
Counseled group:
  Biweekly casework counseling sessions with woman
  Monthly casework counseling sessions with husband
  Obstetrical examinations—Monthly
Control group:
  Obstetrical examinations—Monthly
 	
Seven months (both groups)
Casework interviews—2 for counseled group; 1 for control group
Psychiatric interview—1
Sentence Completion Test—1
Obstetrical examinations—Monthly
 	
Eighth and ninth months (both groups)
Parents' prenatal interview with pediatrician
Obstetrical examinations—Biweekly 8th month
  —Weekly beginning 9th month
Counseled group
  Biweekly counseling sessions with wife
  Monthly counseling sessions with husband
	Obstetrical services and observations
	Caseworker—Hospital visit
	Pediatrician—Hospital visit
		Counseled and Control Groups
		Four weeks
		Infant observation—Home visit by infant observer
		Mother-infant observation—Home visit by caseworker
		
		Six weeks
		Pediatric examination
		Mother-infant observation in office by pediatrician
		
		Twelve weeks
		Infant observation—Home visit by infant observer
		Mother-infant observation—Office interview or home visit by caseworker
		Pediatric examinations and observations
		
		Six months
		Infant observation—Home visit by infant observer
		Pediatric examinations and observations
		Psychiatric examination of woman
		Psychological evaluation of woman
		Casework interview with mother and mother-infant observation—Home visit by caseworker
		Casework interview with husband

Each woman was assigned to one obstetrician for her prenatal care and delivery. From the third to the seventh month, she had an obstetrical examination once a month; in the eighth month, she had biweekly examinations; and in the ninth month, weekly examinations. Medical care in the prenatal as in the postnatal period was the same for both counseled and control groups, and the physicians did not know whether a patient was in the control or counseled group.

During pregnancy, each woman had a minimum of (a) three interviews with the social worker, two at three months and one at seven months; (b) three interviews with the psychiatrist, two at three months and one at seven months; and (c) a two-hour testing session with the clinical psychologist at three months. Husbands of control group members had at least one or, more often, two interviews with the social worker during this period of the study.

In addition to these diagnostic and medical procedures, each woman in the counseled group was engaged in a process of casework counseling on a biweekly schedule throughout the pregnancy, until the date of delivery. Her husband was similarly involved, but on a monthly schedule.

At the eighth month, opportunity was extended to couples in the project to meet with the pediatrician for a prenatal interview.

Postnatal Period of Study. The postnatal study was the same for both counseled and control group members. It included: obstetrical and pediatric observations of mother and infant during confinement; an interview with the mother in the hospital conducted by the social worker on the fourth or fifth day postpartum; pediatric examination, observations and psychological tests of the infant, observations of mother-infant interaction, and interviews with both mother and father at one, three, and six months; psychiatric, psychological, and social work restudy of the woman at the six-months' postnatal period.

Confidentiality and Authorized Use of Data

Subjects were advised that the data would be made available only to the study team for use in the project, and that they would be protected from any disclosure of personal identifying information. The broader use of the data "for professional purposes of medical research, education, or science," inherent in the nature of this undertaking, was authorized by the participants on a form that was signed by both husband and wife.

As background data for the presentation of methods of study and data analysis later, a full description of the research subjects is now given.

DESCRIPTION OF RESEARCH SUBJECTS

Number of Families. The number of families included as the basic sample varies in different reports within this volume. Sixty-four families participated in the project, and data were used from all 64 participating families in some of the reports; for example, all 64 women were included in the analysis of the medical obstetrical aspects of the project. While there were no "dropouts," once the couple undertook the year's collaboration with the research team, two families moved from the city in the latter part of the postnatal period of study, leaving some schedules incomplete on those cases. Postnatal evaluations were not appropriate in a few cases because of deviant outcomes of the pregnancy (stillbirth, for example). In some reports, 62 families are included as the basic group under study; anticipating that this number was to be the final sample, social characteristics were analyzed on that basis. For purposes of statistical estimation and analyses, however, 57 families, for whom data are complete in all aspects and time periods of the study, represent the final basic sample.

In the factual analysis that follows, all figures are based on the sample of 62 cases.

Marital Circumstance. All couples were married and living together when they entered into participation in the project.

Two men but none of the women had been married previously.

Marriages of persons of different faiths occurred in 23 per cent of the sample. Early in the marriage and even during the pregnancy, some of the couples reported minor but continuing conflict over religious issues. However, after the birth of the infant, no situation was reported as problematic because of religious differences. The religious affiliations of the subjects are shown in Table 2.

TABLE 2.

Religion	Women	Men
Protestant	55%	58%
Catholic	21%	21%
Jewish	24%	21%

Social and Individual Characteristics

Race. Seventy-nine per cent of the sample of 62 families were white; 21 per cent were Negro.

Birthplace. Approximately one-third (32 per cent) of the men and women were born in the District of Columbia, Maryland, or Virginia, the area in which the study was made. Approximately one-half of the total sample of men and women were born in the South (including the District of Columbia, Maryland, and Virginia), with the next largest grouping from the Middle Atlantic states, represented by 22 per cent of the total (Table 3).

Education. All the participants had a high school education as a minimum. Beyond this, 74 per cent of the women and 83 per cent

TABLE 3. *Birthplace, ordinal position, education, and occupation*

Variable	Women %	Men %
Birthplace		
Outside USA	3	3
West	10	5
South	50	47
North Central	10	15
Middle Atlantic	23	21
New England	5	10
Ordinal birth position		
Only child	15	13
Oldest	40	40
2nd	18	26
3rd to 8th	27	21
Education		
High school graduation only	26	17
1-3 years of college	31	11
College graduate	37	40
Graduate and professional degree	6	32
Occupation		
Labor	3	6
Clerical, sales, and technical	34	23
Scientific and professional	32	61
Business	—	4
Student	5	6
Housewife	26	—
Occupation of father		
Labor	23	34
Farm	5	3
Clerical, sales, and technical	16	10
Scientific and professional	31	26
Business	23	21
Unknown	2	6

of the men had some college training, ranging from one year of college to varied academic and professional degrees, including the Ph.D. in a few instances (Table 3).

Occupation. Thirty-two per cent of the women and 61 per cent of the men were engaged in scientific and professional work. Thirty-four per cent of the women were engaged in clerical and sales work. The activities of the men were more scattered with 23 per cent in clerical and sales work, and smaller proportions in business and labor (skilled and semiskilled) activities (Table 3).

Factors Specific to the Pregnancy

Age. The women's age range was 18 to 28 (Table 4). Forty-four per cent of the first pregnancies occurred among the group of women who were 20 to 23 years of age, and nearly half (48 per cent) among the group 23 to 28 years of age. Fifty-two per cent of the men were between 22 and 26 at the time of the first pregnancy.

TABLE 4. *Age at time of first pregnancy*

Age (years)	Women	Men
18-20	8%	
20-23	44%	
23-28	48%	
Mean age (women)	23 years, 5 months	
Under 22		6%
22-26		52%
Over 26		42%
Mean age (men)		27 years, 1 month

Interval Between Marriage and Pregnancy. The interval between date of marriage and time of the first pregnancy (Table 5) ranged from less than three months to ten years, with 37 per cent of the pregnancies occurring in the first twelve months of marriage.

TABLE 5. *Interval between marriage and first pregnancy*

1-3 months	6%
4-12 months	31%
1 year (over 12 months to 24 months)	29%
2 years (over 24 months to 36 months)	17%
3-5½ years	15%
Beyond 6 years	2%

Incidence of Problems in Conception. Sixteen per cent of the women reported problems in conceiving before this first pregnancy occurred.

Planned and Unplanned Pregnancies. Seventy-three per cent of the pregnancies were planned; 27 per cent unplanned.

Financial Circumstances

During the period of the pregnancy, all husbands in the study were employed; several were in partial student status in after-work hours, and one devoted himself full-time to his Ph.D. studies. Three-fourths of the women were employed at the time of the diagnosis of pregnancy, and all discontinued work at varying periods of time prior to delivery. For most families, the basic family income from the husband's earnings enabled the family to live in a two-bedroom apartment, often in a new modern garden-type apartment development, and to make payments on one automobile. In some instances, the household furniture was not fully paid for and required monthly payments. Twenty-six per cent of the total, generally representing those who were married longer and had attained better incomes, had purchased homes prior to the pregnancy. These were all in attractive sections of the city or, more often, in the suburbs. At the upper range were a few couples who were able to maintain two automobiles and who had purchased homes which were in communities of upper middle-class status.

Medical Background

Medical History. Over half of the women and a third of the men reported earlier or current medical conditions of some consequence, such as rheumatic fever, asthma, or stomach ulcer (Table 6).

Psychiatric Care. By definition no family was included in the sample if the husband or wife was currently in psychotherapy or had been in treatment within two years preceding the pregnancy. Only a few participants—8 per cent of the women and 10 per cent of the men—had ever been in psychiatric treatment (Table 6).

TABLE 6. *Medical and psychiatric background*

	Women	Men
Medical history		
None	44%	66%
Asthma	6%	5%
Ulcers	0	8%
Other	50%	21%
Previous psychiatric care	8%	10%

Parents of Research Subjects

Parents' Status: Loss of a Parent. In the large preponderance of cases, the parents of the research subjects were living. However, 13 per cent of the women and 26 per cent of the men had suffered the loss of one or, in a few instances, both parents, at widely varying periods in the lives of the participants. For three women and one man, the parent's death had occurred before the child was five years of age; for three men it had occurred between the ages of six and 13.

Proximity to Family. Forty-four per cent of the women and 35 per cent of the men had parents living in Washington, D.C., or its vicinity.

Frequency of Contacts with Parents. The frequency of contacts with family (Table 7) on both sides included personal visits and regular contacts by telephone (local and long-distance).

TABLE 7. *Usual frequency of contacts with parents*

	Women	Men
Weekly (or more often)	47%	32%
Monthly	18%	23%
Every few months	27%	31%
Less frequently	8%	10%
Unknown, not living, or no contact	0	4%

METHODS OF STUDY

Interviews

The clinical orientation of most of the research team influenced the choice of methods in data collection toward reliance on clinical methods: relatively unstructured interviews, observations, and clinical judgment. The interviews of the psychiatric team—psychiatrist, psychologist, and social worker—represented an adaptation between open, unstructured, clinical exploration and direct inquiry to obtain specific psychosocial data for a given research purpose. Interest in individual response of the woman and her husband to their current experience required that they be given as much latitude as possible for initiating discussion of subject matter and for spontaneous expression of feelings and reactions. On the other hand, some direction of the interview was necessary, because the members of the psychiatric team were responsible for obtaining data that would enable them to make discriminating evaluations in rating each subject on a number of variables. Consequently, the interviews of the psychiatrist, social worker, and psychologist were semistructured. The counseling sessions of the psychiatric social worker with each woman in the counseled group and with her husband were essentially unstructured. The interviews of the infant observer with the mother were the only structured interviews in the project.

Psychological Tests

Psychological tests of the woman, administered in the first trimester of the pregnancy and again a year later at the end of project participation, six months postpartum, included the following: Rorschach Psychodiagnostic Examination; Selected Thematic Apperception Test Cards (card numbers 1, 2, 3GF, 4, 7GF, 12F, 13MF, 16, and 18GF); Rotter Sentence Completion Test; Draw a Person Test, plus a drawing of what the woman thought the inside of her body looked like; Wechsler Adult Intelligence Scale (administered only once, in the prenatal period).

The psychological tests of the infant included the Bayley Scales of Infant Development. In addition, the infant was observed at home for periods of approximately two hours each, two days in succession, at age one month, three months, and six months. During these periods, a feeding and bath were observed, the Bayley Mental and Motor Scales administered, and the mother interviewed. All of the activities of the infant observer and most of the postnatal interviews and observations of the social worker took place in the home.

Rating Schedules

The rating schedules were developed as the major measures of the study to permit the qualitative data from the interviews, observations, and projective tests to be quantified. To encompass the several sets of variables (outlined in Chapter I), a number of rating schedules were developed, some of them to be repeated at intervals. The full listing of the rating schedules is shown in Table 8. Their names suggest the relationship of each to the particular body of variables.

TABLE 8. *Rating schedules chart*

		When rated	Raters
Pregnancy period			
Schedule A*:	Prenatal life history, personality, family adaptation; adaptation to pregnancy	3rd or 4th month	Psychiatrist, psychologist, and social worker; obstetrician present at conference
Schedule B:	Adaptation to pregnancy	7th month	Psychiatrist and social worker
Two special forms for medical observations—one on pregnancy-related symptoms; one on psychological attitudes to pregnancy, medical procedures, etc.		At each visit for medical examination, usually 14 in number	Obstetrician
Schedule C:	Adaptation to pregnancy; perspective on pregnancy and delivery	At delivery	Entire research team
Medical staff observations, labor, and delivery; psychological aspects		At delivery	Obstetrician
Schedule D:	Labor and delivery	At delivery	Entire research team
Postnatal period			
Schedules E-I, F-I, and G-I: Infant characteristics		1 month, 3 months, 6 months	Infant observer
Pediatric evaluation of infant		6 weeks, 3 months, 6 months	Pediatrician
Schedules E-III, F-III, and G-III: Maternal adaption		1 month, 3 months, 6 months	Infant observer, pediatrician, and social worker
Schedule G-IV: Personality		6 months	Psychiatrist, psychologist, and social worker
Schedule H: Summary evaluation		6 months	Entire research team

*Each rating period was identified by a capital letter as Schedule A-H.

For some schedules, as Table 8 indicates, several of the research staff members independently rated each subject on each item. The procedure for these ratings was as follows: based on his own data (whether interviews, psychological tests, examinations, observations or any combination of these methods), the staff member completed an independent rating on each item. He then reviewed the narrative recording or analyses of tests of the other two raters. Finally, a staff conference was held at which the raters arrived at a consensus rating.

Consensus was not always achieved without extended discussion and consideration of the whole body of data on the item at issue. Guidelines were developed to facilitate resolution of conflicting views. In cases of difference or indecision, the view of the professional person who had the most information on the particular item was decisive. For example, the psychologist's view was accepted on items defined through psychological tests, such as ease of fantasy production and covert dependency; the psychiatrist's view was determinative if there were differences on such matters as psychiatric diagnosis or emotional adaptation; and the social worker's view prevailed on issues involving overt behavioral adaptations and husband-wife adjustment.

As the Rating Schedules Chart shows, the entire staff participated in the rating conferences at two periods: at the end of the pregnancy, when overall adaptation to pregnancy, labor, and delivery were evaluated (Schedules C and D); and at the end of the intensive restudy six months postpartum when the Summary Evaluation Schedule (Schedule H) was rated. This latter procedure marked completion for that family of their participation in the formal aspect of the project.

A complete set of the rating schedules is reproduced in Appendix B.

DATA ANALYSES

Rater Agreement

Rater agreement for eleven item schedules dealing with the woman's personality (as studied at six months postnatally), her maternal adaptation, the characteristics of the infant, and the overall summary evaluation was calculated from comparisons of independent individual ratings and consensus ratings with independent individual ratings. In the case of infant characteristics and maternal adaptation ratings, both observers rated independently after direct observation or inquiry. An outside psychiatrist with no direct knowledge of the subjects served as an independent rater who rated from the protocols of the team members.

Table 9 shows the percentages of perfect agreements on item ratings between raters. They range from 38 to 69, with a median for the eleven schedules of 56. The criterion of perfect correspondence between ratings was a stringent test of agreement.

TABLE 9. *Rater agreement for postnatal schedule item ratings*

Schedule and comparison made			Number of			
			Subjects	Items rated	Perfect agreements	% Perfect agreements
Infant characteristics	EI	— 6 weeks	8	108	60	56
(rater vs. rater)	FI	— 3 months	9	117	71	61
	GI	— 6 months	10	134	85	63
	Total		27	359	216	60
Maternal adaptation	EIII	— 6 weeks	3	65	42	64
(rater vs. rater)	FIII	— 3 months	5	107	65	61
	GIII	— 6 months	8	170	86	50
	Total		16	342	193	57
Maternal adaptation	EIII	— 6 weeks	3	70	33	47
(rater vs. consensus)	FIII	— 3 months	4	85	59	69
	GIII	— 6 months	9	188	72	38
	Total		16	343	164	48
Current personality (rater vs. consensus)	GIV	— 6 months	8	334	183	55
Summary evaluation (rater vs. consensus)	H	— 6 months	8	132	54	41

Data Reduction

Because of the large number of items (700) involved in the study, reduction of data to retain significant and independent sets of variables was necessary to enhance the reliability of measurement. This need was particularly evident for the rating items which comprised half of the item pool obtained on each subject. Where an occasional observation was missing, the group or individual mean was used to fill in the missing value; where several items in a given schedule or test were missing, correlations were computed only on those subjects who had complete data for the variables involved.

Means, standard deviations, and percentages were the principal descriptive statistics calculated. Product-moment correlation and linear regression analyses were used to relate items and scales with one another. Principal-components factor analysis of correlation matrices with varimax rotation was used to identify sets of variables that were highly interrelated (Kaiser, 1958; Harman, 1960; Cooley and Lohnes, 1964).

In examining differences between counseled and control groups, two-tailed tests of significance generally were used because of the exploratory nature of the analyses (McNemar, 1955). Similarly, two-

TABLE 10. *List of initial factor scales and twelve other variables*

Factor scale no.	Name	Schedule	Factor scale no.	Name	Schedule
1	Perception of experience being mothered	A-I	30	Responsiveness to infant	F-III
2	Interest in children	A-I	31	Acceptance of infant	F-III
3	School and peer relationships	A-I	32	Confidence in maternal role	F-III
4	Ego strength	A-II	33	Acceptance of maternal role	F-III
5	Nurturance	A-II	34	Responsiveness to infant	G-III
6	Husband's responsiveness to wife	A-III	35	Acceptance of infant and maternal role	G-III
7	Husband's responsiveness to pregnancy	A-III	36	Individualization of infant	G-III
8	Adaptation to pregnancy experience	A-IV	37	Husband-wife adaptation	E-III
9	Visualization of self as mother	A-IV	38	Reaction to paternal role	E-III
10	Reaction to characteristic fears of pregnancy	A-IV	39	Husband-wife adaptation	F-III
11	Adaptation to pregnancy experience	B	40	Reaction to paternal role	F-III
12	Confirmation of sexual identity	B	41	Husband-wife adaptation	G-III
13	Reaction to pregnancy fears	B	42	Reaction to paternal role	G-III
14	Visualization of self as mother	B	43	Ego strength	G-IV
15	Response to project experience	C-II	44	Nurturance	G-IV
16	Overall reaction to pregnancy experience	C-II	45	Family adaptation	H
			46	Mother-infant adaptation	H
17	Infant adjustment	E-1		Birthweight (ounces)	—
18	Infant alertness	E-1		DIQ	E-1
19	Infant adjustment	F-1		DMQ	E-1
20	Infant alertness	F-1		DIQ	F-1
21	Infant adjustment	G-1		DMQ	F-1
22	Infant alertness	G-1		DIQ	G-1
23	Infant functioning	E-II		DMQ	G-1
24	Infant functioning	F-II			
25	Infant functioning	G-II		Psychological aspects of delivery (item 150)	D
26	Acceptance of maternal role	E-III		Medical aspects of delivery (item D 151)	
27	Acceptance of infant	E-III			
28	Individualization of infant	E-III		WAIS: VIQ	—
29	Responsiveness to infant	E-III		PIQ	—
				FSIQ	—

tailed significance tests were used to examine differences between repeated measures on the same subjects taken at different time periods.

In analyzing pregnancy-maternity dynamics, the total sample was used, and relationships among variables were calculated. Here, standardization of scores within counseled and control groups could be made to permit pooling them if they differed significantly on the variables involved.

Initial Factor Scales

Twenty separate factor analyses of rating item sets were made, proceeding chronologically from the earliest prenatal schedule to the six-month postnatal summary evaluation. Ultimately, 46 scales were derived containing only items that correlated or loaded at the 0.01 level of significance with a factor (Burt and Banks, 1947). Of these, 16 were specific to the prenatal and 30 to the postnatal period. All cases were scored on the scales using simple additive formulas, since the item variabilities were similar (Gulliksen, 1950). A list of the scales and the schedules from which they come is presented in Table 10.

Superfactor Scales

Because the 46 scales were developed from 20 separate factor analyses of item intercorrelations, the relationships among all items had not been taken into account. Twelve variables which were not rated items had not been included in the factor analyses. (These twelve variables are listed at the bottom of Table 10.) Consequently, a final, overall factorization was made for the 58 variables.[1] The same procedures were followed as in the initial factor analyses, and only loadings of items that were significant at the 0.01 level were interpreted.

Twelve significant factors were rotated. They were named "superfactors" to contrast them with the initial 46 factor scales developed previously. Of the twelve superfactors, eight were interpretable from a theoretical or empirical standpoint. These eight are listed in Table 11, which also shows the initial factor scales and other variables of which they are composed. Then superfactor scores for each subject were calculated by formulas derived through multiple regression analyses of the variables which best predicted each superfactor (Jenkins, 1952).

Two additional variables—total number of stresses (not pregnancy-engendered) and the number of pregnancy-related medical

TABLE 11. *List of superfactor scales and their composition*

Super-factor	Name		Factor scales involved
I	Feminine identification	9	Visualization of self as mother
		45	Family adaptation
II	Infant adjustment	19	Infant adjustment
		31	Acceptance of infant
		46	Mother-infant adaptation
III	Woman's intelligence		None
IV	Infant alertness	18	Infant alertness
	(at 1 month of age)		DMQ
VI	Maternal responsiveness	26	Acceptance of maternal role
		29	Responsiveness of infant
IX	Husband-wife adaptation	6	Husband's responsiveness to wife
	(prenatal)	7	Husband's responsiveness to pregnancy
XI	Husband's responsiveness	40	Reaction to paternal role
	to paternal role	42	Reaction to paternal role
VIII	Woman's self-confidence	1	Perception of being mothered
		13	Reaction to pregnancy fears
		32	Confidence in maternal role

symptoms—were next analyzed in relation to the superfactor scores for each subject.

Finally, the superfactor scores of the women assigned to the three counselors were analyzed. The Mann-Whitney U Test (Siegel, 1956) was used for the comparisons between counselors and between counseled and control groups for two of the counselors (the third counselor had only one control case).

The reader with special interest in the composition of factor scales and detailed statistics is referred to Appendices C, D, and E.

Appendix C. Compendium of 46 Initial Factor Scales.
Appendix D. Initial Factor Analyses.
Appendix E. Supplementary Statistical Tables:
    Table 1. Formulas for Calculating Superfactor Scale Scores.
    Table 2. Composition of Superfactor Scales.
    Table 3. Means, Standard Deviations, and Significant Differences Between Counseled and Control Groups.
    Table 4. Intercorrelations of Superfactor Scores, Stresses, and Medical Symptoms.

The presentation and discussion of findings will appear at appropriate points in each of the chapters dealing with separate aspects of the maternity cycle and in the chapter on counseling. At this point, a series of relatively reliable, well-developed, and parsimonious factor scales were created which, we will see, are useful in explaining the psychodynamics of pregnancy, the early period of maternity, and infant adaptation.

[1]As the subsequent chapters on pregnancy, maternal and family adaptation, and infant adaptation will show, most of the statistical findings are based on interrelationships of these 46 factor scales and the twelve other variables.

REFERENCES

Burt, C., and Banks, C. (1947) A Factor Analysis of Body Measurements for British Adult Males. *Annals of Eugenics,* 13:238-256

Cooley, W.W., and Lohnes, P.R. (1964) *Multivariate Procedures for the Behavioral Sciences.* New York: John Wiley and Sons.

Gulliksen, H. (1950) *Theory of Mental Tests.* New York: John Wiley and Sons.

Harman, H.H. (1960) *Modern Factor Analysis.* Chicago: The University of Chicago Press.

Jenkins, W.L. (1952) An Improved Short-Cut Method for Multiple R. *Educational and Psychological Measurement,* 12:316-322.

Kaiser, H.F. (1958) The Varimax Criterion for Analytic Rotation in Factor Analysis. *Psychometrika,* 23:187-200

McNemar, Q. (1955) *Psychological Statistics.* New York: John Wiley and Sons.

Siegel, S. (1956) *Nonparametric Statistics for the Behavioral Sciences.* New York: McGraw-Hill Book Co.

Psychological Aspects of a First Pregnancy and Early Postnatal Adaptation.
Raven Press, New York © 1974

Chapter III
Background Variables

Pauline M. Shereshefsky and Robert F. Lockman

INTRODUCTION

We set ourselves the task of identifying facets of the woman's personal background, her life experience, past and present, that might bear on her feelings and behavior during her first pregnancy, focusing on these sets of variables: Life History; Current Personality; Marital Adaption; and Current Stresses.[1] We were interested in how these variables related to the woman's handling of the pregnancy and her ability to function as a mother. In addition, we asked whether the mother's life experiences and personality might be predictive of the infant's early adjustment.

OUTCOMES OF STUDY

Three sets of variables, Pregnancy Adaptation, Maternal Adaptation, and Infant Adaptation, were seen as pivotal for understanding the psychodynamics of pregnancy and the maternity cycle. The factor scales comprising each set of variables will be described in the separate chapters dealing with the pregnancy, the woman's adaptation to her maternal role, and the infant (Chapters IV, VIII and XI, respectively).

LIFE HISTORY VARIABLES

The initial study of the woman included an exploration of her life history with reference to:

1. Her family of origin, which included her own experience in being mothered and the degree of disruption or family intactness.
2. Development of identity, a cluster of items which included identification with her parents, school achievement and adjustment, peer relationships, and work performance.
3. Interest in and experience with children.
4. Health, with special consideration of trauma due to ill health and accidents.

The factual data with regard to social background and medical history were obtained in part during the screening interview. Life history data at a deeper level were secured during interviews with the social worker, psychiatrist and psychologist, and through psychological testing.

Family Background

Most of the women were reared in middle-class family homes; a few came from upper middle-class and two from lower-class homes. Most (80 per cent) had been reared in parental homes in which both parents were living.

Many of the women had been exposed to family experiences of a potentially traumatic nature at an early age. For 29 per cent of the sample, life histories revealed deviant family circumstances such as death of a parent during the childhood of the woman (before age

13), separation and divorce of the parents, mental illness of a parent, and prolonged periods of absence of the father for military service (more than a year). Two women had been adopted early in life; two others had not been reared by their own mothers.

Mother-Daughter Relationship

Both psychoanalytic theory and contemporary research in human and animal psychology stress the significance of early mothering influences on the emotional and behavioral pattern of the individual.[2] However, we have been unable to find any studies of mother-daughter relationships that focus on the woman's adaptation to pregnancy and maternal functioning.[3] Although we did not obtain data directly from the mothers of the women in our sample, we did assess the mother-daughter relationships from the perspective of the young adult daughter. Several items rated by the psychiatric team dealt with the woman's perception of her mother, that is, how she evaluated her mother's closeness to her, her empathy, her anxiety level, her intrusiveness, reaction to her maternal role, and, finally, the extent to which to which she satisfied her emotional needs at various periods during her life.

Five of these items—empathy, closeness, reaction to her maternal role, and the extent to which the mother met the emotional needs of the daughter up to age twelve and from age twelve to the time of the pregnancy—were highly intercorrelated. These five items constituted the scale called perception of experience in being mothered. As shown in Table 1, this factor scale correlated significantly with two other prenatal factor scales: ego strength and woman's reactions to fears of pregnancy at seven months. The implication is that women with good experience in being mothered are likely to have adequate ego strength and to handle characteristic fears of pregnancy with minimal anxiety; or it may be that women with adequate ego strength are more likely to evaluate their mothers positively. Perception of experience in being mothered also correlated with several postnatal factor scales: confidence in maternal role, individualization of the infant, and especially husband-wife adaptations as measured at all three rating periods. Perception of mothering experience was highly correlated with the two variables that measured current mother-daughter relationship at three and seven months prenatally and six months postnatally.

The statistical findings on this factor, woman's perception of her experience in being mothered, can be summarized as follows:

The correlates of the factor suggest that women who saw their mothers as close, empathic, happy in the maternal role, and adequately supportive were likely to be less anxious about the pregnancy, better adapted as wives, and more confident in the maternal role. Although the number of significant relationships are few, they are theoretically meaningful.

The quality of the woman's relationship with her mother—the degree of support extended by the mother to meet her daughter's emotional needs—was consistent over time.

While several aspects in the growing-up process were explored in depth, yielding revealing information on personality and current attitudes, the developmental data showed few statistically significant relationships to the woman's adjustments during pregnancy or her maternal adaptation. The one exception was the factor, an early interest in children, which was one of the variables that predicted maternal adaptation.[4]

Health History

Thirty-five women had suffered from an illness or accident of some seriousness prior to marriage. In several instances the illness and recovery period was protracted, necessitating absence from school for many months and sometimes for a year or more. It was our impression that women who had had such an illness history gave evidence of accentuated dependency needs in some cases, and that pregnancy and especially labor and delivery often reactivated concern about body image and anxieties about doctors, medical procedures, and hospitalization.

Observations Regarding Life History Variables in Relation to Pregnancy Adaptation and Maternal Adaptation

Many experiences within and outside the childhood home have important effects on the personality development of the woman, in addition to her experiences in relationship to her mother. The reactions to these events have undoubtedly been tempered, intensified, or otherwise influenced by relationship to the mother or mothering figure. The child's response to these events and her integration of a significant event will itself have modified the underlying pattern that was developed in interaction with her first "environment," the mother (or caretaking person). Encounters in early adulthood and marriage, closer

TABLE 1. *Correlates of woman's perception of experience in being mothered (N = 57)*

Factor scale	Study period involved (months)	Correlation coefficient	Significance level
Prenatal			
Ego strength	3	0.38	0.01
Reaction to fears of pregnancy	7	0.47	0.01
Postnatal			
Individualization of infant	1	0.29	0.05
Confidence in maternal role	3	0.33	0.05
Husband-wife adaptation	1	0.28	0.05
Husband-wife adaptation	3	0.29	0.05
Husband-wife adaptation	6	0.28	0.05

in time to the first pregnancy, require adaptations which may further serve to obscure the impact of earlier relationships and events. Moreover, we were seeing the woman at a time when the pregnancy itself was initiating a re-evaluation of her attitudes towards the mother (Deutsch, 1945; Bibring, 1961).

The observations of another researcher in this field bear on the same issues: "... with increasing understanding of the 'openmindedness of the maturational process,' pregnancy has begun to be seen as one of the later growth phases in young adult life, one taking place within the structure of a developing family. . . .

"This orientation to the experience of pregnancy as significant in its own right, and influential in its impact on the life style of the young adult, is corrective to those notions of maturation that emphasize the primarily repetitive nature of adult experience—the dialogue reflecting only the earlier identifications—and ignore the fact that stimulus and resolution are both aspects of an interpersonal field in which historical factors play a significant but not exclusive role. . . ." (Deutscher, 1970, p. 22). Obviously more research of a penetrating quality, involving methods of validating subjective response, is needed in this area.

PSYCHOLOGICAL STUDY OF THE WOMAN

Sara Saltzman and Toby Schneidman

Introduction

Because the question of the effect of prenatal influences on early mother-infant interaction was a central issue in initiating this research, we undertook to study the personality of the woman early in pregnancy as well as at the end of project participation. We hoped thereby to evaluate the impact of pregnancy, childbirth, and the early mothering experience on the woman's personality and on her interaction with the infant in the first six months postpartum.

Background and Method

Caplan (1961) and Bibring et al. (1961), in their studies on the psychology of pregnancy, suggest a regressive shift in personality during pregnancy. Caplan describes very marked regression in psychological functioning during pregnancy, so that psychological test productions of pregnant women resemble those of severely disturbed schizophrenic patients. Bibring, in a more conservative statement, describes a regressive shift shortly after quickening.

Other writers believe that a woman's reaction to pregnancy is so individual that no generalization can be made. Stechler and Geller (1961) found that women retested three to six years after pregnancy were more primitive and explosive in the non-pregnant period when compared with the pregnant period.

Helene Deutsch (1944) also stresses the individuality of each woman's response to pregnancy, which in each woman, she says, is inseparably connected with her total personality. Dealing largely with analytic patients, her conclusion is that every woman brings to pregnancy emotional factors and conflict situations.

Purpose of Personality Evaluation

The psychological examination had a threefold purpose:

1. To provide insight into the woman's personality strengths as well as her problems so that the counselor would be able to work with her more effectively.
2. To obtain an independent and, it was hoped, more objective picture of the woman's personality from a source other than the ratings on personality variables to help understand the particular psychological problems of pregnancy. (The psychological test materials were also used in rating the personality variables.)

3. To compare the woman's personality characteristics prenatally with her characteristics after the baby's birth, and also to determine whether there were any noticeable changes as a result of counseling. We noted earlier the statements by Bibring et al. (1961) and Caplan (1961) to the effect that pregnant women frequently show psychotic-like, if not actually psychotic, test productions. By comparing the woman with herself prenatally and postnatally, we were able to test whether pregnancy is indeed such a disorganizing experience in a group of normal women as these researchers have found. It would have been preferable to test the women before they became pregnant to determine whether changes occurred, but this was not possible.

Psychological Test Battery

All the women in the project were tested soon after they agreed to participate, usually at three months of gestation; they were retested six months after delivery. The psychologist did not know whether the women were in the control or the counseled group and had only a brief factual summary of the social history before the psychological evaluation.

As indicated in Chapter II, the test battery consisted of the Wechsler Adult Intelligence Scale (WAIS), the Rorschach, Thematic Apperception Test (TAT card numbers 1, 2, 3GF, 4, 7GF, 12F, 13MF 16, and 18GF), the Rotter Sentence Completion Test, the Draw a Person Test, plus a drawing of what the woman thought the inside of her body looked like. These tests were selected on the basis of their known clinical value. From the drawings, we hoped to gain insight into the woman's body perception and the clarity of her image of the baby. The WAIS was added after it became evident that there was a wide variation in I.Q. in this group of women, all of whom were at least high school graduates. All tests except the WAIS were repeated at six months postpartum.

Psychiatric Diagnostic Classification

It was evident from the initiation of the project that our sample, like others from normal populations, would nevertheless represent a spectrum of degrees of mental health (Hollingshead and Redlich, 1958;

Loevinger, 1962; Leighton, 1963). A diagnostic classification was developed by the research team to indicate gradations of normalcy and include classifications for those women who did not fall within the range of normalcy by psychiatric definition. The classification and percentage of the sample in each grouping follows:

Normal-normal	18%
Normal with tendency to psychosomatic disorders	3%
Normal with tendency to psychoneurotic disorders	39%
Normal with tendency to character or personality disorder	18%
Psychosomatic	0
Psychoneurotic	16%
Character and personality disorders	3%
Borderline psychotic	3%

While this is a rough progression from the most to the least healthy, it is not a genuine rank order of psychological health. However, it does serve as a rough method of ranking the group as to current personality on a consensus rating after the history, psychiatric interviews, and psychological testing have been done.

On the basis of this classification, 78 per cent of the group might be considered relatively healthy and normal. The remaining 22 per cent (the psychoneurotic, the clear character and personality disorders, and the borderline psychotic) were more seriously disturbed. This is a group that was originally screened to have no psychiatric problems in the sense of being in, or actively looking for, treatment. Though by gross criteria the women were essentially normal, when examined by psychological tests and psychiatric interviews they were found to exhibit a wide range in personality and integration.

Current Personality Variables—Rating Schedules

At the three months' prenatal period, following psychological testing and psychiatric and social work interviews, the women were rated on 28 items in addition to the diagnostic ratings.[5] Two of these items were rated by the psychologist alone, since they were considered to be almost entirely derived from the psychological tests: covert, underlying dependency pattern and ease of fantasy production. A few items were included which were developed around: responsiveness to husband and to others (giving and nurturant quality), gratification in female sexuality, and sense of success as a wife. The other items were directed to an assessment of the woman's predominant defenses, characteristic way of expressing feeling, sense of her own identity, achievement of an adult role, and a general evaluation of her adaptive behavior (how adequate her defenses were in dealing with her needs).

Following retest six months after delivery, the same set of items was rated. The diagnostic evaluation was not repeated, nor was the WAIS given again.

The 28 individual items concerned with the woman's personality were reduced by factor analysis to two factor scales, ego strength and nurturance. The composition of these two scales and their significant correlation with Pregnancy Adaptation and Maternal Adaptation scales will be presented later.

In the staff conferences at which the ratings were made, there were many discussions on the interpretation of discrepancies between the woman's self-report and the psychological test materials—that is, whether a woman who said she had no problems, was happy in her marriage, delighted to be pregnant, had a happy relation with her mother, functioned well on her job, etc., but who on the psychological tests was inhibited, depressed, anxious, or insecure was, in fact, disturbed. Since denial was a strong defense (noted in 68 per cent of the women), it is understandable that psychological tests often suggested more disturbance than the woman either knew or was able to express to the psychiatrist and the social worker. Even so, the psychiatrist and the psychologist tended to see the women as having more personality problems than did the social worker.

To achieve agreement on personality assessment for the consensus ratings, concessions had to be made. Some of the tests suggested disturbance and, in fact, actually anticipated what happened later in pregnancy or in the postpartum period. A number of women who started out denying problems later showed serious problems. In many instances, test responses were inadequately reflected in the consensus ratings because of contrary clinical impressions. Consensus ratings thus represented compromises between test results and clinical impressions.

The item ratings represent only one body of data available from the psychological study of the woman. A second body of data represented more intensive analyses. These were the case-by-case comparison of test results made of the three months' prenatal study with the retests at six months postnatally.

Findings

Test Responses. Many of the women gave anxious responses prenatally on the Rorschach Test. Nearly three-fourths of the women saw such things as clouds, fog, storms, and a "fetus not in its proper place." One woman, who later developed a depression and felt inadequate in her role of mother, at three months saw a "brain with lots of parts missing" or a "squashed uterus with lots missing," but then also gave resolutely happy responses such as a "garden with sun shining to make it grow." There was a surprising number of women who showed depressive feelings at three months (prenatal period). Forty-one per cent gave gay responses indicating a clearly happy, positive mood. There were women who saw the sun shining or saw sunlight with the clouds, a little brook or children playing pat-a-cake or bears kissing, but these were outweighed by the anxious responses given by a large number of women. For many, all was not so rosy, and there was ambivalence and shadows with the sunlight.

The final comparison of test-retest scores was limited to the TAT. Analysis of both prenatal and postnatal TAT scores showed little correlation with other variables, nor were there many sizable correlations between the same TAT scales administered prenatally and postnatally. For the total group, the number of positive outcomes (happy or constructive endings) given in response to TAT pictures increased ($p=0.001$) as the women moved from pregnancy to maternity, and the theme, nurturance, increased significantly from the prenatal to the postnatal period ($p=0.01$).

Comparison of prenatal and postnatal test codings for the remaining test battery was abandoned as relatively unproductive. By omitting this phase of the detailed analysis of test codings, one purpose that the tests were to serve was partially forfeited: we could not look to the test data as a separate, objective body of data on the personality study of the woman apart from case studies and the consensus ratings.

Case Studies Based on Psychological Test Data

When results of testing at six months postpartum were compared with results at three months prenatally, little significant quantitative or qualitative change occurred in the majority of psychological records. The pregnancy reaction was highly individualized, and it did not appear from our data that pregnancy-engendered stresses lead in a consistent and predictable manner to more regression, introversion, or primitive affect than do the stresses of any other life period. One woman in the group proved an interesting exception to this general finding.

At the three months' prenatal study, Mrs. W. performed, for the most part, quite normally on the Rorschach. But, every now and then, there was a marked break, a response denoting a combination of peculiar reasoning, lack of appropriate emotion and a feeling of deterioration and damage. She saw a brain that has "been deteriorated or eaten away because it hasn't been used very much." Again, she sees two spiders, male and female, spinning a web, everything caught in the web and the spiders working together to spin it. The psychologist observes that "if she were not pregnant ...if she came as a psychiatric patient, one would characterize her as a psychotic." In summary, the psychologist states: "On the Rorschach she gives a number of responses that suggest a breakdown in ego controls. She tends to react in a very flat way emotionally, evidently withdrawing to some extent from the world around her. There is a tendency to paranoid thoughts at times, especially in the more distressing situations when her controls break down. It is hard to know whether she is really psychotic, pre-psychotic, disorganized, or simply pregnant."

At the postnatal testing period, Mrs. W. showed a more benign Rorschach protocol. Bizarre responses seen earlier had dropped out. It was still felt, however, that she had potential for odd sorts of behavior and thinking in difficult and/or emotionally stimulating situations. The psychologist hypothesizes that "The earlier feeling of deterioration may have been related to her anxiety about what the baby would be like, anxiety about something being drained from her in the process of pregnancy, etc."...In terms of Mrs. W.'s emotional response to the child, she was seen as sensitive, affectionate and tender, although an element of detachment was noted at times. She also developed a closer relationship to her husband. Her attitude and mood seemed less inclined to depression.

The psychiatric report at six months postnatally indicates none of the bizarreness that was seen during the early part of the pregnancy and she is pleased and relaxed about her situation.

Personality constriction, as indicated by psychological examination, may sometimes be indicative of subsequent difficulty. All but one of the five women who became depressed in the postnatal period exhibited constriction in the psychological evaluation during the prenatal period.[6]

> Mrs. H. was seen, prenatally, as a very constricted person —immature, vague, passive and stereotyped in her thinking. She showed a lack of fantasy and, in addition, seemed to be uncomfortable in the world which to her seems cold, "a cave, only an ice cave." Life was precarious and she felt insecurely unbalanced. In the postnatal tests, she no longer sees the ice cave on Card VIII which may represent a feeling of some greater warmth in her environment. The more pretentious anatomical answers she saw on the first test have dropped out on the second, suggesting perhaps somewhat less anxiety about body adequacy. If anything, she is more controlled now, though not in a really comfortable way. Mrs. H. experienced and described feelings of depression for which she was able to seek therapy.

A few women who exhibited constriction in the prenatal psychological study were found to have achieved a better level of integration after the birth of the infant.

> Mrs. D. was a very constricted, defensive woman. There was a great deal of anxiety that was immediately denied (dark forests brightened by sunshine). She gave many signs of depression. It was difficult for her to express genuine feeling or fantasy. She persisted in making everything work out right but drained the life from her perceptions in the process. On the basis of this bleak portrait of personality dynamics, a poor pregnancy and maternal adaptation was

to be expected. But Mrs. D., who was still seen at the six months' postnatal examination as rigid and defensive, covering feelings of inner loneliness and depression by exaggerated insistence that everything is lovely, is described by the infant observer as managing well, handling the baby in an alert and sensitive manner. She is also seen as well adapted in her marriage and happy with her current life situation.

Sometimes an occasional bizarre response or a detail of a drawing in the prenatal tests has great meaning in terms of the woman's future adjustment.

Mrs. B., who later had grave psychiatric disorders, gave a realistic and well-integrated picture, save for a flavor of confusion and primitive morbid feeling when she saw a "skinned knee with a lot of dirt in it."

Mrs. S., who drew no baby at any time during her pregnancy, turned out to be a detached, intellectualized mother.

Mrs. G., who saw a "nurse running after a child trying to climb a tree," had a hyperactive child and spent months running after him. Her drawing of her insides at three months prenatal shows a perky baby sitting upright.

Similarites and differences between prenatal tests and postnatal retests are suggestive of the range of response to the pregnancy and maternity experiences.

Mrs. A. has one fewer movement response and a good deal less labile emotion on her second Rorschach. She gives more "hard" responses. She sees many more lungs, ribs, pelvic bones, bugs with pinchers, for instance. She does, however, end up the test by seeing a "rosebud" so that in the end there is some tenderness. On the second test she gives the impression of a certain over-assertiveness. One still has an impression of a young woman who has not resolved competitive feelings with mother.

Mrs. C. appears, on retest, as a woman who brings little of herself into a situation but who sits passively by. Unlike the first time she is able to fill out all of the items of the Sentence Completion Tests, and in this there may be more openness. She admits now that her greatest fear was that she would have an abnormal child. At the earlier period (prenatal) her greatest fear was that she couldn't have children. She continues to show anxiety about her child and one sees it in the Thematic Apperception Test, too, where the blank card produces a story about a woman who lost a child in a fire. She says on the Sentence Completion Test that her mind is always on the baby and his future. She again gives the impression of being somewhat depressed as well as extremely inhibited and possibly also consciously distrustful of the project's motives.

In the case of Mrs. E., one sees somewhat more constriction on the postpartum Rorschach; in analyzing the content of responses, however, it would seem that she is more open in regard to her feelings of anger as well as to her fears. An illustration of the change from a more serene to a more intense response is that on Card V she now sees "charging bison" instead of "leaping deer," and yet on Card IX there is more structure and she now sees a "bud opening" rather than the more diffuse Marin painting. One has the impression of both more control and more tension and also a somewhat more realistic way of perceiving. It may be that the counseling has made it easier for her to express her feelings, to become more open about what she likes and doesn't like, and less affected.

On the whole, these case studies indicate a tendency to more conscious control, more realism, and some greater openness about expressing feeling. The similarity to the earlier basic responses is prominent in all cases.

Some women who "looked good" on the psychologicals turned out to be "good" mothers, satisfied with their current life situations and future expectations. Others who "looked good" did not fare so well. As always, our hindsight is excellent in these cases. We feel that we "should have known" from this or that indicator that something was drastically wrong and that overt emotional maladjustments would result. While psychological tests during pregnancy in themselves do not provide a single reliable predictor of postpartum adjustment, the above cases suggest that careful scrutiny of the content can help us foresee problems in some women.

Our scanning of the test protocols led us to believe that each woman was true to herself in terms of basic perceptual and thought processes. From the tests administered early in the pregnancy, we found no regressive or psychotic-like tendencies in the majority of pregnant women we encountered. What we did find generally was that each woman entered upon, confronted, and dealt with the pregnancy experience and maternity according to the strengths and weaknesses she possessed prior to that experience.

Personality Variables and Outcomes: Statistical Correlates[7]

From the initial psychological study of the woman and the one conducted a year later, two factors were derived through factor analysis. The factors, from the prenatal and postnatal periods, were both entitled ego strength and nurturance.[8]

The factor scale *ego strength* comprises nine items: the degree to which the woman was seen as emotionally adapted; the covert, underlying dependency pattern; the woman's general anxiety; her sense of humor, flexibility, and ability to meet her own needs, including pleasure; acceptance of her own identity; the degree to which she has achieved an adult role; and an overall evaluation of her adaptive behavior. Broadly conceived, this factor describes the woman's maturity and emotional adaptation.

The factor scale *nurturance* brought together several other items of the Current Personality section of the rating schedule: responsiveness to husband, gratification in female sexuality, responsiveness to others, sense of success as a wife, the degree to which the woman was tender and affectionate as part of her characteristic way of expressing feeling, her ability to give help and support, and her sense of success as a homemaker. In obtaining a nurturance score, the number of predominant defenses (denial, repression, reaction formation, regression, and others) was subtracted from the sum of the ratings of the seven items. In general terms, this factor describes the woman's responsiveness and giving quality.

Pregnancy Adaptation and Personality Factors (Prenatal). The correlates of the personality factors from the prenatal period with Pregnancy Adaptation scales are presented in Table 2. Since personality factors were developed from data obtained early in the pregnancy, their close association with Pregnancy Adaptation scales at all prenatal

TABLE 2. *Pregnancy adaptation and personality factors (prenatal)*
statistically significant correlates (N = 57)

Factor Scale		Correlated with	Study period involved (months)	$r*$
No.	Name			
4	Ego strength	Scale 8 Adaptation to pregnancy experience	3	0.56
	(3 months prenatal)	10 Reaction to characteristic fears of pregnancy	3	0.57
		11 Adaptation to pregnancy experience	7	0.28
		13 Reaction to pregnancy fears	7	0.42
		16 Overall reaction to pregnancy	9	0.29
5	Nurturance	Scale 8 Adaptation to pregnancy experience	3	0.44
	(3 months prenatal)	11 Adaptation to pregnancy experience	7	0.25
		12 Confirmation of sexual identity	7	0.31
		16 Overall reaction to pregnancy	9	0.26

$*r = 0.25$ $(p = 0.05)$; $r = 0.34$ $(p = 0.01)$

ratings periods means that they may be viewed as *predictors* of pregnancy adaptation.

Maternal Adaptation and Personality Factors (Postnatal). The personality factors derived from the retesting and study of the woman six months postnatally correlated with Maternal Adaptation factors measured at the three postnatal rating periods. The results are shown in Table 3. The nurturance factor, as evaluated at the end of the study, correlated significantly with ten of twelve Maternal Adaptation scales. Maternal adaptation, in other words, is generally consistent with the level of personality integration represented in the ego strength and nurturance factors evaluated postnatally.

The degree of correlation of the personality factors with family adaptation scales postnatally (correlation coefficients of 0.67 between ego strength and family adaptation, and 0.71 between nurturance and family adaptation, all rated concurrently), statistically confirms common sense observations of the meaningfulness for family living of maturity and giving qualities on the part of the woman. The personality factors, ego strength and nurturance, loaded significantly on the superfactor, feminine identification. Ego strength also moderately related to the superfactor, woman's intelligence, which was dominated by the Full Scale I.Q.

Personality Factors Over Time. The mean for the factor scale, nurturance, was significantly higher in the postnatal period ($p < 0.01$) than in the prenatal period. There was no change over this period for the factor scale, ego strength.

Summary

A wide range of personality health and integration was identified in this normal sample, and the case studies revealed an equally wide range of emotional reactions to pregnancy and maternity. The close association of the personality factors with the two outcomes, pregnancy and maternal adaptation, indicates that the study of the psychology of the woman from which the personality factors emerged is of major importance in anticipating coping strengths and future problems in the maternity cycle.

TABLE 3. *Maternal adaptation and personality factors (postnatal) statistically significant correlates* ($N = 57$)

Scale no.	Schedule—name	Correlated with	r^*
		Scale	
43 G-IV	Ego strength	26 Acceptance of maternal role (E-III)	0.37
		27 Acceptance of infant (E-III)	0.25
		30 Responsiveness to infant (F-III)	0.32
		32 Confidence in maternal role (F-III)	0.40
		33 Acceptance of maternal role (F-III)	0.46
		34 Responsiveness to infant (G-III)	0.47
		35 Acceptance of infant and maternal role (G-III)	0.56
		36 Individualization of infant (G-III)	0.32
		Scale	
44 G-IV	Nurturance	26 Acceptance of maternal role (E-III)	0.49
		27 Acceptance of infant (E-III)	0.34
		29 Responsiveness to infant (E-III)	0.31
		30 Responsiveness to infant (F-III)	0.46
		31 Acceptance of infant (F-III)	0.26
		32 Confidence in maternal role (F-III)	0.26
		33 Acceptance of maternal role (F-III)	0.38
		34 Responsiveness to infant (G-III)	0.46
		35 Acceptance of infant and maternal role (G-III)	0.55
		46 Mother-infant adaptation	0.32

$^*r = 0.25$ ($p = 0.05$); $r = 0.34$ ($p = 0.01$)

MARITAL ADAPTATION

Prenatal Assessment of Husband-Wife Adaptation

In conceptualizing factors likely to affect the woman's attitude towards her pregnancy and her adaptations to it, the husband's impact was considered of major importance. On this assumption, a considerable number of items were developed to evaluate the husband's responsiveness to his wife and the pregnancy, and later to the newborn baby and his wife in her new role as mother. Analysis of items covering the prenatal period resulted in two factor scales dealing with the husband's role:

Husband's responsiveness to wife,[9] composed of nine items: empathy; communication; affection; hostility; sexual adjustment; decision process; extent to which husband allows dependency; husband's fostering of woman's self-confidence as a mother; and overall husband-wife adaptation.

Husband's responsiveness to pregnancy, composed of five items: reaction to wife in regard to pregnancy; reaction to baby-to-be; feelings about sharing wife; congruence of the pregnancy with current way of life; and congruence of the pregnancy with long-time plans.

Husband-wife adaptation was evaluated and rated at every prenatal and postnatal study period.

The assessment of husband-wife adaptation in the prenatal period was found to be a more complex process and to show fewer significant statistical relationships than the evaluation of husband-wife adaptations for the postnatal period. Before presenting the data on the two factors described above, we offer a summary of the marital situations in our population at the time the first pregnancy occurred.

Marital Situation During the Pregnancy

The interval between date of marriage and time of the first pregnancy showed a spread from less than three months to ten years (see Chapter II, Table 5). For 37 per cent of the research sample, the first pregnancy occurred in the first year of marriage indicating that these couples were still largely involved in the task of early marital adaptation, establishing themselves as a family unit emotionally, financially, and socially.

The level of marital adjustment at the time of the first pregnancy, as well as the range in time of its occurrence, showed wide variation. Well-adapted marital relationships were characterized by such factors as an intense degree of affection, empathy, satisfying sexual adjustment, mutuality of goals, and flexibility in decision-making. Less adapted relationships showed negative aspects, such as more conflict than mutuality, considerable hostility, more inhibition than freedom in communication, and decisions arrived at with difficulty and further threat to mutuality. The families in conflict included two quite different patterns and processes: (1) those involved in differences that were essentially related to the early adjustment phase of the marriage—differences that were transitory in nature, and (2) those involved in serious marital disharmony, probably long-time in duration or predictive of eventual disruption of the marriage.

Transitory Problems. In the first group of relatively transient maladaptive patterns, issues were those of achieving a balance in such aspects as a comfortable dependence on each other versus adequate room for independence, or acceptance of assertions of individuality versus movement towards identification as a family unit. Among this group were those who were caught up in the bewilderment of early marriage with its still surprising rewards and demands and in the moments of discomfiture over its disappointments or sharp encounters. Many marital issues were resolved to a considerable extent even within the one year of project participation. "... The difference between a normal and a neurotic family life is that, in the first, unconscious conflicts are worked through without full conscious insight—it happens every day—and in the second the partners neurotically repeat the conflict situation without finding the way out..." (Grotjahn, 1960, p. 284).

Marital Disharmony. Serious marital disharmony was found in 21 per cent of the families in the initial study process. These families were already in considerable trouble when the pregnancy occurred. Marital disharmony is defined here in clinical terms as involving those cases in which thoughts of separation were overt or nearly so, or temporary separation had already taken place, and commitment to the marriage was uncertain for one or both members. In cases of marital disharmony, the pregnancy often became another focus of conflict, or its significance was obscured by the involvement in the marital conflict. The negative impact of a poor husband-wife relationship on the woman's adaptation to pregnancy was clearly evident in individual cases.

The few reported instances of infidelity on the part of the husband during the pregnancy were all in families of problematic marital adjustment. In these instances the woman quite clearly closed her eyes to the occurrence of infidelity. Possibly only men who knew their wives would condone their unfaithfulness involved themselves in extra-marital relationships during the pregnancy. We can conjecture further that the wife feels herself realistically more dependent on her husband during pregnancy, and therefore prefers not to jeopardize her situation by a confrontation. The issue did not always remain suppressed or dormant, as subsequent follow-up (after project participation) revealed, when a few of the families faced further deterioration in the marriage situation.

Where the marital commitment was unclear and anxiety regarding the marriage was added to anxiety regarding the pregnancy, a sad imbalance occurred and a woman could feel herself very much alone and uncertain in this venture of having a baby.

> She's scared about having the baby, scared that her husband won't be there. Once he sees it maybe it will be better, she says, and then very sadly she says that he just doesn't seem to care anything about this baby or about her in her pregnant state. She's tried to get him to go buy baby furniture with her and he keeps putting it off and avoiding it and just once she wishes he would open up the subject of the baby. Sometimes she has what she calls horrible thoughts. She thinks that maybe the baby will die and then he will really be sorry. Or else she thinks that when the baby comes it will be a lineup in which the baby and she will unite against him. But she is ashamed of these thoughts and doesn't like having them.

Only a few couples in the sample were as troubled as the one cited here, but the fearfulness expressed by this woman characterized in varying degrees the attitude of those whose marriages were unsatisfactory. These husbands tended to undermine the woman's confidence in herself as a mother, and both husband and wife usually entered into the first phase of parenthood with little belief in the woman's capacity to function in the role of mother. The obverse side of the picture was that the women in this group of conflicted families were equally lacking in confidence in their husbands' capacities as fathers. Each tended to undermine the other's sense of worth.

Characteristic Marital Adaptations to a First Pregnancy. For husbands and wives to learn to carry a responsible function in the family required sensitive response to each other's strengths, weaknesses, and needs. Where the marriage commitment was clear, the process went on smoothly, almost imperceptibly, with constant give and take in establishing balance.

Normally, there was much that was exciting and gratifying to counterbalance pregnancy-engendered uncertainties and anxieties. We saw in most instances that an emerging sense of common goal seemed to give new depth to the husband-wife relationship. This was expressed in many ways: shared preoccupations about what kind of parents they were likely to be and how they would meet crises and everyday issues, the moments of wonder over the movements of the fetus and what they portended about the sex and the future level of activity of the expected child, practice in acting (and in helping each other act) in more disciplined ways as appropriate models for a growing child. Most husbands and wives found these and related aspects of the pregnancy experience gratifying and, at times, delightful. Moreover, here and there in the project sample were men who were able to sustain their wives with confidence, humor, affection, reassurance— whatever quality was needed at the moment—throughout the changes of the pregnancy, the stress of labor and delivery, and beyond. The nurturant quality, usually associated only with the maternal woman, may at times be found in an equally rich vein in a masculine man.

Statistical Findings

The first factor scale described earlier, husband's responsiveness to wife, was not significantly related to any of the scales which constitute the outcome variable, Pregnancy Adaptation. The second factor scale, husband's responsiveness to pregnancy, correlated with only two of six scales measuring pregnancy adaptation. The means for husband-wife adaptation show improvement between the first and third trimester, implying that the pregnancy generally serves a positive role in family adaptation for this period. This is of special interest in view of the contrary development in the six months following the birth of the infant.

It is somewhat puzzling that there was so little relationship between the husband's impact and the outcome scales measuring pregnancy adaptation. It may be that the statistical relationship of family adaptation to pregnancy adaptation was obscured by the complexity resulting from the interaction of adjustment processes characteristic of (1) early marriage in a substantial proportion of the families, (2) marital stress in another segment of the sample, and (3) the impact of the counseling with half of the sample, the counseled group.

Postnatal Assessment of Husband-Wife Adaptation

The assessments of husband-wife adaptation in the postnatal period resulted in these factors:

Husband-wife adaptation,[10] consisting of: wife's reaction to husband's new role; husband's reaction to wife as mother; responsiveness of husband to wife; responsiveness of wife to husband; overall husband-wife adaptation; effect of infant on family homeostasis.

Reaction to paternal role, consisting of: husband's reaction to his role as father; husband's reaction to baby.

Marital and Maternal Adaptations. The close correspondence between marital adaptation and maternal adaptation is the most outstanding aspect of the series of correlates of the scales measuring maternal adaptation. In each study period, the husband-wife adaptation factor, derived from ratings done concurrently with those evaluating maternal adaptation, correlated with eight to ten of the twelve Maternal Adaptation scales. In addition, the scale, reaction to paternal role, correlated with eight Maternal Adaptation scales at the six-month period and with several scales in the earlier rating periods.

Among the superfactor scales is one called maternal responsiveness. Maternal responsiveness correlated with husband's responsiveness to the paternal role. These results from factor analyses at all postnatal rating periods provide statistical evidence in support of a wealth of data from interviews and clinical observations indicating the crucial role of the husband in affecting the level of mother-infant adaptations.

It is of interest that the postnatal ratings on husband-wife adaptation show a trend downward compared to the evaluation made at the end of the pregnancy, doubtless reflecting the strains introduced into the relationship by the arrival of the infant.

Our emphasis here on family adaptation comes from a commitment to the concept of the family as formative in the development of the child—a concept stated succinctly and meaningfully by Allen (1963, p. 245).

Within the framework provided by the parental figures the ever-recurring drama of self-realization occurs. The child, being a new biological integrate, starts on...a journey he can take only through the help and direction of the significant adults who are the representatives of the new world into which he is born. It is a preformed world the child awakens and walks into and to which he adapts. While the child contains within himself the potential for being an individual, separate and different from those who gave him life, he becomes this in a setting that, in a large measure, determines the kind of individual he is expected to become.

EXTERNAL STRESSES

It seemed clear to us that, if the psychology of pregnancy was to be understood in realistic terms, we would need to concern ourselves with the external events that impinged on the families under study, and to ascertain how external events may exacerbate stresses associated with a first pregnancy. Since many couples were adapting to the early phase of their marriages and all were making adaptations to a first pregnancy, some common psychological problems characterized the whole group. Here our interest is to separate difficult life conditions from physiological and psychological stresses that are primarily pregnancy-engendered and to identify the kinds of problems that were encountered by individual families and not by the total group.

In the first chapter we called attention to the persistent findings reported in large-scale researches conducted in many countries, that reproductive disturbance occurs among women of lower social-economic class to a greater extent than among upper-class women (Richardson and Guttmacher, 1967). This is doubtless due in large part to obvious deficiencies in diet and other basic needs, but may be equally related to a pattern of recurring traumatic events which is also seen as characteristic of lower social class life (Riessman et al., 1964; Dohrenwend and Dohrenwend, 1965; Lewis, 1966).

The criteria for selection of the sample for this study were designed to exclude this vulnerable group—women in lower-class status and families involved in gross trauma, such as serious mental or physical illness or chronic dire poverty. Stresses there were, nevertheless, in this as in any social group, as we recognized from the beginning.

Moreover, some families reacted to a problem by dealing realistically with it, either finding adequate solution to it or quickly coming to terms with the circumstance. Others responded to the same problem as if it were extremely stressful and possibly insoluble.

Specific Stresses

We identified specific problems external to the pregnancy, and the numbers of families who experienced them as stressful, as follows:

Anxiety about financial security—29 per cent
Job dissatisfaction on part of husband—27 per cent
Serious marital disharmony—21 per cent
Isolation related to geographical distance from major family supports—15 per cent
Crises of own parents, and acute relationship problems between couple and their parents—14 per cent
Illness of husband or wife during pregnancy—12 per cent
Illness or death of a member of the extended family—12 per cent

The above listing represents 70 per cent of the sample. During the pregnancy 42 per cent were involved with two or more stresses. The number of stresses ranged from none in 29 per cent of the families to a maximum of four in 3 per cent of the families.

Statistical Findings: Stresses as Related to Other Variables

Except for serious marital disharmony, which was studied and measured in many ways, separate stresses were not analyzed in detail, but the total number of stresses was analyzed with respect to other variables. Statistically significant intercorrelations were found between the total number of stresses and several important variables both in the prenatal and postnatal periods.

Table 4 shows that total number of stresses had its highest correlation with problematic husband-wife adaptation at several periods at which ratings were made, and more stresses correlated with less responsiveness on the part of the husband both to the wife and to the pregnancy. This high correlation was, to some extent, accounted for by the fact that, except in two instances, cases of marital

TABLE 4. *Significant correlations of total overt stresses* with personality, pregnancy experience and outcome, and postnatal family adaptation factor scales*

Factor scale	Study period involved (months)	Correlation coefficient
Prenatal		
5 Nurturance	3	−0.27
6 Husband's responsiveness to wife	3	−0.39
7 Husband's responsiveness to pregnancy	3	−0.41
8 Adaptation to pregnancy experience	3	−0.30
9 Visualization of self as mother	3	−0.27
14 Visualization of self as mother	7	−0.26
15 Response to project	9	−0.28
16 Overall reaction to pregnancy	9	−0.32
Postnatal		
37 Husband-wife adaptation	1	−0.28
39 Husband-wife adaptation	3	−0.39
41 Husband-wife adaptation	6	−0.36
44 Nurturance	6	−0.26
45 Family adaptation	6	−0.43

$r = 0.25$ ($p = 0.05$); $r = 0.34$ ($p = 0.01$)
*The total number of stresses shows a negative correlation with all but one item in the table, since the scale items were rated from low to high, whereas total number of stresses moves in the opposite direction.

disharmony also had at least one other stress as well, and several were among the cases with three or four stresses. The highest correlation was with the overall rating for the factor scale, family adaptation, at the six months' postnatal period. A significant inverse relationship was found between total number of stresses and the superfactor scales, feminine identification and husband-wife adaptation.

These correlations lend weight to clinical observations that, when characterized by mutuality, the husband-wife relationship is itself a deterrent to the development of stresses. The indication is that, through joint effort, a potentially stressful development can be confronted and the problems dealt with before the circumstance becomes crystalized into a persistent, serious stress. Of special interest in terms of the purposes of the study is the fact that both the prenatal and postnatal personality variable, nurturance, is significantly inversely related to the number of stresses (Table 4); that is, more stresses are found in families in which the woman's giving or nurturant qualities are limited.

Correlations were based on the 57 cases included in our final sample, as indicated earlier.[11] In the three cases of reproductive casualties, postnatal data regarding maternal adaptation and the infant were, of course, not available. Overt stresses were in fact prominent in all three families with reproductive casualty. In this connection, it is noteworthy that other investigators have found stressful external circumstances significantly related to perinatal complications (Gordon and Gordon, 1960; Hetzel et al., 1961; Larsen, 1966).

External Stress and Inner Reaction

In each instance of external stress, its psychological meaning is found in the interaction of the particular stress with the particular person or family. In the language of the Menninger Foundation project on psychotherapy outcome, the environmental situation is significant in the degree to which it "resonates favorably or unfavorably with individual autonomous values, interests and characterological styles" (Voth et al., 1962).

Financial Issues. A few families had a realistic problem about finances, in that the income from an unsatisfactory job in one case and from intermittent employment in two other situations left them at or very near the poverty level as commonly defined in government publications.[12] However, anxiety over financial security characterized nearly one-third (29 per cent) of the families prenatally. Much of this anxiety represented a displacement from other aspects of the couple's current reality, such as reluctance to become a one-income instead of a two-income family, concern over varied aspects of the pregnancy itself, or tension between the couple in their overall relationship.

Problems in Relationship to Parents of the Couple. Varied aspects of relationship to parents were found to be problematic for some of the families under study, including: traumatic events in the lives of parents or siblings; unrealistic expectations and demands made of the young couple on the part of parents; and geographical distance from parents, with the resultant loneliness of the pregnant woman.

Preparation for marriage includes a process described in one study as "disengaging...oneself from especially close relationships that compete with or interfere with commitment to the new marital relationship" (Rapoport, 1963). Traumatic event in the lives of the extended family—such as separation of parents, problems of siblings, mental or physical illness or death of a parent—tended to draw our participants back into closer interrelationship with the nuclear family at least for a time. The significance of such involvement in the concerns and needs of the extended family lies in the extent to which the young couples' psychological and physical energies become diverted from their own tasks of planning for and adapting to the pregnancy and later to the infant.

The acute illness or death of a parent stirs feelings of a range and depth to tax the psychological resources of anyone.

> In the case of Mrs. N., whose mother died during her first pregnancy, it was two years after project participation before she could talk to a project staff member of the sense of terrible aloneness that she experienced during the pregnancy. The early postnatal period found this woman persistently low in mood, her difficulty in adjustment complicated by her infant's hyperactivity.

The pregnancy seemed at times to generate undue anxiety in the parents of the pregnant woman, fear for their daughter's well-being bringing to the surface latent conflicts in their own lives. Since parents during pregnancy see their children as more nearly co-equal, visualizing them as parents in their own right, they tend to become somewhat more open and frank in sharing problems, past and present. At times this kind of sharing had an aspect of a too-early or unwise reversal of roles and placed a heavy emotional burden on the pregnant daughter.

The availability of family supports varied greatly. Less than half of the women had parents or siblings in close enough proximity for free interchange of telephone calls and visits, and approximately one-third of the husbands' parents lived in the same community.[13] Living too closely to parents sometimes threatened the independence of the newly married couple. Many couples had difficulty assuming adult roles within the extended family, either because of their own dependence or the parents' inability to see them in any new way.

At the same time, many expectant mothers wanted to be closer to their families. A number of young families had come to the city in recent months, following marriage. For them close family ties had been disrupted. In approximately 15 per cent of the sample, the lack of family ties close at hand was experienced as a stress, and inability to draw on the family remained a void, especially for those who for varied reasons found it difficult to reach out to meet their emotional needs.

Inner State and Outer Stresses—A Case Illustration. To indicate the interplay of environmental factors and inner state of the pregnant woman, some highlights are presented from an interview of the psychiatrist with a young woman at the seventh month. The interviews with the psychiatrist took place initially at the three-month period and not again until the seventh month of pregnancy. The seven-month interview focused on current concerns, such as fears and/or anticipation of the labor and delivery experience, mood changes, relationship to husband and other key figures, and preoccupations regarding the baby-to-be.

In the interview with this 22-year-old woman, the areas listed above were explored, and in the course of the interview a few of the changed factual circumstances were brought to light. She had stopped working at the end of the 6th month. As a result, money was comparatively tight. In recent weeks her parents, whose marital situation had been strained as long as she could remember, had separated for the first time. She talked of feeling edgy and moody, unable to do as much as she wanted to do, impatient and apprehensive about labor and delivery, and worried about her parents' attitude towards her pregnancy. The earlier months of pregnancy had been much better. Summarizing, the psychiatrist states: "Mrs. A. is indeed having a very difficult time. It appears that some physical difficulties have their roots in emotional disorders. In the past she was able to cope with some of these difficulties by extensive social interaction, either at work or in other social situations. The limitations placed upon her by the pregnancy seem to have altered her pattern sufficiently so that the old defenses do not really operate effectively, and she is suffering with a great deal of anxiety that is reflected in insomnia as well as other physical complaints. There are questions about her femininity that also get stirred up by this and the experience seems to be an assault on her narcissism. The baby is, at this point, the focus for a fair amount of hostility, and although she attempts to handle some of this by joking, it is quite apparent that there are some intense hostile feelings towards this fetus and what havoc it is wreaking upon her adjustment."

This woman, in responding both to external stress (her parents' acute problem) and to stresses associated with her pregnancy, reacted with a degree of psychosomatic complaints and psychological distress that was more maladaptive than was characteristic for the majority of the women. For her, the experience of this period "resonated unfavorably with...her characterological style."

SUMMARY

We undertook to identify facets of the woman's background that bear on her reactions to her first pregnancy. We directed ourselves in part to the past, to the woman's life history prior to marriage and pregnancy. We explored as well her current personality and current life situation, including the husband's impact and their family adaptation, and external stresses that may have impinged on the family during the pregnancy. We were interested in assessing the impact of these separate aspects of background on the central concerns of the study—the three outcome variables of Pregnancy Adaptation, Maternal Adaptation, and Infant Adaptation.

Life history variables included the woman's family relationships and circumstance and aspects of personal history that might be formative in the development of a sense of identity, such as school and peer relationships, and interest in children and experience with them from an early age. A variable entitled woman's perception of her own experience in being mothered invited recall of early memories and current experiences that were highly charged emotionally. The variable was designed to obtain the woman's retrospective evaluation of the relationship to her mother and her view of her mother's satisfaction in the maternal role.

While the variable, perception of experience in being mothered, did not correlate with any of the three outcome variables at a statistically significant level, it did correlate with a small number of other variables that were interestingly selective in nature: prenatal factor scales measuring ego strength and reaction to characteristic fears of pregnancy, and postnatal factor scales evaluating husband-wife adaptation. It was also related to the overall superfactor, woman's self-confidence. The statistical relationships imply that women who view their mothers as having been emotionally close and empathic, happy in the maternal role and able to satisfy the emotional needs of the daughter during childhood and in her premarital life, are likely to have little anxiety about the pregnancy, to be confident in the maternal role, and to be adapted as wives. The extent to which the mother met the daughter's changing emotional needs, evaluated at several time periods (retrospectively for childhood, adolescence, and early adulthood, and concurrently during pregnancy and at six months postpartum) was found to be quite constant over time. The implication is that the quality of the mother-daughter relationship does not change essentially over the years.

The factor dealing with an early interest in and experience with young children was predictive of Maternal Adaptation. The other two life history factors—perception of experience in being mothered and school and peer relationships—were not predictive of the woman's adaptation to her first pregnancy or her functioning in the maternal role in the early postpartum period. By the time of the first pregnancy, the impact of the woman's relationships in early life appears, from our data, to have been partially obscured by intervening events and integrated with other developmental phases.

In particular the emphasis in the literature on the crucial significance of the mother-daughter relationship in the woman's adaptations to entering upon motherhood are not borne out in our statistical analyses with any consistency. Our results do suggest an indirect role for the significance of that relationship, expressed especially in the build-up of the woman's self-confidence.

Our interpretation of these findings recognizes that significant aspects of mothering take place in the earliest years of life and are not readily available to memory. An assessment of a relationship in the past is, in any case, subject to vagaries of memory, whether these take the form of maximizing the ideal and minimizing conflict and unhappiness, or the reverse. Whitehead, quoted by Gordon Allport, states one of the obstacles to the assessment involved here: "We do not even have words with which to describe what is always with us; we tend to take the ubiquities of our lives for granted. . . ." (Allport, 1960, p. 22).

In marked contrast to the life history variables, *the current personality of the woman* was highly correlated with a number of variables representative of all phases of the maternity cycle. The psychological study of the woman in the first trimester of pregnancy and a year later at six months postpartum yielded two sets of factors, for the prenatal and the postnatal periods respectively, which were entitled ego strength and nurturance; each set of factors was of pervasive significance for both periods.

The current personality of the woman, as evaluated early in the pregnancy, gave clear indication of her capacity to accept and adapt to the pregnancy experience; the factors, ego strength and nurturance, were in fact predictors of Pregnancy Adaptation. Similarly, the postnatal factors, ego strength and nurturance, were highly correlated with the woman's functioning and attitudes in her role as mother. Thus, personality variables are closely associated with two of the three outcomes of the study. Except for a few correlations with variables dealing with infant characteristics, the ego strength and nurturance factors were less related to Infant Adaptation.

From a comparative study of psychological test results in the prenatal and postpartum periods and the overall evaluation of the woman's adaptations in pregnancy and the early period of maternal functioning, we concluded that the woman's adaptation to pregnancy and maternity tends to be consistent with her characteristic patterns of response and her adaptive behavior in general. Unlike some of the researchers working in this area in the past two decades, we found no psychotic-like tendencies during pregnancy in the majority of women in the study population; this conclusion is largely based on psychological tests and interviews of the first trimester of pregnancy.

Turning to the woman's *current life situation,* we were interested in evaluating *marital adaptation* both during her first pregnancy and after the infant's arrival. The husband's impact during pregnancy was measured by two factor scales entitled husband's responsiveness to the wife and husband's responsiveness to the pregnancy; the former was not significantly related with any of the Pregnancy Adaptation scales, and the latter correlated with only two of the Pregnancy Adaptation scales. We are somewhat puzzled by the lack of a clear relationship between the husband's impact and pregnancy adaptation.

The marital circumstances in the study sample included the fact that, in approximately two-fifths of the cases, the couples had been married rather recently, for a year or less, when the pregnancy occurred, and adjustments characteristic of the early phase of marriage had not yet been stabilized in many instances. Moreover, on initial study during the first trimester, serious marital disharmony characterized approximately one-fifth of the families. It may be that the process of adjustment to the early phase of the marriage, or, in 20 per cent of the families, to serious marital stress were so complex in interaction with the compelling adjustments demanded at the time of the first pregnancy that they tended to mask statistical relationship.

It may also be that the intervention of counseling with part of the sample (the counseled group) played a role in altering the relation of family adaptation to pregnancy adaptation. Another possibility, suggested by our statistical findings on factors closely associated with pregnancy adaptation, is that the woman is responding at this time less to significant relationships in her life than to intrapsychic and physiological developments from within.

In the postnatal period, the husband's impact was unequivocally related to maternal adaptation. The statistical relationships here confirm clinical observations on the vital role of the husband in the transition from a dyadic to a triadic family unit.

The level of marital adaptation for the sample as a whole showed variations over time. During pregnancy the husband-wife relationship improved, the pregnancy apparently drawing the couples closer in feeling. In the postnatal period, the relationship deteriorated in a substantial proportion of the families, doubtless due to the strain of trying to adapt to the infant's needs and to the unfamiliar roles of mother and father.

Although, in the interest of maintaining a focus on normal young families, the research design was planned to exclude families likely to be burdened by traumatic circumstance, a number of stresses —unpredicted circumstances separate from the pregnancy—were found to affect our families intimately. This was true in the current life situation of 70 per cent of the families in our sample. These stressful circumstances ranged from financial anxieties and job dissatisfactions of the husband through illness of the husband or death of a parent. The total number of stresses in a family correlated inversely with a number of variables relating to all phases of the study, especially those involving aspects of husband-wife adaptation and feminine identification. In the families with more stresses, acceptance of and adjustment to the pregnancy was achieved with more difficulty, as was to be expected, and the family adjustments postpartum were also harder. It is clear that even under relatively favorable socio-economic circumstances, many facets of everyday living can be expected to impose special burdens on young families undergoing a first pregnancy.

[1]In Chapter V we consider these same factors in relation to expectant fathers.

[2]Studies concerned with early mother-infant interaction among humans include: Deutsch, 1945; Bowlby, 1951; Brody, 1956; Bell, 1960; Bibring, 1961; Caplan, 1961; Rheingold, 1964; Spitz, 1965; Yarrow, 1965; Moss, 1967; and Wenner and Cohen, 1968, 1969. For animal studies see Harlow, in *Determinants of Infant Behavior,* II, 1963; and Rosenblatt, in *Childbearing,* 1967.

[3]We know of one study recently completed on this issue: Perceived Styles of Mother-Daughter lationship and the Prenatal Adjustment of the *Primigravida* by Ruth T. Green, a doctoral dissertation, George Washington University, Department of Psychology, 1971-1973.

[4]Table 1 in Chapter VIII, Maternal Adaptation, presents the statistical correlates for the factor, interest in children, and Maternal Adaptation scales.

[5]Appendix B, Schedule A, contains the section on Current Personality rated at the time of the initial study of the woman. Schedule G-IV contains the Current Personality items—rated at six months postnatally.

[6]Chapter IX, which deals with postpartum psychiatric disorders, refers to seven, not five, women who suffered a postpartum psychiatric disorder. The apparent discrepancy is accounted for by reason of the difference in time span covered. The later analysis included psychiatric disorders associated with a second pregnancy, whereas the original study was limited to the first pregnancy.

[7]To follow the development of the results, it is necessary to keep in mind the levels of statistical analysis set forth in Chapter II, Research Design and Methodology.

[8]See Appendix C, Compendium, for a list of items in pre- and postnatal factor scales, ego strength (4 and 43) and nurturance (5 and 44).

[9]See Compendium, Appendix C, for complete list of items in factor scales 6 and 7.

[10]See Compendium, Appendix C, for complete list of items in factor scales 37 and 38.

[11]The final sample of 57 cases is used throughout this section. (See Chapter II, Social Characteristics, for discussion of variations in number of cases used in analyses of data.)

[12]$2,992 per year, representing earnings under the Federal minimum wage law on a 40-hour week and a 52-week year, is taken as the "poverty line" in "Guaranteed Income Maintenance," by Helen O. Nicol, Division of Research, Welfare Adm., *Welfare in Review,* Vol. 5, No. 6. June-July, 1967. U.S. Dept. of HEW, Government Printing Office, Washington, D.C.

[13]Chapter II, Social Characteristics, Table 7, presents data on frequency of contacts with parents.

REFERENCES

Allen, F.H. (1963) *Positive Aspects of Child Psychiatry.* New York: W.W. Norton and Co.

Allport, G.W. (1960) *Personality and Social Encounter.* Boston: Beacon Press.

Bell, R.Q. (1960) Relations between Behavioral Manifestations in Human Neonate. *Child Development,* 31:463-477.

Bibring, G.L., Dwyer, T.F., Huntington, D., and Valenstein, A.F. (1961) A Study of the Psychological Processes in Pregnancy and of the Earliest Mother-Child Relationship. I. Some Propositions and Comments. *The Psychoanalytic Study of the Child,* Vol. XVI. New York: International Universities Press.

Bowlby, J. (1951) Maternal Care and Child Health. *World Health Org. Monograph Series,* No.2.

Brody, S. (1956) *Patterns of Mothering.* New York: International Universities Press.

Caplan, G. (1961) *An Approach to Community Mental Health.* New York: Grune and Stratton.

Deutsch, H. (1944) *Psychology of Women.* New York: Grune and Stratton.

Deutsch, H. (1945) *The Psychology of Women: Motherhood,* Vol. II New York: Grune and Stratton.

Deutscher, M. (1970) Brief Family Therapy in the Course of First Pregnancy: A Clinical Note. *Contemporary Psychoanalysis,* 7:21-35.

Dohrenwend, B.P., and Dohrenwend, B.S. (1965) The Problem of Validity in Field Studies of Psychological Disorder. *Journal of Abnormal Psychology,* 70:52-69.

Gordon, R.E., and Gordon, K.K. (1960) Social Factors in Prevention of Postpartum Emotional Problems. *Obstetrics and Gynecology,* 15:433-437.

Green, R.T. (1973) Perceived Styles of Mother-Daughter Relationship and the Prenatal Adjustment of the Primigravida. Doctoral dissertation, George Washington University, 1971-1973.

Grimm, E. (1961) Psychological Tension in Pregnancy. *Psychosomatic Medicine,* 23:520-527.

Grotjahn, M. (1960) *Psychoanalysis and the Family Neurosis.* New York: W.W. Norton and Co.

Harlow, H.F. (1963) The Maternal Affectional System. In: *Determinants of Infant Behavior,* II, edited by B.M. Foss. New York: John Wiley and Son.

Hetzel, B.S., Bruer, B., and Poideven, L.O.S. (1961) A Survey of the Relation between Certain Common Antenatal Complications in Primiparae and Stressful Life Situations during Pregnancy. *Journal of Psychosomatic Research,* 5:175-182.

Hollingshead, A.B., and Redlich, F.C. (1958) *Social Class and Mental Illness: A Community Study.* New York: John Wiley and Son.

Larsen, V.L. et al. (1966) Attitudes and Stresses Affecting Perinatal Adjustment. Mental Health Research Institute, Ft. Steilacoom, Washington. Report to NIMH.

Leighton, D.C. et al. (1963) *The Character of Danger.* New York: Basic Books.

Lewis, O. (1966) *La Vida.* New York: Random House.

Loevinger, J. (1962) Measuring Personality Patterns of Women. *Genetic Psychology Monographs,* 65:53-136

Moss, H.A. (1967) Sex, Age, and State as Determinants of Mother-Infant Interaction. *Merrill-Palmer Quarterly,* 13:19-36.

Rapoport, R. (1963) Normal Crises, Family Structure and Mental Health. *Family Process,* 2:68-80.

Rheingold, J.C. (1964) *The Fear of Being a Woman.* New York: Grune and Stratton.

Richardson, S.A., and Guttmacher, A.F. (eds.) (1967) *Childbearing—Its Social and Psychological Aspects.* Baltimore: williams and Wilkins Co.

Riessman, F., Cohen, J., and Pearl, A. (eds.) (1964) *Mental Health of the Poor.* New York: The Free Press.

Rosenblatt, J.S. (1967) Social-Environmental Factors Affecting Reproduction and Offspring in Infrahuman Mammals. In: *Childbearing—Its Social and Psychological Aspects,* edited by S.A. Richardson and A.F. Guttmacher. Baltimore: Williams and Wilkins Co.

Spitz, R.A. (1965) *The First Year of Life.* New York: International Universities Press.

Stechler, G.S., and Geller, H. (1961) Psychological Evaluation of Pregnancy—A Follow-up Comparison. Presented at APA, New York.

Voth, H.M., Modlin, H.C., and Orth, M.H. (1962) Situational Variables in the Assessment of Psychotherapeutic Results. *Bulletin of the Menninger Clinic,* 26:73-81.   d Cohen,

Wenner, N.K., and Cohen, M.B. (eds.) (1968) Emotional Aspects of Pregnancy. Final Report of Washington School of Psychiatry Project. Washington, D.C.

Wenner, N.K. et al. (1969) Emotional Problems in Pregnancy. *Psychiatry,* 32:389-410.

Yarrow, L.J., and Goodwin, M.S. (1965) Some Conceptual Issues in the Study of Mother-Infant Interaction. *American Journal of Orthopsychiatry,* 35:473-481.

*Psychological Aspects of a First Pregnancy
and Early Postnatal Adaptation.*
Raven Press, New York © 1974

Chapter IV
Pregnancy Adaptation

Pauline M. Shereshefsky, Harold Plotsky, and Robert F. Lockman

INTRODUCTION

There are times in the life cycle of women when physical events become the focus around which other aspects of their lives are organized. This is true of the girl when she begins to menstruate; emotional changes are precipitated by the menarche and patterns organized which become characteristic ways of response (Kestenberg, 1956; Shainess, 1960). At the time of the menopause also, intensified psychological reaction is interrelated with biological developments (Bibring, 1959, 1961; Huntington, 1961). Something of the same sort, but more far-reaching in its interpersonal and social consequences, takes place during a first pregnancy. Physiological changes become the focal point around which emotional patterns and relationships become organized. The relation of the physiological changes to the emotional or intrapsychic aspects of adaptation to the pregnancy, and the impact of outer social circumstance in that adaptation, is the focus of our exploration in this chapter.

Our sample of some 60 normal families were undergoing a first pregnancy. The meaning of the experience and their reactions to it were necessarily highly individual and varied. Our interviews, psychological tests, medical examinations, and observations were directed to determining characteristic adaptations to this experience and the elements that entered into these varied ways of adapting and coping.

In ordering the substantial body of data covering the period of the pregnancy, it seems appropriate to begin with the major findings that emerged from statistical analysis of the data on these sets of variables. The non-statistically minded reader may find it fruitful to move directly to the sections of the chapter that follow, as this section will concern itself with statistical relationships of items, factors, and superfactors involved in Pregnancy Adaptation.

STATISTICAL FINDINGS

As indicated in the previous chapter, three variables were viewed as outcomes: Pregnancy Adaptation, Maternal Adaptation, and Infant Adaptation. Our concern here is with the first of these, Pregnancy Adaptation.

The pregnancy experience was evaluated with specific reference to some 22 items which were either checked or rated on a five-point scale at two periods during pregnancy, the third and seventh months.[1] Pregnancy Adaptation as an outcome variable is represented by six factor scales covering the three prenatal rating periods:

Factor scale[2]	Description[3]	Schedule*	Rating period (months)
8	Adaptation to pregnancy experience	A-IV	3
10	Reaction to characteristic fears of pregnancy	A-IV	3
11	Adaptation to pregnancy experience	B	7
12	Pregnancy as confirmation of sexual identity	B	7
13	Reaction to pregnancy fears	B	7
16	Overall reaction to pregnancy experience	C-II	9

*The letters identifying the schedules from which the items are drawn are guides to the time periods involved: Schedule A = 3 months; Schedule B = 7 months; Schedule C = 9 months (pregnancy termination); Schedule D = 9 months (labor and delivery).

Table 1 indicates that four variables, all of them representing characteristics of the woman, significantly correlated ($p < 0.05$) with Pregnancy Adaptation scales at all three rating periods. They include the two personality factors derived from the initial psychological study of the woman at three months, ego strength and nurturance; and a factor, visualization of self as mother, evaluated in the context of studying the reactions to the pregnancy experience which was assessed at the three-month prenatal period. A variable with the same

TABLE 1. *Prenatal scales that correlate significantly with pregnancy adaptation (N = 57)*

No.	Name	Correlated with	Rating period (months)	r^*
4	Ego strength (3 months)	8 Adaptation to pregnancy experience	3	0.56
		10 Reaction to characteristic fears of pregnancy	3	0.57
		11 Adaptation to pregnancy experience	7	0.28
		13 Reaction to pregnancy fears	7	0.42
		16 Overall reaction to pregnancy	9	0.29
5	Nurturance (3 months)	8 Adaptation to pregnancy experience	3	0.44
		11 Adaptation to pregnancy experience	7	0.25
		12 Confirmation of sexual identity	7	0.31
		16 Overall reaction to pregnancy	9	0.26
9	Visualizing self as mother (3 months)	8 Adaptation to pregnancy experience	3	0.40
		10 Reaction to characteristic fears of pregnancy	3	0.26
		11 Adaptation to pregnancy experience	7	0.36
		12 Confirmation of sexual identity	7	0.32
		16 Overall reaction to pregnancy	9	0.27
14	Visualizing self as mother (7 months)	8 Adaptation to pregnancy experience	3	0.29
		11 Adaptation to pregnancy experience	7	0.44
		16 Overall reaction to pregnancy	9	0.39
	No. of medical symptoms during pregnancy	8 Adaptation to pregnancy experience	3	−0.26
		10 Reaction to characteristic fears of pregnancy	3	−0.30
		11 Adaptation to pregnancy experience	7	−0.47
		16 Overall reaction to pregnancy	9	−0.59

$^*r = 0.25 \; (p = 0.05); \; r = 0.34 \; (p = 0.01)$

name, assessed later in the pregnancy, is the fourth variable closely associated with Pregnancy Adaptation. In addition, the number of pregnancy-related medical symptoms throughout the prenatal period was found to be significantly related to Pregnancy Adaptation at all rating periods.

Personality Variables

The factors that are closely associated with pregnancy adaptation draw heavily on the data obtained in the initial psychological study of the woman at three months and evaluated by the multidisciplinary team of psychiatrist, psychologist, and social · worker.[4] (The composition of the two personality factors, ego strength and nurturance, has been set forth in Chapter III, Psychological Study of the Woman.) Here we are interested in the central importance of the woman's personality as an indicator of the way the adaptation to pregnancy may be expected to go.

Visualization of Self as Mother

The analysis of items dealing with the pregnancy experience resulted in two factor scales entitled visualization of self as mother, one rated at the three-month and the other at the seven-month period. While they are not identical, in both the two items having the highest correlations with the factors were clarity in visualizing self as mother and confidence in visualizing self as mother.

The factor scale, *visualization of self as mother,* derived from the *three-month* ratings, includes the woman's clarity in visualizing herself as mother, confidence in seeing herself in the maternal role, and degree of anxiety in respect to infant feeding and in respect to infant care.

The scale, *visualization of self as mother,* at *seven months* is made up of clarity in visualizing self as mother, confidence in visualizing self as mother, and an item on significance of the pregnancy as an extension of self.

Tables 2 and 3 present the correlates of the factor visualization of self as mother at three months and seven months, respectively. In regard to prenatal variables, the factor related highly to the factors ego strength and nurturance; it also correlated with performance I.Q., the life history variable, interest in children, and, inversely, with total number of stresses. These correlations indicate that women who visualized themselves with confidence and clarity as mothers even early in pregnancy (three months) were likely to make a good adaptation throughout pregnancy.

Visualization of self as mother, especially as rated at three months,

TABLE 2. *Significant correlates of visualization of self as mother (3 months) with pre- and postnatal variables (N = 57)*

Time period	Prenatal factor scale	Correlated with	Time period (months)	r*
		Prenatal variables		
		Performance I.Q.	3	0.25
3 months	Visualization	Scale 2 Interest in children	3	0.48
	of self	4 Ego strength	3	0.60
	as mother	5 Nurturance	3	0.50
		8 Adaptation to pregnancy experience	3	0.40
		10 Reaction to characteristic fears of pregnancy	3	0.26
		11 Adaptation to pregnancy experience	7	0.36
		12 Confirmation of sexual identity	7	0.32
		14 Visualizing self as mother	7	0.45
		16 Overall reaction to pregnancy	9	0.27
		Total stresses	3	−0.27
		Postnatal variables		
		Scale 18 Infant alertness	1	0.26
		22 Infant alertness	6	0.30
		26 Acceptance of maternal role	1	0.34
		33 Acceptance of maternal role	3	0.40
		34 Responsiveness to infant	6	0.31
		35 Acceptance of infant and maternal role	6	0.34
		37 Husband-wife adaptation	1	0.28
		39 Husband-wife adaptation	3	0.28
		41 Husband-wife adaptation	6	0.35
		43 Ego strength	6	0.52
		44 Nurturance	6	0.46
		45 Family adaptation	6	0.45
		Birthweight		0.25
		DIQ	6	0.28

*r = 0.25 (p = 0.05); r = 0.34 (p = 0.01)

was also significantly related to the Maternal Adaptation scales at all postnatal ratings ($p < 0.05$). In addition, the visualization of self as a mother factor correlated with a number of other postnatal variables, including: infant alertness at one month and at six months, birthweight (one of the very small number of variables that showed any correlation with either of these variables), husband-wife adaptation at all study periods postnatally, and with the family adaptation scale of the final overall rating schedule. Moreover, in the composition of the superfactor scales described in Chapter II (Research Design

TABLE 3. *Significant correlates of visualization of self as mother (7 months) with pre- and postnatal variables (N = 57)*

Time period	Prenatal factor scale	Correlated with	Time period (months)	r*
		Prenatal variables		
7 months	Visualization	Scale 5 Nurturance	3	0.42
	of self	8 Adaptation to pregnancy experience	3	0.29
	as mother	9 Visualizing self as mother	3	0.41
		11 Adaptation to pregnancy experience	7	0.48
		16 Overall reaction to pregnancy	9	0.39
		Subjective reaction to labor and delivery	9	0.28
		Total stresses	3	−0.26
		Postnatal variables		
		Scale 35 Acceptance of infant & maternal role	6	0.26
		37 Husband-wife adaptation	1	0.27
		44 Nurturance	6	0.37
		45 Family adaptation	6	0.26

*r = 0.25 (p = 0.05); r = 0.34 (p = 0.01)

and Methodology), visualization of self as mother had the highest correlation of the five prenatal variables included in the comprehensive superfactor scale, feminine identification.

Medical Symptoms

The number of pregnancy-connected medical symptoms was compiled from the obstetricians' set of charts for each patient. On each visit (usually totaling 14 to 16 visits from the third month to the time of delivery) the obstetrician noted medical complaints of enough seriousness for him to prescribe treatment.[5] He did not record very slight and highly transitory physical discomforts of pregnancy as symptoms. The number of symptoms by cases ranged from none to 19 and covered the whole course of the pregnancy.

The number of pregnancy-connected medical symptoms was inversely related (p < 0.05) to Pregnancy Adaptation at all three periods. Thus, a large number of medical symptoms related to poor adaptation in overall reaction to the pregnancy. Since the final sample of 57 cases included only those with healthy infant outcomes, it is clear that the number of symptoms was not related to reproductive difficulties.

The correlation of medical symptoms and difficult pregnancy adaptation leaves unanswered the basic question of cause and effect, that is, whether physical symptoms were primarily causative of psychological adaptation or the reverse. This is a problem with which other investigators have concerned themselves (Grimm, 1967). However, a case-by-case review of the 9 per cent of our sample with eleven or more medical symptoms showed that psychological conflict and personality problems were prominent in every instance.

General Observations on Variables Closely Associated with Pregnancy Adaptation

Of special interest is the fact that three of the five variables closely associated with Pregnancy Adaptation came from the initial study of the woman at three months—the two personality variables and one of the factors on visualization of self as mother. Since they are based on data obtained and assessed early in the course of the pregnancy, they can be viewed as *predictors* of Pregnancy Adaptation. Of equal interest is the fact that all of the variables that were closely associated with pregnancy adaptation throughout the course of the pregnancy represent psychological and physiological aspects specific to and intimately involved with the woman in relation to herself; two derived from the psychological study of the woman delineating current personality, two from the study of her attitudes and reaction in the pregnancy experience, and one medical variable. They add up to highly important aspects of the immediate reality of the woman at this period.

In the grouping of all factor scales into eight superfactors, the same emphasis emerges. The superfactor, feminine identification, contains several scales from the prenatal period, all of them specific to the woman: visualization of self as mother, nurturance, ego strength, adaptation to pregnancy experience (all of these from the evaluations at three months), and overall reaction to the pregnancy experience, related to the whole period of the pregnancy. Of the ten variables from the *postnatal* period that also correlated with the superfactor, feminine identification, four of them involve husband-wife and family adaptation, that is, the woman in relationship to others. These findings imply an overriding significance during pregnancy for the woman's psychological health and adaptive capacity.

THE EXPERIENCE OF A FIRST PREGNANCY

The statistical findings on the outcome variable, Pregnancy Adaptation, taken together with the data on background variables presented in Chapter III, indicate that the woman's readiness and capacity to cope with her first pregnancy is a function of her personal strengths and weaknesses. If, by the time of the first pregnancy, she has developed strong personality characteristics of nurturance and ego strength and has a strong feminine identification as evidenced by her confidence and clarity in visualizing herself as a mother, it can be predicted that her predominant mood and her adjustments during pregnancy are likely to be good.

The composition of the personality characteristics involved has already been presented—ego strength and nurturance factors in Chapter III, Psychological Study of the Woman; and the two variables entitled visualization of self as mother, in the preceding section of this chapter. We will now look at the varied ramifications of current experience and try to see the woman as a whole—in relation to her new experiences, in relation to significant other persons in her life, basically in relation to herself.

Psychological Adaptations to Pregnancy

Earlier it was reported that, on the psychological tests at three months prenatally, nearly three-fourths of the women gave anxious responses while only 41 per cent gave responses indicating a clearly happy mood.[6] In analyzing the psychiatric interviews, we found that approximately 40 per cent of the women noted a tendency to moodiness or depressive attitudes, whether occasionally only, or fairly persistently throughout the pregnancy. A large proportion of the women spoke of tempers more easily aroused, a tendency to be "edgy," tense, nervous or "touchy," to "snap" more easily, to be more demanding of their husbands, to dissolve in tears more often—general indications of greater vulnerability and heightened emotionality.

The women were responding to many currents both in their external circumstance and inner experience. Practical problems, internal physical developments, changing body image and shifts in relationship to significant persons in their lives precipitated intensified psychic activity. In looking at the impact of the realities of this period, internal and external, it is understandable that "childbirth at every level and at every stage proceeds on a groundwork of anxiety" (Chertok, 1969, p. 35).

Planned and Unplanned Pregnancies

Seventy-three per cent of the pregnancies were reported as planned. These included the 16 per cent of the group who had had some problem in conception and had obtained medical advice and treatment in connection with it.

Investigators interested in the issue of motivation to have a child call attention to the healthy conscious and unconscious wishes that enter into the decision to become pregnant and also to the varied neurotic bases for the decision (Menninger, 1943; Greenberg et al., 1959; Wenner, 1967; Flapan, 1969). Unconscious motivation to have or not have a child is difficult to assess. "A healthy and creative family is a family with a free-flowing communication between the conscious and the unconscious of all family members" (Grotjahn, 1960, p. 287).

> One woman said the pregnancy was planned, it is true, but the circumstances were that she had been feeling lonely and depressed, and it had occurred to her that having a child would make her feel better by giving her a new interest and outlook. She knew that her husband had always wanted children, but that he was concerned about his graduate studies and their financial obligations. It was because he sensed her need and urged her to go ahead with the plan for starting their family now, that she discontinued taking the contraceptive pills.

Many families who had not planned the pregnancy had an easy, happy acceptance of this development in their lives. None of this group had made the conscious choice not to have a child at all, but some had wished that the first pregnancy had been delayed until they were more firmly established.

Whether the pregnancy was planned or unplanned was not clearly related to adaptation to the pregnancy. There were some interesting correlations, statistically, between unplanned pregnancy and other variables that suggest greater difficulty for this group of families in adjusting to the reality of the pregnancy. Unplanned pregnancy correlated with youthfulness of husband and wife, shorter interval of marriage, lack of congruence with the current family situation, the husband's dissatisfaction with his job, his lack of response to the pregnancy, and a less positive mood on the part of the woman at the three-month prenatal period.

An example of a characteristic situation of an unplanned pregnancy, in which the rejecting side of the ambivalence was prominent, follows:

> This 20-year-old woman who worked as a nurses' aide in a public institution conceived within the first three months of marriage. She verbalized much enthusiasm about having a child of her own. She had difficulty stating any ambivalence, but her husband, speaking for himself in part, said, "She is quite worried about the financial end and the additional responsibility. She is deathly afraid of the labor because of things that she knows about from the mothers of the defective children that she cares for." Like some of our other young women, this woman dreamed that suddenly the baby had been born in a sort of painless process, and later that her own mother had had the baby and had given it to her.

Rarely was a pregnancy totally unwanted, although we thought we encountered this situation at least once.

Pregnancy-engendered Practical Changes

Early in the pregnancy, the women needed to be quite active in organizing themselves for impending changes in everyday living. Three-fourths of the women were working at the time of the pregnancy and were soon faced with decisions about whether and when to stop work. Some were in student status and had to discontinue schooling; most of them had to decide with their husbands about new housing, since 74 per cent were living in apartments, many in one-bedroom units. Husbands, too, had to decide whether their earnings in the present job would be adequate, faced as they were, in most families, with the simultaneous loss of the wife's earnings and the need for increased financial outlay. Many of the women were in conflict about discontinuing work or schooling. Some were as yet less sure of themselves in the role of wife and homemaker than in that of teacher, secretary, or student.

Qualities of personal resilience and emotional readiness for, as against reluctance to, taking on the role of mothering entered into the woman's adjustments at this time and made the process satisfying and ego-enhancing or the reverse. Among these qualities were her capacity to make important decisions in a limited period of time, her resourcefulness in adjusting everyday living arrangements in practical ways, the relative amount of eagerness she felt in anticipation of the birth of the child, and the degree of anxiety engendered in confronting change and new use of self.

Reaction to Physiological Developments

All the women reacted to physical aspects and changes, some with eagerness to "show" early and with pleasure in their new bodily appearance, others with more mixed feelings. Many of the women seemed to be continuously aware of their bodily processes even before quickening and fetal activity brought special reminder. A few needed to minimize or deny any importance attaching to this as to other aspects of the pregnancy.

Bewilderment at what was going on internally was a common reaction, and even otherwise knowledgeable young women at times showed confusion at frequency of urination, breast enlargement, or the need for frequent napping. A number of women found symptoms of the first weeks of pregnancy hard to deal with because they did not immediately connect the symptoms with the possibility of pregnancy, or they were doubtful about the diagnosis and ashamed to have so many complaints without apparent cause. Nausea might mean the need to turn over the cooking to husbands, which sometimes brought on guilt feelings on the part of young wives or engendered misunderstandings if the husband saw the behavior as evasion of responsibilities.

In pregnancy the physical and psychological states are indeed inextricable:

> An older primigravida, aged 28, was painfully lonely because of geographical distance from family. Pregnancy had occurred during the first month of marriage, at the time the couple had just moved to this city. This was a case in which nausea persisted until the eighth month. The project staff, seeing the woman as shy, untrusting, lonely and nauseated for so many months, could not know how much the physical discomfort contributed to a failure to make friends and develop a life for herself in the new community, nor how crucial was the fact of strangeness and isolation in prolonging the symptom of nausea; that they were interrelated for the woman was entirely clear.

Not knowing what to expect in a specific way tended to leave the woman feeling out of control of herself and her situation. This was particularly true of cases of delay in experiencing quickening, and also of the few cases in which a special problem existed such as Rh incompatibility or inability to gain enough weight—the latter more anxiety-provoking as to outcome of the pregnancy than the typical anxiety over excessive weight gain.

Reaction to Medical Aspects of Pregnancy*

As members of the prepaid health plan of the Group Health Association, the women, characteristically, would have been under the care of a rotating panel of obstetricians. However, in this project each patient selected who agreed to participate was under the care of one and the same obstetrician during her prenatal course, labor, and delivery.

Medical observations were recorded by the obstetrician at each visit, in addition to the standard medical records noting physical aspects on examination. These observations ranged from noting the patient's general appearance to indicating her questions about conduct of labor and delivery and method of feeding the baby. The emotional state of the patient was noted: whether she was depressed, anxious, or content. Her general relationship to the obstetrician was assessed as resistant, demanding, dependent or cooperative. A form was completed which contained a list of pregnancy-related physical symptoms, the degree of complaint, and the treatment prescribed. On the following visit a note was added as to the patient's acceptance of the previously prescribed therapy.

Most of the symptoms about which the patient complained were those which would normally be expected; they were consistent with the period of gestation. Frequency of urination was a common symptom seen early in the pregnancy and in a few instances just before delivery. Early in pregnancy nausea and/or vomiting was a common complaint, usually disappearing by the third month. Two patients of the group failed to respond to therapy, continuing to have severe nausea and vomiting up to the eighth month of gestation.

"Swelling of the feet," edema, was high on the list of complaints, especially in the third trimester. Fifty-four of the patients noted some swelling on one or more occasions, especially in the evening. Twenty patients had edema which was considered marked on the occasion

---

*This section on medical aspects is adapted from the report written by John Lukasik, M.D., and Josiah Sacks, M.D.

of at least one of the visits to the obstetrician. Constipation was another common complaint. For eleven of the patients, marked constipation was noted which, with prescribed remedies, was changed to mild or moderate. One patient continued to have marked constipation despite prescribed remedies.

Other symptoms frequently noted were abdominal pain or pressure, backache, and weight gain. Less commonly expressed complaints were heartburn, vaginal discharge, sleepiness and constant fatigue, and leg cramps. One patient complained of dyspareunia on only one occasion. Vulvavaginitis was noted in six patients, and all responded well to therapy. The total number of symptoms reported by the patients varied from none to 19 for one patient.

The pervasiveness of the physiological aspects and their close correlation with difficulty in adapting to pregnancy is indicated by the statistical finding presented earlier: the number of medical symptoms associated with the pregnancy was found to be inversely related to Pregnancy Adaptation at a statistically significant level at all three rating periods.

Quickening

Reactions to quickening sometimes revealed how uncertain the woman had been that the pregnancy was real. Several women would not let themselves believe their own sense of something alive stirring within them until the physician said that he could now hear the heart beat. For the most part, the women reacted with an admixture of relief at the relative certainty and excitement and gratification at the newness of the experience. A characteristic reaction to quickening was that it first felt "fluttery." One woman added that she couldn't quite tell whether anything was happening at first, but then added, "It was awfully nice to realize that something was really there." A shy, anxious young woman rather startled us by the keenness of her response: "I felt as if I was sparkling all over."

Some women, however, raised anxious questions throughout the remainder of the pregnancy about whether so much activity would result in a hyperactive or damaged infant. A few were constantly irritated by the activity and found it more fatiguing than gratifying. For most women, whatever the degree of ambivalence, quickening gave the pregnancy a dimension of reality. Now it could be and must be taken into account in terms of practical planning.

Visualization of Self as Mother: Case Studies

Two of the five factors most closely associated with Pregnancy Adaptation relate to the woman's clarity and confidence in visualizing herself as a mother. The statistical analyses presented at the beginning of this chapter indicate the wide ramifications of the variable we have called visualization of self as mother in its interrelation with Pregnancy Adaptation, its significance as a predictor of Maternal Adaptation, its close correlation with prenatal personality factors and with postnatal factors of family adaptation and infant alertness. Because of these wide ramifications, this factor scale may be worth looking at, in the varied, highly individual, homely ways in which attitudes were actually presented.

Women with much clarity in visualizing themselves as mothers were often those who had seen themselves as mothers since early childhood. Several recalled wanting a child from the age of three or four. Some women could say directly, as one did, "It's easy to see yourself as a mother—I've imagined myself as one ever since I was a little girl," and another could react explosively, "Who, me as a mother? No, I think of my *mother* as a mother!"

Two women who felt confident about child care are presented below:

> Mrs. A. at the 7th month interview says she is confident that she can learn to care for a baby. She notices people with babies more and the women look happy with the children. She looks forward to being a mother with a sense of "good things to come." She adds, "Of course, we won't be as free."
>
> Mrs. B. reports, at 3 months, that she feels comfortable and confident about the early postnatal period; she has taken care of many children including many infants. Her friends often come to her to ask questions about baby care. At the seventh-month interview she says that she thinks about the baby most of the time. The baby has been very active, and she has been very comfortable. She is never without awareness of the baby's movements; often she can feel various parts of the baby, and because of this she is quite apt to think of the baby as an individual.

These two women enjoyed their pregnancies. The next three women were unsure of themselves and troubled during the pregnancy:

Mrs. G., a 27-year-old woman, said in the initial study period that her main worry was whether she would be able to take care of the baby the first day they bring him home from the hospital. "He'll be so tiny and I don't know if I'll know how to give him a bath safely, fix the formula and all that, by myself." This woman never considered breast-feeding as she felt she was too nervous. At seven months and again at nine months and after the infant's birth, the same anxieties are expressed. She impresses the interviewer as a person "who feels herself to be a very young child in a baffling, strange and formidable world."

Mrs. H., coping with serious marital difficulty, cried when questioned about the expected baby. Sometimes she pictures herself singing to the baby, but most of the time it frightens her to think of herself as a mother.

Mrs. I. wonders whether she will know whether to pick the baby up or let it cry. Mrs. I's. marked enthusiasm for the pregnancy persisted against considerable odds, including her husband's ambivalence about the pregnancy, and her mother's characteristic belittling attitude towards her. To evaluate her level of confidence and clarity in visualizing herself as a mother it was necessary to take into consideration a complex body of data, summarized in this statement of the psychiatrist: "She wants to produce something very worthwhile in this pregnancy and she wants people to become aware that she could become pregnant and give birth to a child. She has cathected this experience with a great deal of feeling and of hope, and at the same time there is a fair amount of apprehension about the outcome of her pregnancy."

In varying degrees and manifestations, these three women carried over the anxiety and lack of confidence of the prenatal period into the first months of infant care.

In evaluating this factor of clarity and confidence regarding maternal functioning we were apparently tapping a complex of attitudes closely related to feminine identification. Researchers in this field of inquiry have generally concerned themselves with this issue, a recent study still in process, reporting the use of imaginative new tools for eliciting retrospective data on life history and psychosexual development (Flapan and Schoenfeld, 1972). Certainly this aspect of our findings, indicating the significance of ascertaining how the woman sees herself in the role of mother, suggests a productive area for further study.

Husband-Wife Relationship

We have already indicated that we found little statistical relationship between the woman's adaptation to the pregnancy and her husband's responsiveness to her and to the pregnancy (Chapter III, Marital Adaptation). Clinical evidence points in another direction, most apparent in instances of poor marital adjustment, in that the strains in the relationship were seen to affect the woman's predominant mood and accentuate the negative side of her ambivalence about the pregnancy. We also saw two different tendencies clinically. On the one hand, the pregnancy seemed to draw the couple closer as they shared in planning and sustaining each other at times of anxiety, and also in projecting themselves into the new roles they would be carrying in the near future. At the same time we noted a tendency on the part of the woman to shut her husband out from her inner preoccupations. Husbands, in turn, were not always ready to be patient and supportive over the long months of waiting, and many women were left to their own resources in handling their conflicting feelings and their fantasies.

Because we initially saw the husband's role as central, we have presented our data about husband-wife relationships at various points throughout this volume, including Chapter III, already noted, a chapter on Expectant Fathers (Chapter V), and sections in Chapter VII on Techniques in Prenatal Counseling.

Mother-Daughter Relationship

The women were responding to many conflicting feelings arising from a changed relationship to their childhood families, and especially to the woman's mother. On the one hand there was usually a need on the part of the woman to see herself as separate from her childhood family, a need and process that had been particularly marked at the time of her marriage. The pregnancy in part accentuated the striving for independence since now the woman was facing the assumption of responsibility for a child of her own. At the same time pregnancy stirred up many regressive feelings; physical discomfort and anxiety about the unknown, relating most acutely to labor and delivery, brought on moments of longing for maternal comforting.

Most couples were eager to share their "news" with their parents as soon as the pregnancy diagnosis was made. Even in an urban setting where many people live far from their childhood families, pregnancy is still an experience that generally involves the nuclear family (the young couples, in our sample) and the extended family in new closeness.

Women with good mother-daughter relationships were soon making practical plans together, with a new sense of the privileges of "women's talk." This included shared accounts of pregnancy and delivery experiences; advice about layettes, diaper service, nursery decor, and the varied needs of a newborn infant; details about what to expect in the way of night-time routines, etc.

All of the women were preoccupied with the psychological task of working out the relationship to their own mother on a new or different basis, whether the mother was living in the same community or far removed from the woman geographically, or was no longer alive. We saw, in "good" mother-daughter relationships, the relaxation of some anxiety on the part of the daughter about her capacity to be mature and to "hold her own" with her mother as a woman. On the part of the woman's mother, we saw a new readiness and freedom to share the facts of her life with her daughter, sometimes for the first time. An open tenderness, specific to the young woman's physical and emotional state, could be displayed, as often it could not in recent years, when tenderness could be mistrusted as possessive overprotection by an adolescent and young adult.

One phase of the mother-daughter relationship dealt with in our study focused on the woman's conscious effort to decide how much she would be like her mother in her own pattern of mothering. The more mature woman tended to define herself in the ways in which she wanted to be like, and those in which she would want to be unlike, her own mother.

A number of the women were somewhat let down by the initial reactions of their parents; they were surprised that the announcement of confirmation of the pregnancy was not met with unalloyed joyous response. Like the couples themselves, the parents of the couple appear to have had mixed feelings, compounded of some anxiety for their daughter especially, or for the couple, with some uncertainty as to their readiness for the experience of pregnancy and parenthood. We can only surmise that memories of their own past experiences, past conflicts and satisfactions were possibly reactivated.

In instances where the pregnancy did not meet with the approval of the parents, the woman generally continued to be troubled by this fact throughout the pregnancy and kept trying to obtain favorable response from her parents or struggled to come to terms with their lack of response. The need for some warmth and closeness from their own mothers was apparent, even (or especially) among women with difficult mother-daughter relationships.

We had earlier indicated the special stress of crises in the prenatal families as they affected the young family—illness, separation, death of a member of the extended family. In some instances the parents leaned heavily on the young couple for emotional support and were certainly not available to the pregnant daughter at this time when she was herself in need of special understanding or reassurance.

The Pregnancy Experience: Rating Changes over Time

To determine the shifts in attitude that occurred in the course of the pregnancy for the total group, comparison was made of the 22 item ratings in the section of the schedule, the Pregnancy Experience. The statistically significant changes that occurred for the group as a whole, between first and second trimesters, reflect better adaptation to the pregnancy in these aspects:

> Lessened anxiety regarding infant care.
> Clarity and confidence in visualizing self as mother.
> Effect of pregnancy on feeling of well-being.
> Adaptability to changes of pregnancy.
> Evidence of growth towards new family identification.
> Pregnancy as confirmation of feminine identity.
> Validation of couple in their identity.
> Husband-wife adaptation.

It may be of interest to follow in more detail one of the items which reflects the changes that have been presented, the effect of pregnancy on the feeling of well-being. In the initial study period at three months, 51 per cent of the women were rated as having "diminished vitality," whereas by the seventh month only 33 per cent were so rated. At three months, only 23 per cent were rated as having "enhancement of feelings of well-being" while 49 per cent were so rated at the seventh-month period.

It is particularly noteworthy that favorable change occurred for the group in two items regarding the marital situation: husband-wife adaptation and pregnancy as validation of couple in their identity. Finally, anxiety in regard to infant care lessened between the first and second trimesters.

Anxiety was high in the first trimester but had substantially subsided by the second trimester. By the eighth and ninth months, the anxiety level was generally intensified as we learned from the obstetricians' records and from the women in the counseled group (we did not see the women in the control group between the seventh and ninth months).

A comparison was made of the changes over time of the three factor scales measuring Pregnancy Adaptation: no significant change occurred between the first and second trimester scales, but definite change occurred between the first and third trimester and between the second and third trimester ratings. In other words, the psychological movement in adaptation to the pregnancy was not clearly defined for the period between the first and second trimesters. However, by the end of the pregnancy, the group as a whole showed improvement in adaptation to the pregnancy experience. By the time of childbirth, accommodation had generally been made to the reality of the anticipated birth

Planning for Help on Homecoming with the Newborn Infant

The matter of help for the new mother immediately on homecoming from the hospital was prominent among items for planning. In making their plans during the pregnancy, many women needed to deny the possibility that they would need help at all, and yet there was uncertainty and anxiety in the denial in most cases. Many women were not sure they would or should want to use help from anyone other than the husband. Sensitivity to her husband's wishes sometimes vied with concern on the part of the woman over the reliability and competence of his help.

The woman more often than not wanted "her own womenfolk" at hand (usually her mother and sometimes her mother-in-law, sister, or grandmother) at the time of bringing her first-born child home from the hospital and undertaking his care. Many women wanted their mothers to initiate the offer of help at this time. In several cases in which a mother did not come or, if close at hand, failed to offer her help, the woman was invariably clearly disappointed and, at times, confirmed in doubts about herself, her mother, or the relationship.

A First Pregnancy—A Time of Aloneness

Depressed states are so variously reported and observed during pregnancy and postnatally that they tend to be minimized as "natural" or to be entirely denied. In the group sessions both men and women described the drastic change in activity patterns that occurred in the latter part of the pregnancy, when they were not as free to come and go as they had been previously, indicating that there were times of enforced inactivity and many hours of actual aloneness for the woman. This inactivity accentuated the tendency to daydream about past, present, and future.

In general, we gained the impression that a first pregnancy may be a lonely time for a woman. This was acutely so for 15 per cent —those who had no close family nearby and had fairly recently come to the city. For many more, however, loneliness was self-initiated in the sense that they seemed to need time for themselves. A researcher, interpreting this mood and attitude in psychoanalytic terms, states: "The woman turns in upon herself, loving and confusing her body and her foetus, whose anabolism demands all her energies. Some pregnancies are thus experienced as extremely gratifying in a thoroughly narcissistic fusional way. At the other extreme, some women whose narcissism is too centered upon an unimpaired and unalterable body have difficulty in accepting these changes and suffer with respect to their body-image" (Chertok, 1969, pp. 31-32).

Much of the need for aloneness concerns itself with the matter of looking ahead—daydreaming, weaving fantasies about the infant, seeing themselves in the new role of mother. The women were in process of giving up much that had been meaningful in the past and at the same time reorganizing their psychological resources to look toward the future. This was work for the woman at this period of her life: relinquishing her hold on an earlier phase of her life, to some extent mourning the loss of the old self, and looking to the new phase and tasks ahead—work of the pregnancy period that seemed meaningful and necessary to many of the women. Possibly it yielded dividends in adaptability during the time of waiting and, later, in achievement of psychological readiness to meet maternal responsibilities.

LABOR AND DELIVERY

It was clear throughout that great personal significance was attached to the confinement. Much of the psychological preparation in the nine months of gestation had been directed toward the event. This was true even on the part of the women who had tended to deny the meaningfulness of the pregnancy.

The labor and delivery experience is presented in two parts: the psychological meaning of the experience, reported by two members of the psychiatric team, and medical aspects, reported by the two obstetricians associated with the project.

The attitudes of the woman prenatally and postnatally toward labor and her actual experience in childbirth were explored in the course of four interviews with the psychiatrist during the year's collaboration and in other phases of project activity, including obstetrician-patient relationship and reports, psychological tests, social work interviews, and home observations.[7]

Psychological Meaning of Labor and Delivery Experience*

Harold Plotsky and Pauline M. Shereshefsky

Characteristic Reactions

Each woman brings into her pregnancy experience and, equally, into the labor and delivery experience, certain emotional characteristics, a certain personality style with which she tends to deal with new experience. Conflicts, anxieties, the impact of earlier relationships, and characteristic ways of coping and of expressing feeling enter into her way of reacting and adapting to the pregnancy experience, particularly so at the time of its culmination in the delivery experience.

We found that, universally although in varying degrees, the women were preoccupied with labor and delivery all through the first pregnancy. Researchers have reported the increased stress of the last month or two of pregnancy (Grimm, 1961; Jessner, 1964, 1966; Chertok, 1969). Anxiety became intensified in the last weeks of the pregnancy in the group of women included in this study. In the eighth and ninth months of pregnancy, "emotional status" was reported as "anxious" by the obstetricians for one-half of the sample, representing a distinctly larger proportion of the patients reported as "anxious"

---

*This section, which appeared as a separate paper entitled "Psychological Meaning of Watching the Delivery," in *Child and Family*, Vol. 8, No. 3, Summer 1969, has been slightly modified for presentation here. It is used with the permission of *Child and Family*.

than at previous periods. With labor and delivery looming near, and physical awkwardness and discomfort more marked, most patients became more open with the obstetrician in showing anxiety and expressing eagerness to have the pregnancy over. Equally suggestive of mounting anxiety is the fact that approximately one-fourth (23 per cent) of the women had some degree of false labor and several had to be admitted to the hospital for observation, sedation, and rest.

Women readily give evidence of the importance attached to their experiences in labor and delivery. For example, in group sessions which took place as long as one to three years after the experience, each woman referred to the exact day of the week, hour and minute of various events—the first identified labor pain, the time of arrival at the hospital, the move to the delivery room, and the actual birth. To state underlying feelings and associations to the event was more difficult.

As in other aspects of pregnancy and childbirth, the physiological and psychological aspects were tightly interwoven and the reactions varied widely. "It was not much worse than bad cramps during the menstrual period," several women reported, in some surprise and relief. The note of wonderment was doubtless related to the "build-up" to psychological readiness for a heroic or at least demanding struggle which had somehow been averted. A number of women were happily exhilarated, finding the experience easy and satisfying in reality.

Characteristically, many covered over the painful aspects and perhaps actually "forgot" them quickly. However, revealing glimpses frequently came out with questioning.

> Mrs. G., reporting at the six-month postnatal period, stated that labor and delivery were wonderful; it was so easy, she is afraid she won't be so lucky next time. The baby was born at 6:10 on a Saturday. She had some discomfort while she was having dinner at her parents' home on Friday evening, but she did not go to the hospital until the next morning and it was some hours later, at 2:30, that she began to have serious pains. She doesn't remember the pains but she remembers crying. She was afraid about the anesthesia mask; she remembered the story of a girl who was being anesthetized and the tank exploded. When she awoke she had a hard burning pain. Somebody told her she had a baby.

Two women describing their experiences used the same phrase but with widely varied reactions. "It felt as if everything inside of me was exploding." The first woman had an unusually prolonged labor and delivery process due to medical complications. She was an impulsive young woman who had had varied uprootings in her earlier, premarital life. Besides feeling labor and delivery as cruelly painful, she felt it was "the loneliest time of my life." The second woman, with more ego strength and a more secure life situation both currently and prior to marriage, also spoke of the "exploding" effect; she added, "I felt calm inside, however, and very much a part of what was happening." One of the patients in our group said: "I thought before-hand that this would be a wonderful time to have my husband with me, but I found that when the labor pains came I was all wrapped up in *me*."

We had limited opportunity to observe reactions in natural childbirth as most of the women who planned to undergo the necessary prepara-tions failed to carry out the program. One woman did so, and her reactions were suggestive of the findings by Newton (1955) on similarity in the physiology of some types of childbirth and sexual excitement.[8]

Watching the Delivery

The inherently anxiety-provoking nature of the delivery experience, especially during first pregnancies, has been well established by other researchers (Klein, 1950; Newton, 1963; Heinstein, 1967; Chertok, 1969). From this viewpoint, the experience of the women who chose to watch the delivery was of particular interest and led to an attempt to sort out our observations and speculations.

Almost one-third of the total group (30 per cent) in this project had a type of anesthesia which permitted the women to watch the delivery. The obstetricians followed the woman's preference as to type of anesthesia, except in a few instances when their medical judgment contraindicated doing so. If the woman wished to watch the delivery, the obstetrician arranged for her to do so through the mirror available for the purpose. Even among those women who had a form of anesthe-sia which would have permitted them to watch the process, some chose to be participant and awake but without watching through a mirror. One woman said, "I felt it would make it seem unreal if I watched through a mirror, as if it were not happening to me."

Those who did make the choice to watch through the mirror usually reported favorably on their experience, as, for example, in the following account of one woman on the fourth day after childbirth:

> At no time were the pains very intense; she said she had been saving her yelps and yells until later and never did need them because when the doctor examined her after being "prepped" he said that she was ready to deliver, and then she received Demerol and a caudal (as agreed upon prior to labor), and she felt no pain. She told the doctor she would like to watch the delivery, but only parts of it; she did not want to see the incision. She said she would close her eyes until he told her it was time to look. He did tell her when the head was beginning to appear, but at the point when he had to pull she closed her eyes again. They put the baby on her stomach and he looked all red and white.

The act of watching the delivery has different meaning to different women. Many women who wish to see the birth do so, apparently out of a desire to participate more actively in the delivery process by being aware of the happenings during the birth of the child. For these women the experience is constructive, giving them a heightened sense of involvement and adding the dimension of completion to the pregnancy experience.

Some of the women wanted to be awake because they felt the need to have control over their own behavior. It was common for a woman to worry that she would not conduct herself in ways that were consonant with her image of herself: she was afraid that she would become "wild," would scream, become hysterical, say foolish or untoward things. To be awake during delivery may have meant that she had more control in the experience.

The women who feared to be unduly dependent on others and tended to be controlling, similarly seemed to feel uncomfortable in submitting to the obstetrician's handling of the delivery and to find that it was important to see and have something to say about what the obstetrician was doing. In this way they could a avoid surrendering themselves to him passively. By following the process actively, they could feel themselves in control.

Watching the delivery could yield some satisfaction in cognitive or heuristic terms. We heard from some of the women how much meaning it had to them to see and understand the birth process.

One of our women told excitedly about learning a new term ("crowning") and other medical facts unknown to her before. It seemed to us this had two different aspects—the procedure itself became a highly cathected experience, and the emotional aspects of childbearing were thereby minimized, converted from an emotional to a cognitive experience or even an intellectual achievement. When it was actually witnessed, labor and delivery could become less mysterious; delivery became less separated from other physiological processes and from other more ordinary events. Moreover, in getting something from the experience, taking in knowledge or learning, an element of replacement may have occurred for some sense of loss. This sense of loss in childbirth is recognized as a pervasive reaction on the part of many or possibly most women (Deutsch, 1945; Greenberg et al., 1959).

Another way in which watching the delivery has psychological meaning is in regard to the emotional investment in the act of seeing, possibly in the sexual significance in watching and seeing. Women who have such voyeuristic tendencies may find some sexual need gratified in seeing the birth process. We were not clear that this kind of emotional gratification was in fact sought by any of the women in our sample. Whether watching the process had a sexualized meaning for any of the women in our group or not, it may be important to examine the possibility as an area for further study in achieving more differentiated understanding of women during childbirth.

For still other women, a counterphobic quality may be involved in this wish to watch the birth process. A woman may be impelled by a strong desire to see what is happening in the course of the delivery because of her very dread of the event. The dread may be compounded of fears that are in her awareness or, on the other hand, that are deeply repressed and defended against.

An unusual occurrence in the delivery room in one case in our group possibly exemplifies this counterphobic quality. This was a woman who, throughout the period of her pregnancy, had been specific about wanting to witness the delivery. The medical report states: "At 9:00 P.M. the patient was quite comfortable and had been for the past hour or so. She had reached the second stage of labor and was ready to go to the delivery room. The nurse asked if she would like to witness the delivery and her reply was in the affirmative; therefore, a mirror was set up so that she could watch the delivery. Under caudal anesthesia the patient very seldom crowns as in a spontaneous delivery and it is almost always necessary to use forceps; therefore, a pair of forceps was obtained from the nurse. However, because of the mirror the patient saw the forceps and asked if they were going to be used and she was given an affirmative answer. She remarked at this time that she still had scars because she was a forceps delivery, and I believe at this point the patient panicked a little because as the forceps were applied and traction was made on the forceps she complained bitterly of pain, yet had a good level of anesthesia. The patient, all of a sudden, lost her anesthesia entirely. I asked her if she would like to be put to sleep for the delivery and she answered yes. We put her to sleep with general anesthesia. She delivered a living term male infant without difficulty at 9:22 P.M."

This patient later recalled the many stories of her own difficult birth, including the markings by the use of forceps. The long-suppressed anxiety about her own birth broke through, as well as her fears for her baby, to the extent that she suddenly and unexpectedly lost the effect of the anesthesia.

All through pregnancy a woman experiences changes in her body image. Once in the process of labor and delivery, she may be faced with an experience that could be threatening, disorganizing, or damaging. We wondered what effect it might have on a woman's body image to have a part of her body numb which she could see but not feel, as if she were watching someone else. Could it produce a fragmentation of the body image, or some sense of depersonalization? Would this experience not represent a stress to the ego?

That the impact of the experience is deeply felt became clear as we noted increase in anatomical responses in psychological tests administered at the six-month postnatal period. Two examples are quoted, both from psychological retesting at six months postpartum:

Mrs. F. is a woman who gives a very high proportion of pure form responses, namely, the conscious control, and then when she meets the red color, she immediately collapses and gives a very primitive type of response in which she sees "blood" and the birth process...She seems very much preoccupied with sexual anatomical responses. There is a compulsive repetition of responses about the birth process, the birth canal, the vagina...She sees on Card II the birth process with the blood, etc. Yet, interestingly enough, she sees the womb in the white space on Card VII as a "cavern" where the baby is, a "borning" place. It is interesting that she sees this void not as something warm and protective but rather as a "cavern," an empty place.

Similarly, Mrs. G.'s response to Card II, which looks to her like a perforation for a "baby to be born," may be related to the caudal she had. There is a feeling of shock in this response, also a conversion of her hostility into an anatomical answer which probably reflects both her anxiety and effort to intellectualize it.

The responses in these two cases are noted especially because, in comparing prenatal and postnatal tests, it was found that these women had not given the same kind of responses in the prenatal period.

The significance of this exploration is that for some few women, watching the delivery may be experienced as an anatomical assault. Fears regarding body intactness precipitated throughout the earlier months of bodily changes during pregnancy may thus be intensified. If the delivery procedure is, indeed, experienced as assaultive or damaging, this would evoke concerns about body intactness and bring about more drastic changes in body image than those already suffered during pregnancy. It may be that a reorganization of the defenses takes place which makes it possible for the woman to accommodate to the impact, such as through more repression, suppression, or hypochondriasis.

Medical Aspects*

John Lukasik and Josiah Sacks

The following observations on labor and delivery were made of the 64 patients participating in this study:

Nature of Delivery

The term "normal delivery" refers to either spontaneous delivery

*This section on medical aspects is adapted from the report written by John Lukasik, M.D., and Josiah Sacks, M.D.

or outlet forceps. There were 60 normal deliveries. Of the remaining four, there were two mid-forceps, one mid-forceps with rotation, and one Caesarean section. The indication for Caesarean section was a breech presentation with contracted pelvis confirmed by x-ray pelvimetry.

Timing of Delivery

The estimated date of confinement was calculated by employing the rule of Nagele. A patient was considered "overdue" when her pregnancy continued beyond 42 weeks. Premature labor and delivery was determined by the weight of the infant; any infant weighing under five pounds was considered premature.

In this series there were 54 deliveries considered to be "on time," seven deliveries overdue, and three infants were premature. One of the prematures was delivered at 21 weeks' gestation and died shortly after birth.

False Labor

Fifteen patients had some degree of false labor. The extent of this false labor ranged from 24 hours prior to the onset of true labor up to five weeks before delivery. The false labor was so severe in several patients that they were admitted to the hospital for observation, sedation, and rest. One patient was hospitalized on three occasions prior to her delivery because of painful uterine contractions. This particular patient experienced false labor for about five weeks prior to delivery.

Stimulation of Labor

Stimulation of labor, either by the intramuscular injection of sparteine (Tocosamine®) or the intravenous infusion of oxytocin (Pitocin®), was used in 24 of the 64 patients delivered. The reasons for stimulation of labor were elective induction, induction for postmaturity, premature rupture of the fetal membranes without contractions, desultory labor, and primary uterine inertia.

There were no complications as a result of using the uterine stimulants. X-ray pelvimetry was obtained in all cases of questionable cephalopelvic disproportion prior to the use of these uterine stimulants.

Onset of Labor and Stage of Admission

During the prenatal course the patients in this series were instructed as to what to expect at the onset of labor. As they were all primigravida they were encouraged to remain at home as long as they felt they could. The general advice was to the effect that they try to remain at home for at least one hour after the uterine contractions occurred at five-minute intervals.

The patients were examined vaginally immediately on admission. The dilatation of the cervix was used to determine if the patient was in the early, midpoint, or late first stage of labor. Early was defined as 1 to 3 centimeters, midpoint as 4 to 6 centimeters, and late as 7 to 10 centimeters, dilated. In this series 43 patients were in the early first stage, 16 patients in the mid-first stage and five patients in the late first stage of labor on admission.

Reaction to Pain and Procedures

Also during the prenatal course the patients were informed as to what would happen to them once they were admitted to the hospital. This information included such things as the history and physical examination by the house physician, perineal preparation, enemas, etc. The patients were scored by their obstetricians as to normal reaction, overreaction, and little reaction to pain and procedures. They scored as follows: normal reaction, 36; overreaction, 18; little reaction, 10.

Duration of Labor

Duration of labor was recorded for this group. The results were as follows:

a) Very short (less than 6 hours) 18
b) Short (6 to 12 hours) 33
c) Average (12 to 15 hours) 11
d) Moderately long (15 to 18 hours) 0
e) Prolonged (over 18 hours) 1

There was one elective Caesarean section for feto-pelvic disproportion.
There was no direct relationship between the "very short" and "short" groupings and those who received some type of uterine stimula-

tion as compared to the number of patients in these two groups who did not receive any uterine stimulants.

There was definitely a relationship between those patients who showed little anxiety at the time of their admission to the hospital and the length of labor, the less anxious patients generally falling into the shorter-duration groupings.

Complications of Labor and Delivery

The complications immediately postpartum (while in hospital) and those occurring at home until the time of the six weeks' checkup were recorded. The following complications were noted:

Endometritis	2
Atony of the bladder	2
Acute cystitis	2
Premature rupture of membranes and resulting premature labor at 21 weeks' gestation	1
Insomnia, requiring medication	1
Constipation	1
Postpartum depression	1
Postpartum psychosis	1
Stillborn antepartum, death cause unknown	1
Hematoma of episiotomy	1

Administration of Analgesia and Sedation

The administration of analgesia and sedation was charted as to dosage and also the stage of labor administered. The previously described criteria were used throughout for recording the stage of labor. Three patients received no analgesia because of immediate regional or general anesthesia. One patient received no analgesia because of desire for "natural childbirth." Twenty-two patients received meperidine (Demerol®) alone. Thirty-four received meperidine and pentobarbital sodium (Nembutal®) and three pentobarbital sodium alone.[9]

Types of Anesthesia

During the antepartum course, the various types of accepted obstetrical anesthesia were discussed with each patient. After some understanding of the modalities the patient's desire was recorded, with the understanding that this could be changed either by her desire at the advent of labor or for obstetrical reasons. Of the anesthetics used, 43 patients received general anesthesia; 17, caudal or epidural, and two, spinal anesthetics. Ten of the epidurals were administered in mid-labor and seven in late labor. Two patients received no anesthesia—the one who had the premature birth at 21 weeks and the one natural childbirth patient.

Physical Complaints During Postpartum Stay in Hospital

The patients' complaints during their postpartum stay in the hospital were recorded. Complaints concerning the episiotomy were the largest in number, 47. Two of these were of severe discomfort, while the remaining were slight. Three patients complained of severe headaches, one attributed to spinal anesthesia; the others followed general anesthesia. Seven patients complained of severe hemorrhoids, three patients of breast engorgement, and one patient of a severe toothache. Fourteen patients had no physical complaints.

In summary, 64 primigravida women were cared for during their prenatal, intrapartum and postpartum course. From a medical and obstetrical point of view this "study group" fared quite satisfactorily.

Attitude Toward Obstetrician

Most patients presented themselves as favorably as possible to the doctor in terms of personal appearance, desire to cooperate and win his approbation, and the tendency to minimize personal problems (if they were presented at all). The obstetricians recorded what issues were discussed on the patient's initiative. The following subject matter, apart from medical symptoms, was found to have been most frequently considered with the obstetrician: problems in weight control, breast feeding versus bottle feeding, fears regarding giving birth to a defective infant, sexual activity and its effect on the fetus, quickening, and the nature of labor and delivery.[10]

The obstetrician was the authoritative source of medical information. However, when he explained medical facts that were emotionally charged for a particular woman, she was at times too disturbed to hear what he had to say. The woman's exhaustive questioning on these issues in her interviews with the counselor, following upon the opportunity to explore them with the obstetrician, indicated how much anxiety the physical aspects engendered and how much was needed in some cases to bring a measure of reassurance and trust.

The patients in this setting clearly did not see the physician as one with whom special stresses that they were experiencing should be discussed apart from specific physical complaints and medically related issues. Even patients with acute personal problems (as disclosed to the psychiatric team) showed little of their anxiety about their personal situation to the medical staff. It was, in fact, the obstetricians who noted that these patients, although given the opportunity to do so, rarely talked about their non-medical problems. At the same time, the importance of their trust in the obstetrician was such that several patients subsequently left the prepaid medical program in order to have the care of the same obstetrician in later pregnancies, when his services could only be obtained on a private basis.

SUMMARY

A first pregnancy, despite its social ramifications and interpersonal meanings, appears from our results to be essentially an intrapsychic experience, one in which the woman is responding less to significant persons and events in her life than to immediate physiological and emotional developments from within. This statement is based on the fact that, in this study, only variables involved with the woman herself were found to be closely associated with Pregnancy Adaptation: her qualities of nurturance, ego strength, and confidence and clarity in visualizing herself as a mother. In addition, an inverse relationship was found between Pregnancy Adaptation and the number of medical symptoms the woman had during the course of the pregnancy.

The predictive significance of the personality factors, ego strength and nurturance, with respect to Pregnancy Adaptation has been emphasized in the preceding chapter. Of at least equal significance to personality for adaptations throughout the maternity cycle and specifically for Pregnancy Adaptation was the factor entitled confidence and clarity in visualizing self as a mother. This variable seems to tap the elusive quality of "feminine identification;" in its pervasive significance throughout the maternity cycle, it appears to confirm commonly held assumptions about the importance to the woman's adjustment in pregnancy of her capacity to find gratification in nurturant roles.

Thus, the statistical findings indicate that if by the time of the first pregnancy the woman has developed nurturant qualities, considerable ego strength, and a strong feminine identification, as evidenced by the clear and confident attitudes she holds with respect to herself in the role of a mother, it can be predicted that she will make a good adjustment during pregnancy. Our results also emphasize the close relationship between physical well-being on the one hand and predominant mood and emotional adaptations on the other.

Characteristic of all of the women during this first pregnancy were emotional states consisting, in varied combinations and degrees, of ambivalence, anxiety, and eager anticipation. We found that the woman generally experienced some heightening of emotional sensitivity and more lability than usual, especially in the first period of the pregnancy. Almost one-half of the women gave indication of moodiness and depressive states at intermittent periods. At the same time, there was a definite movement in respect to physical and psychological adaptations at varied stages of the pregnancy. As between the first and second trimesters, a marked decrease occurred in the proportion of women suffering from diminished vitality, and a marked increase (twice as many women, approximately half of the group) in the number reporting an enhancement of feelings of well-being over the same time span.

Anxiety was high in the first trimester and tended to subside during the second trimester. Towards the end of the pregnancy, in the eighth and ninth months when labor and delivery was imminent, a definite increase in anxiety was noted.

Changes in terms of psychological preparation for childbirth and maternity occurred in several major aspects defined by a number of items, among them those involving clarification and confidence in visualizing self as mother, effect of the pregnancy on the feeling of well-being (already noted), husband-wife adaptation, evidence of growth towards new family identification, and an overall variable identified as adaptability to changes of pregnancy. Comparing the changes over time of the Pregnancy Adaptation scales, we found definite change between the first and third and between the second and third trimesters in the direction of favorable adaptation to the pregnancy. By the time of childbirth, accommodation had generally been made to the reality of the anticipated birth.

There was indication of improved husband-wife adaptation during the pregnancy, and, except for the most acutely discordant families, there were many times of mutuality and keen enjoyment in this major venture. At the same time that the woman tended to draw heavily on the husband to sympathize and reassure with respect to physical aspects of the pregnancy, she tended to exclude him in relation to inner emotional reactions and concerns. His own emotional needs and doubts prevented his full response to his wife at various times, as the later presentation on expectant fathers will indicate.

In many instances we were aware oɪ much spontaneity and pleasure in the woman's wish to share her experience with her mother, and, equally, to enjoy the evolving co-equal woman-to-woman relationship. The women with a history of difficult relationships with the mother were almost always those who met with fresh disappointment in attempting to establish themselves on a different basis now. All of the women tended to examine their mothers' patterns of mothering at this time, in searching for those attitudes and methods that they would like to emulate and, equally, the ways in which they hoped to function differently and establish new ways vis-a-vis their own children.

Although each of the women had her own obstetrician and was given full opportunity to discuss problems with him, medical or otherwise, the women saw the physician as their medical advisor and kept other concerns from him. Looking toward possible supportive resources—parents, husband, the obstetrician—we found that for many, if not most women in this sample, these sources of emotional understanding and response were only partially available or minimally so.

All through pregnancy a woman experiences varied bodily changes and is involved in accommodating to them and to changes in her body image. This process is often most acute at the time of delivery and especially so during delivery of a first-born infant. The study revealed some psychological reactions to the delivery that led to an exploration of the impact on the woman of the experience of watching the delivery process. Most of the women who chose to watch the delivery were apparently motivated by the desire to participate in this significant event. Watching the delivery appeared to provide a sense of involvement, completion, and discovery in some instances; in other cases, it was apparently experienced as an anatomical assault, intensifying fears regarding body intactness precipitated throughout the earlier months of the pregnancy.

A first pregnancy tends to be a time of inwardness and aloneness, during which the woman may be doing the psychological "work" involved in accommodating to physical aspects and changes, relinquishing past gratifications, and anticipating those of the future. It may be assumed that, to the extent that she accommodates to the physical aspects and evolves constructive adaptive patterns to cope with changes within herself, she undergoes development that enables her to undertake the active nurturant tasks of the adult woman—an assumption supported by the findings that will be presented on the relation of pregnancy adaptation to maternal adaptation.

[1]To follow the development of the data, it is necessary to keep in mind the various measures developed for obtaining and assessing our data and the levels of statistical analysis which are set forth in Chapter II, Research Design and Methodology. The process of factor analysis is also presented in that chapter. Appendix B, Schedules A and B, contains the section on the Pregnancy Experience for rating at three and seven months, respectively.

[2]The original items and rating definitions involved in the composition of each factor scale is contained in a Compendium of the Factor Scales, Appendix C.

[3]Factor scales 8 and 11, Woman's Adaptation to Pregnancy Experience, are identical in name and contain the same items but the data are drawn from schedules for different rating periods; factor scales 10 and 13, Reaction to Characteristic Fears of Pregnancy, are composed of four items, three of them identical but rated at different time periods. The composition of each of the scales is in the Compendium of the Factor Scales, Appendix C.

[4]Appendix B, Schedule A, contains the section on Current Personality rated at the initial study of the woman. Schedule G-IV contains the Current Personality items rated at six months postnatally.

[5]Seventeen physical symptoms of pregnancy were available for checking in this way. See Schedules, Prenatal: Medical Observations, Appendix B.

[6]See Chapter III, Psychological Study of the Woman.

[7]The psychiatric interviews from which the observations in this section are drawn were conducted by the senior author of the presentation on the Psychological Meaning of Labor and Delivery.

[8]John Lukasik, M.D., obstetrician member of the research team, first called our attention to similarities between behavior during natural childbirth and orgasm. For an intensive and also comprehensive view of natural childbirth, see Kitzinger (1972).

[9]See article on "The Relationship of Antenatal and Perinatal Psychological Variables to the Use of Drugs in Labor," by Walter A. Brown, M.D., Tracey Manning, M.A., and Jay Grodin, M.D., 1972, for a full analysis of these data.

[10]Data obtained from the form "Prenatal: Medical Observations " were analyzed on a sampling basis only—that is, for visits in the fourth, seventh and eighth months of each patient's pregnancy. This form is contained in Appendix B, Set of Schedules.

REFERENCES

Bibring, G.L. (1959) Some Considerations of the Psychological Processes in Pregnancy. *The Psychoanalytic Study of the Child,* Vol. XIV. New York: International Universities Press.

Bibring, G.L., Dwyer, T.F., Huntington, D., and Valenstein, A.F. (1961) A Study of the Psychological Processes in Pregnancy and of the Earliest Mother-Child Relationship. I. Some Propositions and Comments. *The Psychoanalytic Study of the Child,* Vol. XVI. New York: International Universities Press.

Brown, W.A., Manning, T., and Grodin, J. (1972) The Relationship of Antenatal and Perinatal Psychological Variables to the Use of Drugs in Labor. *Psychosomatic Medicine,* 34:119-127.

Chertok, L. (1969) *Motherhood and Personality.* Philadelphia: J.P. Lippincott.

Deutsch, H. (1945) *The Psychology of Women,* Vol. II, *Motherhood.* New York: Grune and Stratton.

Flapan, M. (1969) A Paradigm for the Analysis of Childbearing Motivations of Married Women Prior to Birth of the First Child. *American Journal of Orthopsychiatry,* 39:402-417.

Flapan, M., and Schoenfeld, H. (1972) Procedures for Exploring Women's Childbearing Motivations, Alleviating Childbearing Conflicts and Enhancing Maternal Development. *American Journal of Orthopsychiatry,* 42:389-397.

Greenberg, N.H., Loesch, J. and Labin, M. (1959) Life Situations Associated with the Onset of Pregnancy, *Psychosomatic Medicine,* 21:296-310.

Grimm, E.R. (1961) Psychological Tension in Pregnancy. *Psychosomatic Medicine,*   23:520-527.

Grimm, E.R. (1962) Psychological Investigation of Habitual Abortion. *Psychosomatic Medicine,* 24:369-378.

Grimm, E.R. (1967) Psychological and Social Factors in Pregnancy, Delivery and Outcome. In: *Childbearing—Its Social and Psychological Aspects,* edited by S.A. Richardson and A.F. Guttmacher. Baltimore: Williams and Wilkins Co.

Grotjahn, M. (1960) *Psychoanalysis and the Family Neurosis.* New York: W.W. Norton and Company.

Heinstein, M.I. (1967) Expressed Attitudes and Feelings of Pregnant Women and Their Relations to Physical Complications of Pregnancy. *Merrill-Palmer Quarterly of Behavior and Development,* 13:217-236.

Huntington, D.S. (1961) Pregnancy and the Immediate Post-partum States. Presented at the American Psychological Association Meeting in New York.

Jessner, L. (1964) Pregnancy as a Stress in Marriage. *Marriage Counseling in Medical Practice.* Chapel Hill: The University of North Carolina Press.

Jessner, L. (1966) *On Becoming a Mother. Conditio Humana: Erwin W. Straus on His 75th Birthday,* edited by W. von Baeyer and R.M. Griffith. New York: Springer-Verlag.

Kestenberg, J.S. (1956) On the Development of Maternal Feelings in Early Childhood: Observations and Reflections. *The Psychoanalytic Study of the Child,* 11:257-291.

Kitzinger, S. (1972) *The Experience of Childbirth.* Baltimore: Penguin Books.

Klein, H.R., Potter, H.W., and Dyk, R.B. (1950) *Anxiety in Pregnancy and Childbirth.* New York: Harper and Bros.

Menninger, W.C. (1943) The Emotional Factors in Pregnancy. *Bulletin of the Menninger Clinic,* 7:15-24.

Newton, N. (1955) Maternal Emotions. A Psychosomatic Medicine Monograph. New York: Paul B. Hoeber, Inc. (Medical Book Department of Harper and Bros.).

Newton, N. (1963) Emotions of Pregnancy. *Clinical Obstetrics and Gynecology,* 6:639-668.

Shainess, N. (1960) A Re-Evaluation of Some Aspects of Femininity Through a Study of Menstruation: A Preliminary Report. Presented at the Midwinter Meeting of the Academy of Psychoanalysis, New York.

Wenner, N.K., and Ohaneson, E.M. (1967) Motivations for Pregnancy. Unpublished manuscript, delivered at American Orthopsychiatric Association Conference, March 1967.

Psychological Aspects of a First Pregnancy
and Early Postnatal Adaptation.
Raven Press, New York © 1974

Chapter V
Expectant Fathers*

Beatrice Liebenberg

"The most important thing that can happen to a man is the birth of a child," James Joyce wrote after the birth of his son, an event that "staggered and delighted" him (Ellman, 1965, p. 211).

Lincoln Steffens, on becoming a father, wrote, "I don't know yet why I wanted what I wanted, but I believe that in my bones, all my life, I have wanted what I have now—a child!" (Steffens, 1936, pp. 4-5).

Studies of the male parent have been largely eclipsed by literature describing maternal behavior. Animal research describes the mother care of bees and nesting birds more often than the role of the male parent, largely because the male takes little part in family life. Some animal fathers, however, do play a primary role (Michelmore, 1964, pp. 29, 32).

Margaret Mead reports that among some peoples the father's contribution to his child is regarded as even more important than that of the mother who only shelters the new life, treating the unborn child like an honored guest (Mead and Heynan, 1965, p. 47).

Unlike the biological origin of mothering, fathering is social in origin and thus permits the fantasy: "Is this my child?" A routine question asked fathers in our research study as to previous paternity is frequently answered, "Not to my knowledge." The motivation for fatherhood is manifold. In the Virgin Islands men gain more fulfillment in the role of parent than in that of husband. The child is proof of virility and manliness (Weinstein, 1962, p. 76).

"They are so proud when they get you pregnant," says one of the young mothers in our study, revealing at the same time her own

*This chapter, initially presented at the American Orthopsychiatric Association Conference, Washington, D.C., March 1967, was published as an article in a somewhat expanded version in *Child and Family*, Vol. 8, No. 3, Summer 1969. It is included here with the permission of *Child and Family*. The author wishes to express her gratitude to Dr. Gene Gordon, who illuminated various aspects of the clinical material in discussions.

strong need to have children. Just as early marriage has been used by many couples as a way of achieving quick maturity (Beukenkamp, 1959, pp. 532-538), the child also may be an instant stepping-stone into the adult world.

Ackerman (1958) points out that the young father's emotional identity with his own father in the years of his childhood profoundly patterns his self-image as he moves into adult life. Ackerman depicts the image of the father in our society as that of a weak, immature, dependent person frightened of competitive injury by stronger men, in contrast with that of the mother who is seen as strong, self-sufficient, and aggressive.

John Nash (1965, pp. 281, 285, 289), in reviewing the literature on fathers in contemporary culture, emphasizes the need for a close father-son relationship in order for the developing boy to acquire a self-concept as a male person. There is considerable evidence that in the boy's complex development paternal deprivation can be as serious as maternal deprivation, and that the process of identification with the father may be seriously impaired if the father is not present during the preschool period.

Over half of the men in our study were separated from their fathers during early childhood because of illness and death, divorce and army service. In a study of doll play aggression in children, Sears (1951, pp.32, 33) found that the boys whose fathers were absent had lessened total aggression and a less clear discrimination between males and females. Fifty-three per cent of the project fathers report feeling closer to their mothers and estranged from their fathers even now. Although the men in the project present no serious pathology, the absence of the father did occur at an age when hostile feelings and unconscious death wishes against the father are high (Zilboorg, 1931, p. 934), and we feel with Peter Neubauer (1960, p. 308) that the stimulus of both parents is required for the unfolding of all the complexities of the oedipal organization.

Most of the men expressed pleasure on having the pregnancy confirmed. At the same time many worried about whether they could carry the increased emotional and financial responsibilities. A project husband describes his feeling on learning of the pregnancy: "I was happy, or at least I wanted her to think I was happy; actually, I was sad because I knew we weren't ready financially—but I always wanted a child." Another husband admits he is "scared to think of the care another human being will require."

"For the father, the newborn represents survival and also the hope of self-realization" (Benedek, 1959, p. 412). The hope of self-realization is intensified in the fathers who had a poor relationship with their own fathers. "I still can't accept the fact that I will be a father," reflects Mr. A., who was reared by grandparents. "But I want to be close to the baby from the beginning.... From the point of birth on I'll be very close to him. I'll be living with him most of the time. It's important that we develop a relationship."

Pregnancy is a period of heightened dependency for the man, a time when he needs mothering for himself, but the wife, self-absorbed, may include her husband in the pregnancy through a recital of her pains and her fatigue, through descriptions of her urination, constipation, morning sickness, leg cramps, and contractions. She may request that he take over certain household chores, gratify bizarre food cravings, and, above all, that he reassure her about her fears. He may appease her or fly from her demands, but through all of it he feels very lost (Ackerman, 1958).

Husbands who do not have an opportunity to play an active part during the pregnancy are in trouble, Gerald Caplan (1959, p. 55) writes. Many of them identify with their wives. This is partly a rivalry situation because little boys have fantasies about having children just as little girls do. Karen Horney (1926, p. 330) feels that the boy's intense envy of motherhood has hardly received due consideration. Out of her analytic experience, she is impressed with masculine envy of pregnancy, childbirth, motherhood, and breastfeeding. Van Leeuwen (1947, p. 323) also sees pregnancy envy in men who are essentially masculine in their choice of love object but who long to usurp the place of the woman, based upon their inability to magically create a baby.

The fathers in our study have expressed their envy of pregnancy all the way from vigorously denying the pregnancy to almost fusing with the wife in an attempt to experience the pregnancy biologically. A number of husbands found it difficult to accommodate to their wives' fatigue and arranged long motor trips or camping expeditions, insisting that their wives must lead a "normal life." One husband demanded that his wife help paint the nursery, mow the lawn, and prune shrubbery. A number of men have urged their wives to nurse "because it would feel so good." In a joint interview in which a wife explained that if she were to breastfeed the baby her husband would be unable to participate in the feeding, the husband looked down at his chest and said slyly, "I don't know about that."

Mr. D. was one of the fathers who described the minutiae of his wife's pregnancy as if he were joined to her anatomically. He knew the details of every doctor's visit, every project interview. He would measure her abdomen and describe the protrusion of her navel with a kind of bliss. He took innumerable pictures of her in every stage of pregnancy.

Other men in the study, however, expressed a feeling of uneasiness about the pregnant figure. "Every man feels funny around a pregnant woman," explains Mr. C. "He doesn't want to be seen with her." Like the preadolescent, he sees the pregnancy as public evidence as to what he has been doing. Indeed, his wife does remind him laughingly about his "little dirty work." The intense feeling the husband brings with him from his childhood and a passive femininity seem to be reactivated at this time. Latent homosexuality is not as easily contained. Husbands resist sharing their wives' interest in pictures and diagrams of the changing pregnant figure. The woman's genitals are seen as frightening. Her larger breasts and body give rise to incestuous fantasies and anxieties about sexual adequacy. One husband, repulsed by his wife's shape, demanded that she stand in profile before him while he expressed disgust with her swollen body. When he talked about his feelings with the counselor, he was like a young boy overwhelmed by a leonine matriarch.

James Curtis (1955, pp. 937-950), in a study of normal expectant fathers, found the frequent occurrence of psychosomatic symptoms to be the most important distinguishing feature in the psychiatric reaction of the men he studied. They developed complaints which were very similar to the complaints of pregnant women. Sixty-five per cent of the expectant fathers in our study developed "pregnancy symptoms." There were reports of unusual fatigue in the first trimester of pregnancy as well as gastrointestinal symptoms, nausea, backache, headaches, vomiting, and peptic ulcers. A surprising number of fathers gained weight, from ten to twenty pounds, which they lost shortly after the birth of the child. Just as with the women, there was intensified oral craving. One expectant father, who was substantially overweight, would talk repeatedly about his hunger. "I'm so hungry and weak I can't seem to stay on a diet." His wife reported that he seemed to feel he had to eat every time she ate. The preoccupation with food may serve unconscious libidinal tendencies in the man, as with the pregnant woman (Deutsch, 1965, pp. 54-56).[1]

Several men who had previously neglected their teeth now made dental appointments. A number of men stopped drinking coffee and began to drink milk. Several stopped smoking, not at their wives' request, but "for the baby." Trethowan (1965, p. 58), in a discussion of the dietetic couvade, states that the observance of dietary restrictions in other cultures assumes an intimate relationship between father and child in which the child can be affected by the father's activities.

Toward the end of the pregnancy, certain men reported great difficulty in sleeping and general restlessness and anxiety. In several instances the husband took to bed.

The fear of passivity is countered in some of the men by recklessness and physical daring (Blos, 1965, p. 147).[2] We find much concern about body intactness and several auto accidents. A number of men became physically overactive; one husband brought evidence of a new soccer injury to almost every interview. Men related stories of past glory on the athletic field and of heroic encounters with fierce animals. This accentuated masculine behavior did seem to represent over-compensation for castration anxiety and homosexual fears (Fenichel, 1954, p. 188). Several husbands began to drink heavily and became involved with other women.

We noted that many husbands began to work frantically during the second and third trimesters of the pregnancy. Van Leeuwen (1947) suggests that the increased work energy may be explained by the envy of the wife's creativity.

Fifty-two per cent of the project husbands were largely unavailable to their wives because of heavy work or class schedules. Many of these husbands used the job defensively, discharging tension through an action-flight behavior pattern, and the frenzied work activity seemed a protection against the outbreak of serious neurotic phenomena (Abraham, 1948). Twenty-nine per cent of the project fathers expressed job dissatisfaction. Several left their jobs, only to fail in their new endeavors. Mobility was increased as well; 44 per cent of the project population moved to different dwellings within the prenatal and early postnatal period.

Almost half of our sample report a sharp decrease in sexual activity during the pregnancy (Newton, 1963, p. 645).[3] The wives express disinterest in the first trimester because of excessive fatigue, but there is marked disinclination on the part of the husband with the beginning of the fetal movement. Some men describe their fear of hurting the baby, crushing the head. A wife reported in the fifth month that her husband complained of feeling sore and unduly tired because of sexual activity. Mr. G. felt so "awed by the pregnancy" that he could not approach his wife for intercourse; she was unable to convince him that he would not hurt the baby. Even in the cases in which the wives feel they have initiated abstinence, they comment on how understanding and acquiescent their husbands are. Some husbands complain that they cannot sleep next to their wives because the kicking of the fetus disturbs their sleep.

Men who unconsciously see themselves as very aggressive express such thoughts as: "I've really messed her figure up." "Do you think she's big enough?" "How can such a big baby get out from such a little place?" Towne and Afterman (195S), in a paper on psychosis in males related to parenthood, report on the patients' concern about the wife being torn in delivery as masking aggressive and destructive feelings. Mr. H. had a bizarre fantasy that his wife might need surgery at the same time as she was delivering. Toward the end of his wife's pregnancy, another husband wondered if his wife were really pregnant, whether it might not be a tumor. Fear of stillbirth and of postnatal psychosis preoccupied other men.

Fear for the child was more often expressed postnatally; husbands would admit, once it was safe, that they had worried about deformity or retardation during the pregnancy. Certain reality factors intensified their anxiety. Several couples had a history of birth defects in their families. Incompatibility in Rh factor was another concern. Publicized drug hazards made couples uneasy about prescribed medication.

Probably the only man to believe himself pregnant was Boccaccio's Calandrino, who recovered without being delivered. The couvade, however, has been ritualized in many cultures. The Mohave Indian is ceremonially delivered of stones, and the Arapesh husband shares his wife's taboos and childbirth bed (Mead, 1949, p. 129).

> Like an Arapesh father, Mr. L. in the first trimester suffered extreme fatigue and muscle pain. He continued to have gastric distress and "bad nerves." He talked about a "little muscle that sticks out from my stomach that I can feel." In the sixth month he stayed home from work. He slept a great deal and drank only milk. He began to talk anxiously about premature babies, and in the eighth month Mrs. L. awoke to find her husband stumbling across the room. He fell across the bed, gasping for breath because of a pain in his abdomen. He was dispatched to the hospital, but X-rays and examination revealed no physical basis for his symptoms, nor could the doctor detect the alleged lump.

Almost all the fathers expressed anxiety about getting their wives to the hospital. Many made dry runs. Mr. M. was equipped with flares and emergency equipment should the baby be born in the car. The relief at reaching the hospital is forgotten, however, during the bleak period of waiting. "You're the lowest form of life," says Bob Newhart. "Even the maintenance men will have nothing to do with you" (Newhart, Warner Bros. Records, 1517).

Several fathers were able to describe their feelings of abandonment and desertion. They expressed anger toward the obstetrician who did not keep them sufficiently informed during the process of labor. One father describes his wife's labor with such empathy that husband and wife become indistinguishable:

> It seems as if she is deserted. You are on your own now; no one is with you. A nurse comes by, but she is very busy.... There she is at the end of the hall just deserted. You could reach out but what could you do.... It was a symbol of you're on your own.

The obstetrician separated one husband and wife earlier because the husband seemed to be in much more anguish than his wife. A wife asked her husband during labor what he was thinking. "I'm feeling guilty," he replied. "You're having this pain and there is nothing I can do." Several fathers fainted in the hospital.

Dr. Schaefer's manual (1965, p. 19) warns the fathers of disappointment, even shock, when they see their babies after birth. Several fathers do express the sense of shock with phrases such as "incredibly ugly," "looks like a newborn rat," "ghastly," "I thought he was cute but I had no real glandular emotion." With few exceptions, however, the response to the baby is a very positive one.

The men were quite open in stating their overwhelming preference for a male child. This is, of course, not unique to our culture (Thekaekara, 1966).[4]

Margaret Mead (1949, p. 45) states that the father's desire for immortality, whatever form it may take, is essentially embodied in his son. In the project group it was common for the wife to select the name for the girl and for the husband to name the boy. The birth of the child, particularly if it is a male, brings a resurgence of old conflicts, and postnatally a number of men vie with their infants in terms of physical needs (Wainwright, 1966).[5] Mr. K. has been ill a good deal since the birth of the baby. He suffered from a terrible headache that lasted several weeks and left him too debilitated to work. Mr. Q. complained that his wife was lazy because she refused to take off his shoes. A number of husbands quit their jobs during the six-month postnatal period. Some went back to school.

Irritation is expressed toward the child as well. Mr. T. attributes malefic motives to the infant's crying. He hits it when it holds its head a certain way. Many husbands complain that the baby is picked up too much. Mr. W., still competitive with his own father, perceives his life when the baby is one month old:

> Now we're no longer husband and wife but parents. When I come home, first thing is what we need to do for the baby. Here we've both worked hard, saved money for a home and now at last we're able to enjoy some things and we have to stay home and take care of a baby. I don't think about having any more. Maybe one baby is enough. By having one we've given our parents pleasure and now, from here on, we are free to do what we want.

Most husbands help with the housework and infant care during the early weeks. This falls off markedly by three months. Bernstein and Cyr (1957), reporting on a prenatal and child health program, also find a drop in the level of participation of husbands at the two-month period.

More often the rivalry with the child is unconscious and breaks through into consciousness as a fluctuant fear that something will happen to the child—that he will die, that he is not normal, that he will be neglected (Zilboorg, 1931, p. 950).

> In a group meeting, Mr. X. confesses a fear that permeates the entire group. "At the very beginning I would worry about whether the child would survive or not. There was no physical ground for this; there was nothing wrong with the child.... The fear that I had most was that he might choke."
>
> "I have that fear," responds another father. "It's not very strong, but I've had it all along, ever since the baby was born." "It is interesting," notes Mr. Y., "that all of us here have had the fear of choking. That's one of the things I'm really afraid of, is that kid choking to death."

Coleman, Kris, and Provence (1953, p. 26) suggest that the fear for the child's welfare may repeat early aggressive impulses against siblings. Eighty-seven per cent of our fathers have siblings; 40 per cent are first children.

Twenty per cent of the mothers were back at work before six months, with their husband's accord. A number of husbands began to push their wives to go back to work or to begin to prepare for a career. "You can't let the baby run you," one man admonishes his wife. And Mr. K., after describing how the infant nurses at his wife's breast, goes on to express concern about her vocational needs. He insists that she needs a job in order to get a sense of fulfillment.

There is frequent mention in the postnatal records that the husband appears depressed, distant, pale and wan. A number of husbands continue their frantic work pattern. Several fathers have auto accidents in the early postnatal period. Some talk about unfair working conditions and colleagues who compete underhandedly for promotions or commissions. Zilboorg (1931, p. 959) comments that depressive reactions in male parents frequently have a paranoid coloring and that the suicidal drive appears stronger than in women.[6]

A most interesting phenomenon in our project is the father who competes with his wife to see who can be the best parent. Competitive behavior was noted in 41 per cent of the fathers, but was most dramatically illustrated in the husbands whose wives had maximum difficulty in the adjustment to motherhood. Five women in our sample suffered from a depressed state of some intensity.[7] The following characteristics were observed in their husbands. The husbands offered minimal support during pregnancy. All had considerable anxiety in the last trimester of the pregnancy, thus intensifying their wives' fears. Only one of the five husbands stayed with his wife after delivery. All five husbands were often absent from home because of work, study, and travel during the prenatal and postnatal periods. Four of the men were closely involved with their mothers; two insisted on visits to their parents' homes when travel was medically counterindicated for the wife. All five husbands were more competent and tender in handling the baby than were their wives. Their treatment of the child was described by the woman as "wonderful," "better than I," "saintly." Unlike the women described by Caplan, who expressed irritation with their husbands' competition, the project wives seemed helpless when confronted with their husbands' greater competence. These women were invariably able to make contact with their husbands by arousing their anger through willful neglect of the child.

Esther Bick (1964, pp. 559-560), in a paper presented to the British Psycho-Analytical Society, cites the case of a depressed mother who, like the five project women, felt burdened and drained by her infant. It was the supportive behavior of the father that was most important in her improvement and in her growing closeness and tolerance for the baby. The husbands we have described suffered too much anxiety themselves to be able to give such support.

> Husband V, for example, was completely absorbed in his doctoral program and left his wife much alone. Despite her rising agitation and the recommendation of the physician he continued with his study and insisted that they travel to see his parents during her illness.
> Verbally he was most supportive. The counselor noted in the record that he protected the wife from any questions that might embarrass her. She handled the baby so roughly that it would cry, but he would brush his lips tenderly against the baby's forehead. He cared for the child during the night. He refused to consider birth control measures and planned for a family of six to ten children.

It is important to keep in mind the variety of adaptational patterns which may fulfill a couple's mutual needs. John Fearing (1966) emphasizes the need for husband and wife to manage enough closeness to decide what they want and that the conventionalized system of obstetrics be flexible enough to assist them in carrying out their wishes within the limits of medical safety. Fearing also mentions that in his own practice it is not uncommon for the guilt and frustration of the helpless member to make it appear that the spouse is competing in child-rearing.

Parenthood did not precipitate mental illness in any of the project fathers, yet the symptomatology and serious disorders described by Wainwright (1966) and Zilboorg (1931) are reflected to some degree in the transitory difficulties we have observed. A first pregnancy is a time when feelings about separation are intensified, when infantile conflicts between the father and his own parents are reactivated, and dependency needs are heightened. Our study of 64 normal fathers confirms the notion that pregnancy and parenthood are crucial for the male as well as for the female.

---

[1]Deutsch points out the infantile wish of devouring the desired object. She discusses also a male patient who, feeling soft and effeminate, uses food as a strengthening of masculine forces.

[2]Blos discusses the counterphobic role of physical daring in the male adolescent to assuage castration fear.

[3]Newton reports that 20 to 49 per cent of clinic women in a New York City sample reported their husband's fear that sex would lead to loss of the baby.

[4]In a conversation in August 1966 with George Pothen Thekaekara, educator from Karala, India, and cross-cultural studies consultant for VITC Peace Corps, he emphasized the desire for the male child in his country. In the villages a local mendicant predicts the sex of the unborn child by holding a chain over the pregnant woman's head. Invariably he predicts the sex as male. Later if the infant proves to be female he cleverly defends himself by producing a palm leaf hidden in the eaves of the house on which the correct sex is written. His explanation is that he did not have the heart to disillusion the family during the pregnancy.

[5]The birth of a son, says Wainwright, can reawaken homosexual conflicts. He describes the birth of a male child as having been the decisive stimulant in one patient's symptomatic upheaval.

[6]Zilboorg describes rivalry with the child also.

[7]Chapter IX, which deals with postpartum psychiatric disorders, refers to seven, not five, women who suffered a postpartum psychiatric disorder. The apparent discrepancy is accounted for by reason of the difference in time span covered. The later analysis included psychiatric disorders associated with a second pregnancy, whereas the original study was limited to the first pregnancy.

REFERENCES

Abraham, K. (1948) Observations on Ferenczi's Paper on Sunday Neuroses. *The Psycho-Analytic Reader*, edited by Robert Fliess. New York: International Universities Press.

Ackerman, N.W. (1958) Behavioral Trends and Disturbances of the Contemporary Family. *The Family in Contemporary Society*, edited by Iago Galdston. New York: International Universities Press.

Benedek, T. (July 1959) Parenthood as a Developmental Phase. *Journal of the American Psychoanalytic Association*, 7:389-417.

Bernstein, R., and Cyr, F.E. (1957) A Study of Interviews with Husbands in a Prenatal and Child Health Program. *Social Casework*, 38:473-480.

Beukenkamp, C. (1959) Anxiety Activated by the Idea of Marriage as Observed in Group Psychotherapy. *Mental Hygiene*, 43:532-538.

Bick, E. (1964) Notes on Infant Observation in Psycho-analytic Training. *International Journal of Psycho-Analysis*, 45:559-560.

Blos, P. (1965) The Initial Stage of Male Adolescence. *The Psychoanalytic Study of the Child*, 20:145-164.

Caplan, G. (1959) Concepts of Mental Health and Consultation. U.S. Department of Health, Education and Welfare. Social Security Administration, Children's Bureau Publication, No. 373, p. 55.

Coleman, R.W., Kris, E., and Provence, S. (1953) The Study of Variations of Early Parental Attitudes. *The Psychoanalytic Study of the Child*, 8:20-47.

Curtis, J.L. (1955) A Psychiatric Study of 55 Expectant Fathers. *U.S. Armed Forces Medical Journal*, 6:937-950.

Deutsch, H. (1965) *Neuroses and Character Types*. New York: International Universities Press. pp. 54-56.

Ellman, R. (1965) *James Joyce*. New York: Oxford University Press. p. 211.

Fearing, J.M. (November 1966) Anxiety: How, Not Why. *Medical Opinion and Review*, Vol. 2.

Fenichel, O. (1954) The Counter-Phobic Attitude. The Collected Papers of Otto Fenichel. New York: W.W. Norton and Co. p. 188.

Horney, K. (1926) The Flight from Womanhood: The Masculinity-Complex in Women as Viewed by Men and Women. *International Journal of Psycho-Analysis*, 7:324-339.

Mead, M. (1949) *Male and Female*. New York: William Morrow and Co.

Mead, M., and Heynan, K. (1965) *Family*. New York: MacMillan Company. p. 47

Michelmore, S. (1964) *Sexual Reproduction.* Garden City, New York: The Natural History Press. p. 29, 32.

Nash, J. (1965) The Father in Contemporary Culture and Current Psychological Literature. *Child Development,* 36:281, 285, 289.

Neubauer, P.B. (1960) The One-Parent Child. *The Psychoanalytic Study of the Child,* Vol. XV. New York: International Universities Press, p. 308.

Newhart, B. *Bob Newhart Faces Bob Newhart (Faces Bob Newhart).* Warner Bros. Records, 1517, USA.

Newton, N. (1963) Emotions of Pregnancy. *Clinical Obstetrics and Gynecology,* 6:639-668.

Sears, P.S. (1951) Doll Play Aggression in Normal Young Children: Influence of Sex, Age, Sibling Status, Father's Absence. *Psychological Monographs: General and Applied,* 65:32-33.

Schaefer, G., and Zisowitz, M. (1965) *The Expectant Father.* New York: Pocket Books. pp. 19, 97.

Steffens, L. (1936) *Lincoln Steffens Speaking.* New York: Harcourt, Brace and Co. pp. 4-5.

Towne, R.D., and Afterman, J. (1955) Psychoses in Males Related to Parenthood. *Bulletin of the Menninger Clinic,* 19:19.

Trethowan, W.H., and Conlon, M.F. (1965) The Couvade Syndrome. *British Journal of Psychiatry,* 111:57-66.

Van Leeuwen, K. (1947) Pregnancy Envy in the Male. *International Journal of Psycho-Analysis,* p. 323.

Wainwright, W.H. (1966) Fatherhood as a Precipitant of Mental Illness. *American Journal of Psychiatry,* 123:40-44.

Weinstein, E.A. (1962) *Cultural Aspects of Delusion.* New York: The Free Press of Glencoe. p. 76.

Zilboorg, G. (1931) Depressive Reactions Related to Parenthood. *American Journal of Psychiatry,* 87:927-962.

Psychological Aspects of a First Pregnancy
and Early Postnatal Adaptation.
Raven Press, New York © 1974

Chapter VI
The Dreams of Pregnant Women and Maternal Adaptation*

Robert D. Gillman

INTRODUCTION

This is a study of the manifest dreams of 44 normal young women during their first pregnancy and in the early postnatal period. We are interested in whether dreams can contribute to our understanding of psychological stresses during pregnancy and whether they reflect capacity and readiness for motherhood.

During the four psychiatric interviews in the course of the year's participation in the study, the women were routinely asked to report dreams. A few additional dreams were spontaneously reported during interviews with the psychiatric social workers. Three major questions were studied in these dreams. (1) How is the experience of pregnancy reflected in the dream content? (2) Is there a relationship between intensity of adaptational difficulty—as measured, for example, by hostility and masochism in the dreams—and independent ratings of maternal adaptation? (3) To what extent is the manifest dream related to important personality characteristics?

---

*Presented at the 1967 annual meeting of the American Orthopsychiatric Association, Washington, D.C. Published in the *American Journal of Orthopsychiatry,* Vol. 38, No. 4, July 1968. Copyright, the American Orthopsychiatric Association, Inc. Reproduced by permission.

The author wishes to express his indebtedness to Dr. Harold Plotsky, project psychiatrist, for anticipating the usefulness of dreams and painstakingly collecting them during his interviews.

THE MANIFEST DREAM CONTENT

The manifest content of dreams can be studied in its own right. Recent impetus to such study has been the vast research in REM sleep and dreams. In psychoanalytic treatment dreams are studied chiefly through the patient's associations, but the psychoanalyst gets many clues from the dream content, context, form, symbolism, and affect. The use of the manifest dream in psychoanalytic thought and practice was reported in a recent psychoanalytic panel (Panel Report, 1966). Phillips (1964) reviews psychological research in manifest dreams. McReynolds (1966) reports ongoing research correlating manifest dreams with personality traits.

Ella Freeman Sharpe (1959) has stated: "Dreams are a means of exploring present-day stimuli and current conflicts through the elaboration of pre-conscious thoughts." ("Although," she adds, "to understand the unity of psychical life the interrelation of the pre-conscious with the unconscious must be known.") In this study the working assumption is made that the experiences of pregnancy and motherhood are significant factors in the formation of the reported dreams.

In the course of the psychoanalysis of women during pregnancy, Helene Deutsch (1945) found that dreams of the unborn baby can represent ego-ideal fulfillment. A baby girl dream can embody all the qualities that made the dreamer valuable in her own childhood. A baby boy dream can represent the mother's masculinity and over-valuation of her father. These narcissistic representations are opposed by masochistic and guilt-ridden dreams expressing the painful idea that the child will be crippled. Deutsch also suggests that fetal development provokes dreams that parallel individual libidinal development: oral dreams in the first stage, then anal representations of crawling dirty creatures, then human whole-objects in which the baby is more mature than a newborn infant. She reports dreams near term in which labor and delivery are pictured as falling, climbing, slipping through narrow places, striving for a goal. As curiosity sharpens, the sex of the baby is more definitely stated. A dream of an ugly boy at this time represents ambivalence toward the husband. The child may be dreamed as already born, already walking and talking, free from the dangers the mother fears. In some mothers the bodily sensations of pregnancy produce persecution dreams: the mother dreams she is surrounded, caught, in danger of being clawed by a wild beast. In others, projection is evident: the dreamer is represented as the child, or the dreamer witnesses another woman as the mother.

Arthur Colman (1966) in an unpublished paper studied the dreams of 15 primigravidae in group therapy during their pregnancy. He found: (1) repeated nightmares of harm to self or the baby; (2) dreams of delivery in which labor is bypassed; (3) dreams in which the mother is excluded—someone else is holding the baby. Colman theorizes that the mothers' chief concerns were over loss of control, pain, the baby's needs for care, and hostility to the intruder.

Turning now to our own dream series, let me first clarify my own role in the research. As a consultant to the project I did not interview any of the mothers or collect any of the data, but I did have an opportunity to read the recorded dreams.

In our series of 50 women, six reported no dreams, leaving 44 women who reported a total of 132 dreams. The content of these dreams was compared with a tabulation of the dream content of non-pregnant college women in the same age range reported by Hall and Van de Castle (1966). Forty per cent of the dreams were about the baby, compared with 1 per cent in the dreams of the college women, leaving little doubt that the pregnancy experience is reflected in the manifest dream. Almost 90 per cent of our dreams are short, less than 50 words, and tend to omit elaboration of detail found in longer dreams. For example, a dream at three months: "I dreamed about fish, so I knew I was caught; I was pregnant."

It is rare for these women to dream of the process of labor—there were only four such dreams—or to represent a description of a newborn baby. In six dreams the baby was "just there," specifically bypassing labor. For example, at three months: "I was given a baby and didn't have to go through labor. All of a sudden I had the baby and wasn't pregnant." Of 20 dreams which specified sex, it was boys two to one. Ten were mature, past infancy. These are Deutsch's wish-fulfillment dreams in which the anticipated dangers and fears of childbirth and early infancy are bypassed. For example, at seven months: "I dreamed once about the baby, a brown-haired, blue-eyed boy of about 15 pounds."

While the incidence of aggressive acts in these dreams is no greater than the norms of non-pregnant college women, the incidence of misfortunes, harm, and environmental threats is high: 40 per cent of the total and over 50 per cent of longer elaborate dreams, compared with 10 per cent in the college women group (for whom only dreams longer than 50 words were analyzed). In 12 per cent the babies are crippled, deformed, or threatened. These are Deutsch's guilt-laden or masochistic dreams. For example, in the ninth month: "The baby was born with only the head. The body was a stick, but this was considered normal." In most of the misfortune dreams the dreamer herself is trapped or in danger. In the third month: "I was swimming down a muddy river through black reeds and somebody was after me, maybe more than one person. I kept swimming, finally reaching a swimming pool. There were waterfalls or reefs on both sides and I couldn't get by. I woke." These contents, consistent with Deutsch and Colman, may represent fear of the intruder projected as a persecutor, fear of the childbirth process itself, or awakening of old rivalries anticipated in the new arrival. Less than one-third of the dreams explicitly state apprehension, compared with 37 per cent in the college group, but this may be an artifact of brief dreams where the affect is implied rather than stated. Of the stated emotions in our series, over 75 per cent denote apprehension.[1]

Surprisingly, direct references to orality, such as eating or drinking, occur in only 4 per cent of the dreams, and references to talking or singing in 16 per cent, a total less than the non-pregnant norms. Regression in time, to a former period of the dreamer's life, is rare, occurring in only 5 per cent. There was no evident pattern in the dreams of libidinal growth along with pregnancy such as Deutsch found in some of her patients. Nor was the process of childbirth symbolically represented by escape through openings. Perhaps this last kind of dream is more common in subsequent pregnancies, where childbirth has already been experienced.

HOSTILITY AND MASOCHISM DREAMS RELATED TO MATERNAL ADAPTATION AND TO PERSONALITY CHARACTERISTICS

The group of new mothers that make the poorest adaptation to childbirth, those who suffer postpartum psychotic reactions, are characterized by depression, hostility, and sado-masochistic fantasies. The hypothesis was tested that the representations of hostility and masochism in the dreams would correlate with certain personality characteristics and with less adequate maternal adjustment.

The dreams were scored for the presence or absence of masochism on the scale devised by Beck and Hurvich in 1959. This scale has been found to differentiate depressed patients from other neurotic patients. In general, a dream is scored for masochism when the dreamer is explicitly represented as undergoing unpleasant affects or experiences. For example: "I had a helpless feeling. I was trying to reach someone but couldn't. It's a barrier dream. I felt frustrated and unhappy trying to get somewhere, but couldn't quite do it."

Hostility in the dreams was measured by the Saul-Sheppard 1954 scale in which dreams are given a numerical rating according to the degree of hostility contained in their elements. The highest score, for example, is given to death of a person, a lesser score to injury or discomfort. For example, a rating of four on a six-point scale was given for this dream: "I dreamed of an accident in which somebody is hurt or torn up."

After each dream was scored, the women were rated for both masochism and hostility on three-point scales: for the absence, presence, or marked presence of each trait. The intercorrelation between the masochism and hostility ratings was $r = 0.27$, indicating that they measure largely independent factors.

Maternal Adaptation

The masochism and hostility ratings were correlated with overall maternal adaptation measured by five items taken from the final pooled ratings (on a five-point scale) made by the project staff at six months postnatally.

1. The mother's coping with the physical needs of the infant.
2. The mother's coping with the emotional needs of the infant.
3. The mother's predominant mood.
4. The mother's satisfaction with the current situation.
5. The husband-wife adaptation.

Results: Neither of the dream scales showed a significant correlation with any of the five items measuring maternal adaptation. Insofar as these ratings were representative measures of maternal adaptation, we can conclude that masochistic and hostile elements in the dreams of pregnant women are not predictive of adaptation to the maternal role.

Personality Characteristics

The masochism and hostility ratings were correlated with certain personality variables measured by items taken from project staff ratings made at the seventh prenatal month. (Nine additional records were available for these ratings, making a total of 53 cases.)

1. Degree of emotional disturbance (on a five-point scale based on diagnostic classification).
2. Presence or absence of denial as a predominant defense.
3. Presence or absence of repression as a predominant defense.
4. Overall evaluation of the woman's adaptive adequacy.
5. Ability of the woman to meet her own needs, including pleasure.
6. A strong—not a rigid or deficient—superego.

Results: (1) The absence of masochism in dreams correlates significantly with:
No. 4. Overall evaluation of the woman's adaptive adequacy.
$r=0.37$, $p=0.01$
No. 5. Ability of the woman to meet her own needs, including pleasure.
$r=0.35$, $p=0.02$
No. 6. Presence of a strong—not rigid or deficient—superego.
$r=0.26$, $p=0.10$

(2) The presence of hostility in dreams is associated with the presence of repression as a defense, but not significantly: $chi^2 = 4.66$, $df = 2$, $p = 0.10$.

(3) Neither scale correlated significantly with degree of emotional disturbance or with presence of denial as a defense.

These preliminary findings suggest that masochistic dream elements in pregnant women are correlated with personality ratings involving adequacy, ability, and strength; that is, measures of ego strength or capability.

SUMMARY

The manifest dreams of 44 normal pregnant women, who were interviewed and tested psychologically during and after their first pregnancy, clearly represent the impact of pregnancy: almost half of the reported dreams are about the baby, and almost half of the dreams represent misfortune, harm, or environmental threat to the baby or mother.

In a preliminary statistical study the dreams were rated for masochistic and hostile elements. These elements were found nonpredictive of adaptation to the maternal role as judged by independent ratings, nor did they correlate with degree of emotional disturbance based on diagnostic classification. However, those women who were judged most adequate in adapting to their current life situation, those judged able to meet their own needs, including pleasure, and those judged to have adequate superegos, had significantly fewer masochistic elements in their dreams.

The dreams of pregnant women and new mothers occur in problem-solving settings and can be thought of in terms of delineating how the individual comes to grips with her new adaptive tasks. In this study the absence of masochism in dreams correlates with ratings signifying greater ego strength. It is suggested that manifest dreams can offer clues in personality assessment.

[1]Dreams elicited in psychiatric interviews are not completely comparable to dreams written down and submitted by college students, or to dreams volunteered in a psychoanalysis.

REFERENCES

Beck, A.T., and Hurvich, M.S. (1959) Psychological Correlates of Depression. I. Frequency of "Masochistic" Dream Content in a Private Practice Sample. *Psychosomatic Medicine,* 21:50-55.

Colman, A.D. (1966) First-Baby Group: An Investigation into the Psychology of Pregnancy and Mothering. (Unpublished).

Deutsch, H. (1945) *The Psychology of Women,* Vol. 2. New York: Grune and Stratton.

Hall, C.S., and Van de Castle, R.L. (1966) *The Content Analysis of Dreams.* New York: Appleton-Century-Crofts.

McReynolds, P., Landes, J., and Acker, M. (1966) Dream Content as a Function of Personality Incongruency and Unsettledness. *Journal of General Psychology,* 74:313-317.

Panel Report. (1966) The Manifest Content of the Dream. *Journal of the American Psychoanalytic Association,* 14:154-171.

Phillips, R.M. (1964) The Manifest Content of Dreams. *Ohio Medical Journal,* 60:758-761.

Saul, L.J., Sheppard, E., Selby, D., Lhamon, W., Sachs, D., and Master, R. (1954) The Quantification of Hostility in Dreams with Reference to Essential Hypertension. *Science,* 119:382-383.

Sharpe, E.F. (1959) *Dream Analysis.* London: Hogarth.

*Psychological Aspects of a First Pregnancy
and Early Postnatal Adaptation.*
Raven Press, New York © 1974

Chapter VII
Prenatal Counseling

TECHNIQUES IN PRENATAL COUNSELING

Beatrice Liebenberg

Three Methods Used in Counseling

This chapter describes psychotherapy with expectant mothers in the one-half of our project population who were in the counseled group. As Chapter II indicates, the women were initially referred to the prenatal project by the clinic obstetrician in the second or third month of pregnancy, and counseling was undertaken by the psychiatric caseworker with the counseled group after the diagnostic evaluation by the psychiatrist, psychologist, and caseworker.

The prenatal counseling was basically ego-supportive. The particular supportive techniques varied according to the woman's personality and response, the counselor's clinical appraisal, and her technical approach. Since three methods were used in counseling, we were able to study which techniques were more effective in influencing adaptation to the pregnancy and parenthood. The clinical observations of the entire team were useful in delineating these methods of preventive intervention.

Dynamic and genetic interpretation was the predominant technique in twelve cases in which psychotherapy aimed at insight. The treatment technique in eight cases was the clarification of feelings and object relationships, particularly with regard to the marital relationship. Anticipatory guidance, a psychological preparation for future stress, was the primary approach in nine cases.

Response to the Initial Study

The women differed in their expectations of the psychological study. One patient said with satisfaction that the doctor was just the way she had imagined him, like a movie psychiatrist. Some of the women believed that a psychiatrist worked exclusively with psychotic patients. "I don't think I like psychiatrists," reported a patient. "I never really got comfortable. He would ask you simple things but he seemed to get so much out of it. He would grab one word..." A woman might feel defensive and frightened about exposing her anxiety or she might feel angry because the doctor did not reassure her about her concerns. One patient's mother accompanied her to the clinic and demanded that the receptionist tell her what was wrong with her daughter that she needed to see a psychiatrist.

The psychiatric interview included a routine question about dreams (Gillman, 1968).[1] Several women denied any recall of their dreams, and for the more unsophisticated women the questioning brought back their own worries that dreams can mark a baby. Although these were anxiety-provoking situations for many women, the anger served also as a displacement for negative feelings against the counselor.

The response to the psychological testing varied also. Many women were deeply interested and gratified to be learning about themselves under the guise of research. Others were disquieted, fearful of what they might reveal.

> Mrs. F. said there was so much emphasis on whether responses were normal or not, whether one picks the right answer. She laughed about having muffed the arithmetic. She remembered a psychological test she took at college. There were questions like, Do you hate old people? She wonders how valid a question like this is. The counselor asked whether she was worried about whether she would come out normal and she said it was just a passing worry. She does think she is normal. However, she remembers a friend who was hospitalized but thought everyone else was crazy.

Test findings were frequently discussed with the subject in order to point out problems that could be explored during the counseling period.

> Because I felt that she was frightened about the psychological, I said that we saw her as a healthy, well adjusted person but that we thought that in her attempt to underline the positive she covered all the anger that she felt. She replied that this was true, that when she gets angry she only gets more miserable and so she tries not to feel too much anger.

Where the ego structure seemed particularly fragile, the test report was used to fortify the woman's self-image.

> The psychological test was frightening to her and she felt very depressed after leaving. She thought that perhaps the psychologist had discovered something very abnormal. I emphasized her normality and that we felt she had a very realistic expectation of the baby. She was extremely relieved and flushed, and then was able to confess her worry that on one card she saw pelvic bones.

Since the women knew that the project design called for a normal sample they regarded the diagnostic evaluation as an objective measure of their normalcy.

Rationale and Special Problems in Prenatal Counseling

The counseling was envisioned as strengthening the woman in her psychological preparation for motherhood so that she might cope more effectively with the stress of pregnancy and parenthood. There is general agreement on the need for emotional preparation for motherhood. The techniques for such intervention are more obscure. How can we help women to cope with situations still unknown to them? How can we encourage mature mothering in women who may not regard themselves as mothers for months or perhaps several years to come—or help them solve problems that do not yet exist? Does the pregnant woman need a unique therapeutic experience?

Robert Knight (1954, p. 54) points out that there is a continuous internal interaction and a constant external adaptive attempt throughout a person's life with normal crisis periods and stressful life experiences. Pregnancy may be viewed as such a developmental crisis. The woman's adaptation to her pregnancy will vary according to her personality structure, but even the woman who appears well adapted may have certain areas in which she is psychologically more vulnerable to stress. Many of her behavior patterns are an intensification or reactivation of earlier traits and her attitude toward her own body. These underlying neurotic problems as well as the reality of the pregnancy will influence the course of psychotherapy.

We found it extremely difficult to establish a theoretical framework for preventive therapy during pregnancy. A mother's response to her infant may be determined by innumerable factors outside her awareness, and our knowledge of the unconscious determinants of maternal behavior made us doubt at times the value of educative and supportive techniques. Conversely, we sometimes recognized our own unrealistic goals of wanting to build into the young expectant mother all the maturity and wisdom of a grandmother, and, what is more, to accomplish this in twelve to fifteen sessions.

The project patient was aware that the project was dependent on her continued cooperation. Several women verbalized a feeling of obligation to continue treatment for the therapist's sake. The absence of a fee further complicated the therapeutic situation by permitting a parent-child interaction. Some of the women were impressed by how much money was spent on them.

The ideal therapy patient, according to Stieper and Wiener (1965, p. 17), is one who wants to change some specific aspect of his behavior and has faith in a system for doing so. The patient who has no "therapeutic motivation" presents a problem for the therapist. In our prenatal project we had evidence that the research subjects did not lack psychological motivation, but the need was masked by more acceptable reasons—to have one obstetrician and to help science.[2] However, the willingness to undertake long trips to the medical center by public transportation, to be responsive to intimate and intrusive questions, and to submit to a battery of psychological tests cannot be explained by scientific altruism alone.

Whatever the expressed motivation, the counselor needed to stimulate the subjects' trust and interest in sharing feelings. It was difficult for the research patient to put herself in the position of accepting help.

Inquiry in the first interviews was fairly circumscribed in order that major aspects of interaction and content could be rated by the investigators.[3] Communication was indirect in these first interviews.

"It will be fun to be on the other side, to receive, and not just give," says Mrs. C. referring to her work as a psychiatric nurse. She digresses then to describe her younger brothers who were "spoiled rotten." She always wanted to be "spoiled sweet."

The following excerpts from an initial interview point to the woman's unconscious motivation for counseling and indicate early psychological conflicts which may be reactivated during the pregnancy. The counselor was attentive to the patient's non-verbal communication as well as her language and associations. The parenthetical comments below reflect the counselor's observations and questions. Brief psychotherapy at two-week intervals calls for diagnostic understanding as well as empathic understanding.

A number of women stated their interest in the project as purely intellectual.

One such woman was Mrs. D. who experienced considerable anxiety in the initial interview and denied in her final psychiatric interview that the project had meant anything to her.

Mrs. D. was a 24 year old housewife married to a government statistical clerk. She expressed her interest in the project as purely scientific. She volunteered no information and gave terse evasive answers to questions. Initially controlled she became increasingly anxious. Her smile was tight. She was close to tears.

She enjoys cooking, sewing, knitting. She has a fixed routine and is not comfortable unless she can keep herself busy, so she always finds something to do. (She handles her anxiety by being active.)

Her parents are wonderful understanding people. Her sister was born with a congenital defect but it was overlooked by everyone. She is amnesic about any events up to the age of twelve but has clear recall of an incident that occurred when she was about two years old—she bit the finger of a relative who tried to look at her toy. She never went to college because she did not want the chumminess of dormitory life.

Her health is perfect. Pointed questioning reveals that she had anorexia nervosa during early adolescence and a severe injury before the age of five which left her with a slight limp. She denies that the accident or illness were of any concern to her or to her parents. (The surgery following the accident could be interpreted by the child as punishment.)

She describes her husband with real warmth. She depends on him; he is the only person she trusts. They are both looking forward to the baby. Her only worry is that she knows so little about the physical care of a baby. Also she feels her new figure is ugly. She hates the look of this hump in the middle. (She describes it as a growth rather than a foetus. The reaction seems related to her attitude towards her body in the past.)

She describes herself as a person who sets high standards for herself and others. She does not approve of women who wear tight dresses and who are not moral. Very few people are acceptable to her; she cannot tolerate difference.

Mrs. D. is very busy with day to day living. This leaves her little room for introspection. Everything in her early life is covered over, including her illness, her surgery, and the sister's handicap. She has little clarity about her problems and is frightened that the counselor may be perceiving something she herself does not perceive. She does not want the idyllic picture she presents to be scrutinized too closely.

The counselor did not confront Mrs. D. with her resistance. Her pregnancy brought to the fore anxieties about body image that had not been resolved. Her fear of a damaged child was realistically enforced by her physically damaged sibling. These fears were never expressed nor wholly acknowledged to herself.

The counselor's decision was to treat Mrs. D. as if the fears had been expressed. She cared for the young woman by feeding information about pregnancy and the project and by affirming her more adult behavior. She talked with Mrs. D. about her house and activity, helping her to verbalize feeling. She was aware that Mrs. D. was playing out early passivity with her mother in having thoughts extracted from her and forcing the counselor-mother to feed her. This was never interpreted. Nor was her transfer of affectional needs to her husband interpreted. Their neurotic reinforcement of each other's needs was not questioned. The goals were limited: to establish trust, to make psychological help seem less frightening, to help Mrs. D. anticipate some of the problems of motherhood. In short, the decision was to offer Mrs. D. something she could count on without bringing her underlying conflicts into awareness. Interpretation to Mrs. D. would have been more threatening than curative.[4] It was the counselor's nurturing quality, her maternal acceptance and emotional support, that seemed most meaningful in the treatment.

Therapists and patients do not necessarily share the same goals (Stieper and Wiener, 1965, p. 58). Mrs. L's goals were markedly different from those of her counselor. Mrs. L. anticipated that counseling would be an educational experience and that the project members would teach her all about the care of the baby. The counselor hoped to modify certain behavior patterns and attitudes in Mrs. L. which she felt would stand in the way of good mothering.

> Mrs. L. was a simple, naive, immature woman, reality-oriented and without much conflict. She gave her life story willingly. Her family was extremely close and she never felt resentment toward either parent. The counselor felt that Mrs. L. handled conflicts by covering them over and suspected that the conflict with her parents was suppressed. The counselor tried to interest Mrs. L. in developing new activities, but Mrs. L. insisted she was content with life as it was.

The counselor tried to make Mrs. L. more sympathetic to her husband's needs.

> I reminded Mrs. L. that she was to discuss anything that was of concern to her, either past or present. Mrs. L. said she knows this and she does try to think about what she might discuss but really there are no problems.
>
> Were there any sexual problems as a result of the pregnancy, I asked. Mrs. L. replied that she has less sexual interest but that it was no problem. Did it not concern her husband? No, said Mrs. L. Her husband did not press the issue. When I persisted in questioning what kind of problem it could present for him, Mrs. L. said reluctantly that she would talk this over with him and I would know if it backfired because she wouldn't come back.

The counselor and her patient never did get together on goals. Mrs. L. wanted to learn about baby care. The counselor wanted her to explore her feelings, to become more introspective. By suggesting feelings of ambivalence toward parents and by opening up negative feelings she hoped to prepare Mrs. L. for the ambivalent feelings she would have for her child as well. She had a most resistant patient.

In a follow-up group session[5] two years later Mrs. L. reported that her whole pregnancy had been a breeze, but that she had not been prepared for the new demands on her.

> I don't think you can tell a person what it's going to be like to have a child. Just like during pregnancy you can't really tell them. How can someone prepare you for this feeling? Everyone knows that a mother loves a child. But this thing. Sometimes I was so tired I didn't even want to touch her. I just wanted to be able to sleep. But she would cry and I'd have to feed her. Now how much love can you have when you ache from head to toe and you want to sleep?

One staff member was aware of a vague anxiety when she began to work with the expectant mothers and realized that certain aspects of her own maturational crisis were being intensified. The expectant mother reflected an early aspect of the counselor's own life, and in one instance her own feelings unconsciously impinged on a patient who worried that her husband might be away on Reserve duty when it was time for her delivery.

> Mrs. P. reports: "When I was talking with Dr. G. she said she had her baby when her husband was overseas during the war and she managed just great. She felt absolutely marvelous and she thought everybody could—well, she didn't say everybody. But how do I know I could do it? Maybe I would panic and scream where she was so brave."

Problems of Identity

Certain women avoided facing painful feelings and some of their psychic conflicts were transferred to the body (Deutsch, 1945, p. 127). Mrs. C. says, "Everything hurts me more." Mrs. H. explains her headaches as allergic reactions to foods because she is pregnant. Blitzer and Murray (1964, p. 91) attribute the hypochondriasis during pregnancy to the increase in narcissistic cathexis at this time.

For certain women the period of pregnancy was one of heightened vulnerability and sensitivity in which the struggle to work out problems of identity was intensified. A woman who is still involved in acute identity struggles uses the pregnancy as closing off all possibility of becoming a person, not infrequently the person Mother wanted her to be.

In several cases an attempt was made to help the woman resolve the ambivalence of feminine identification through insight-producing techniques.

> Mrs. A., a pretty doll-faced young woman, whose carefully made-up face and grooming was marred only by bitten nails, expressed her fear of losing her identity and admitted that she felt unprepared for the care of the child. The psychiatrist noted the separateness and distance in her attitude toward the pregnancy and the baby. Projective tests revealed her anxiety about her feminine identification. Men were seen as monsters. Her attitude toward being a woman was more negative than positive.
>
> She expressed much boredom in the middle trimester, resented her husband's insufficient earnings, ruminated about what it would be like if she were not pregnant. She talked superficially about child rearing but refused to discuss breastfeeding. She continued to express disappointment and anger with her mother and husband. In her eighth and ninth months of pregnancy she was discussing a former boy friend and questioning whether the marriage was really what she wanted. Mrs. A. thought the counseling helped her to realize many things about herself, but, far from experiencing relief at ventilating anger, she became more depressed and guilty.

In a follow-up group meeting she considered whether the counseling had helped her to anticipate the resentment she felt toward her child.

> I don't think so. For one thing, when you're pregnant you think more about things that are immediate. I didn't think about the child, actually, until he was born. I had to go back to work. When I'm with him all day it bugs me. I felt guilty because I was cheating myself and because

I wanted stimulation and a different king of atmosphere. Before the baby was born I wasn't working and I was very depressed. I felt guilty.

Mrs. B. is another young woman with unresolved identity problems.

In a crisp casual manner she reviewed her life story which included early separation from her parents. In a flat well-guarded series of interviews she talked of the research she would do after the baby was born. She left the counselor off balance by diverting and misunderstanding questions, and used the interviews to discuss religion and politics. In the psychiatric interviews she mentioned her fear of losing her individuality. The psychological tests pointed up her fear of loss of control if she were to give up her intellectual pursuits.

Slightly hysterical she was ready to look to authority for support, making a heuristic approach very difficult. In her sixth hour she pressed the counselor to interpret a dream. The counselor suggested the meaning of certain symbols. Mrs. B. was silent, but later in the interview she commented that her confidence in doctors was destroyed when they said something even slightly wrong.

She was reluctant to come in for the next interview. "What are we going to hash over today?" She was frightened of the delivery, but explained her fear in terms of her high expectations of her behavior. In the last trimester she was not sleeping well, worried about "losing herself." She was bored, bored with being pregnant, bored with her clothes, bored in general. She jumped from a discussion of the *Feminine Mystique* to her fear of pain and her concern that she might harm the baby because she knew so little about infant care.[6] She said sadly in evaluating the counseling, "I have been reminded of things I suspected about myself."

In a follow-up group she discussed the first months after the baby was born and her feeling of resentment toward the child because she could not get herself organized.

I just felt incapable of handling anything. With my type of personality I have to be very organized. You begin to feel that although you're thrilled and happy to be a mother,

you're wondering if you couldn't be just as good a mother
and go out to work and do something productive in another
field. I feel guilt about always being home.

Both Mrs. A. and Mrs. B. were rated low on the Maternal Adaptation
scales.

One of the most challenging and difficult problems was that of
strengthening the defenses and reducing the anxiety of the extremely
anxious woman so that she might be able to look at herself. This
was of particular concern in a time-limited treatment and with women
whose contract did not include psychotherapy.

These interviews were characterized by a great deal of insecurity
and the use of primitive defenses on the part of the woman to ward
off anxiety, sometimes by verbal denial, sometimes by silence and
increased body tension. Patients like Mrs. B. talked loquaciously,
digressed, misunderstood questions, and succeeded in circumventing
counseling. It was difficult to reassure the very anxious patient. One
woman, in considerable anguish over her cousin who had been hurt
in a street fight, recounted the event many times but her fear and
distrust precluded the exploration of her deeper anxiety. In part, the
anxiety of these patients related to the fear that drawing closer to
the counselor would mean a loss of identity. The counselor's warmth
seemed engulfing and threatening. Sullivan (1954, p. 232) discusses
the need for distance in working with certain neurotic or paranoid
individuals.

Authority problems were reactivated during pregnancy. Many of
the women talked about job difficulties. Still dependent on "adults,"
they feared the control of supervisors and rebelled against what were
felt to be parental demands. These young women were struggling
to solve dependency needs with a great outward show of independence
and it was important not to bind them too closely by gratifying their
longing for the omnipotent parent.

The more successful cases were those in which the counselor
provided reality testing, gave support for adaptive gratification but
discouraged regression (Knight, 1954, p. 80). Particular care had to
be taken with the women who lacked sufficient ego strength not to
attack important defenses. In some cases the communication of pathological material led to a sharp increase in anxiety rather than insight.

A comparison was made between twelve cases in which
interpretation was used to stimulate insight and cases in which this
technique was not employed. The women were rated at the beginning

of pregnancy and at the six-month postnatal period for "insight into self." Although differences are noted in ratings for insight between prenatal and postnatal evaluations, they are very slight and statistically non-significant—which in itself supports the recognition that the effort to uncover conflict is inappropriate in working with a group who have not contracted for psychotherapy and who are involved in active tasks of pregnancy adaptation.

An examination of recorded interviews during the seventh and eighth months of pregnancy reveals a higher incidence of depressive affect in those cases (1) in which the counselor addressed herself to the woman's anger, (2) when she promoted regression by encouraging catharsis, and (3) when she continued to explore past relationships despite increased anxiety. The depression was at times impenetrable. Mrs. R. expressed boredom and fatigue after an interview in which she poured out her feelings of rivalry with her mother. The fatigue served as a defense against intense feeling. Mrs. F. felt a sharp pain in her back when she disclosed her resentment over her mother's travels when she was a child.

The women who were most fragile comment on their counseling in follow-up group discussions:

> *Mrs. T.:* I feel in a way that they dug a little too deeply psychologically. There was a little unnecessary digging. I cried for weeks after the baby was born. Maybe I would have had the blues anyway, but I'm wondering if a lot of things may not have been brought out by the counselor. I think they were digging for facts rather than to advise you.
>
> *Mrs. W.:* I too feel that maybe something should have been left alone. In my family for instance...It was the main topic of discussion quite often. My mother and I had a terrible relationship and there is no closeness, nothing, and this was brought up as if maybe your pregnancy will improve the situation. My mother didn't want me to have a baby. It's a situation that I doubt will ever improve. We will never be any closer. It doesn't bother me, but to keep having it brought up—Well, have you talked with your mother? I felt, oh, Gee...

During the prenatal therapy we learned more about the patients than we could practically use. The dreams, fantasies, speech, dress of the patient were all important indicators of unconscious feelings and defense mechanisms. Certain women revealed a more fragile personality structure as counseling continued. Failures in their own child-parent and sibling relationships colored their feelings toward the coming child.

> Mrs. Z. talked sympathetically about her sister who is an unmarried mother, but it was clear that her unconscious impulses were very much at variance with her altruistic motives to help her sister. She talked angrily of a co-worker who gave her terrible headaches. The co-worker got special favors from the supervisor despite her lax attitude and inefficiency. The neurotic problem with her sister was masked by the reality problem at work.

The counselor was careful not to verbalize the connection but by careful questioning and continued support led Mrs. Z. to a partial understanding of her anger and contributed to her increased self-esteem so that the danger that the sibling relationship would be imposed on the mother-child relationship could possibly be lessened. Insight is still beyond her grasp. An interpretation can be effective only "if it is given at the moment when the distance between what is said and what is meant is at a minimum" (Fenichel, 1945, p. 27).

The depressed patient had to learn to ally part of her ego and its reality testing with that of the therapist (Bellak, 1952, p. 333). The therapist helped in this process when she discouraged catharsis and supported feelings of competence and adequacy.

How Pregnancy Determines the Nature of Therapy

The therapist who treats a neurotic patient who becomes pregnant may regard the pregnancy as a point in time. Therapy which begins with the diagnosis of pregnancy and is terminated by the delivery is inextricably tied to pregnancy as a process. This biologic process is always partly unreal to the woman. "The child is a fantasy which will be realized in the future" (Deutsch, 1945, p. 138). When the counselor permits the woman in the few weeks before delivery to question her marriage and to explore career fantasies, she is also denying the reality of the pregnancy. It is important to talk with her about present activities rather than to encourage speculation about how life would be if she were not pregnant. The woman's defenses need to be renewed so that she can mobilize herself for motherhood. Negative feelings must be handled in such a way that the guilt does not become overwhelming.

Nor is it sufficient in prenatal counseling to analyze fears about deformity or pain. The counselor needs to make clear that these are fears that other women share. She dispels with her professional authority such statements as, "All babies born in the eighth month die," or "If you reach above your head the cord will strangle the baby." Fears more deeply rooted, such as, "I do not deserve to have a child—something will go wrong," are also countered by the counselor's involvement in the woman's practical planning and her affirmation of the woman's developing pregnancy.

> She mentioned again that time was flying by and she had done nothing yet. I asked her where the baby would sleep. She thought they would buy a crib when the baby was two months old and borrow a bassinet when the baby was born. I wondered why they had to wait. Could they buy it now and avoid the inconvenience of buying it later? I added that we would schedule an appointment for her with the pediatrician so that she might discuss with him some of the things the baby would need. I noted her excitement and relief at my encouragement to go ahead.

Grete Bibring defines the developmental process of pregnancy and parenthood in terms of the relationship of the woman to her sexual partner, to herself, and to the child. She needs also to resolve her relationship to her own mother before she can move toward motherhood itself. "The positive attitude of a motherly figure toward the patient's pregnancy is an important factor in the patient's acceptance of her pregnancy" (Bibring, 1961, p. 11, 15).

Identification with the counselor was for some of the project women their first real acceptance of themselves as women. The fear and ambivalence in becoming a woman like her mother is more easily explored through questioning past rather than current feelings.

> I asked Mrs. H. whether she had ever worried about her ability to have a child and she said that she had when she was about fourteen, because of her mother's difficult pregnancy. It was her grandmother who reassured her that she would be able to conceive. Mrs. H. thinks maybe a

man is also concerned about whether he is masculine enough to have a child.

Mrs. F. confessed that she used to worry about whether she could have a baby. The counselor said that most women had difficulty assuming the role they associated with their own mothers, and Mrs. F. said it was hard to believe she was pregnant. She talked about how many problems there are in bringing up children. The counselor pointed out that just as a child grows, parents grow also, and that problems which seem insurmountable now would not feel so overwhelming at a later point in their lives.

There was a longing in most of the women for a supporting relationship with a mother substitute during the period of pregnancy. This was a difficult time for the women who had poor relationships with their mothers. The angriest, most deprived women in the project revealed a poor relationship with their mothers and both begged and defied the counselor to set it right. The increased orality in pregnancy increases the need for mothering in therapy.

Mrs. F. is a young woman who suffered narcissistic hurt from her mother and older brother. Only her father encouraged her femininity but his interest was too seductive. She denied her mother's preference for her brother, proclaimed her mother's warmth and loving nature, but increasingly displaced her anger with her mother onto her husband.

Only as she identified herself with the counselor was she able to express some of her feeling of deprivation ("You care what happens to me") and concomitantly she began to meet the needs of her husband. There was a growing understanding of her mother and a deepening of their relationship as she was helped to reach out to her mother in a more adult way.

Daydreams were seldom revealed. Deutsch (1945, p. 137) indicates the healthy woman's desire to hold such fantasies to herself. One woman referred to her pregnancy as her secret. It was as if talking about the feeling would change it or spoil it. Sometimes the counselor elicited such expressions.

The counselor showed Mrs. J. a copy of a magazine featuring a story on pregnancy. A photograph showed the expectant mother pushing her abdomen out with pride. Mrs. J. giggled, "I never would have told you because it seemed so silly but when I was only three months pregnant I used to walk with my stomach sticking out as far as I could. I was so proud."

A joking query to an expectant mother as to her prediction about the baby's sex and appearance was frequently much more informative than the direct question, "How do you visualize the baby?" Unfortunately the clues were not always picked up. A mother who held her hands ten inches apart to show the diminutive size of her baby was deeply disappointed in her nine-pound daughter who looked "too huge" and "too old."

Husband-Wife Adaptation During Pregnancy

The stresses that a pregnancy may impose on marriage have been described by marriage counselors (Jessner, 1964). The relationship between marital partners is important in determining their receptivity to the child. The competitive relationship between certain husbands and wives was so intensified that they were unable to help each other with their increased fears about themselves and their sexual adequacy. Several immature young couples used their sessions to prepare for mature parenthood. When the treatment approach emphasized clarification of feelings with regard to the marriage, the counselor focused on the stress of pregnancy on the marriage and worked intensively with the husband to help him give his wife emotional support.

Mrs. R. began counseling in her second month of pregnancy. A slim, boyish-looking young woman, she presented a history of being cared for by several families during childhood and her speech was colored by bitterness and sarcasm. There was a regressed quality to her behavior and she expressed considerable conflict about dominance and submission.

When she talked about her husband's abuse the counselor was supportive but questioned her own provocation in the arguments. Mrs. R. was reluctant to work on internal problems. She continued to ventilate anger against her husband and father. She complained about her husband's drinking, his insults about her skinny figure. The counselor broke into a long recital of complaints by questioning why Mrs. R. minimized her pregnancy. Mrs. R. replied that it was not fashionable in her circle of friends to want a baby.

With the counselor's support she enrolled in a child care course. She became less aggressive and argumentative and more accepting of the pregnancy. She reported that the marriage was better. In the tenth session Mrs. R. laughingly referred to her husband's drinking as a last fling, but the therapist confronted her with her need to keep her husband weak and pointed out that she could work toward a more responsible pattern in her family than she had experienced in her parental family. The therapist used support consciously to help Mrs. R. resolve her own deep feelings of abandonment by her parents and to accept the pregnancy.

The N.'s were another couple who needed help in weaning themselves from their parental families before they could establish their own family unit.

Mr. N. exploded that his mother-in-law knew where to find things in the house that he didn't even know they owned. His in-laws want to take over completely on buying all the furniture for the baby. He resents their taking over.

In an interview with Mrs. N. in her seventh month of pregnancy she doubts very much that her husband will want to take time off from work after the baby is born. She says very happily that her mother will stay with her.

Joint Interview: Mr. N. is very frightened that she will allow her parents to take over. He feels that her mother sees the baby as hers and it is not. Her parents still want to provide the entire nursery. He feels they are moving in and taking over. He resents very much that his wife and her mother have worked out plans for the mother to stay after the birth of the baby. He wanted to take the week off and help her. Mrs. N. looks very startled and says she did not think he would be able to take time from work and she did not want to be let down. She would certainly prefer him to her mother. Mr. N. with relief says that her mother may come in for visits. She will be able to see the baby in the years ahead but this first week is really theirs.

She thought that she might want to nurse her second child but not this baby. She knew that it would not be easy for her husband to see the baby at her breast. His wanting her to breastfeed the baby was really his own desire to feed the child and she had decided that it was far better for him to share this pleasure than for her to do anything which might jeopardize their relationship.

The women were uniformly pleased with their husbands' involvement in the project. One woman stated:

My husband had never been around babies. I think it really helped him because he learned something about babies that you just don't learn from everyday conversation. I think he got a lot from the project.

Several husbands regarded the counseling as parental interference.

Mr. T. urged his wife to skip appointments and expressed the same distrust of the counselor as he did of her parents.

Most husbands, however, made optimum use of the counseling.

He said quite quickly that he was not going to bother her with sex for now. He worked from early morning to late in the evening and both of them were too tired to do anything but just flop into bed at night.

I said I could understand this but suggested that frequently husbands are frightened of damaging the child in some way. He listened very intently, then said this was his fear also, and that if he did anything to cause a miscarriage he knew she would never forgive him. Although he could accept the fact that the foetus was well protected he still felt that his weight might hurt it in some way...I wondered whether he thought of himself as someone who could cause hurt and he said it was because his wife has accused him of hurting her. He talked with great difficulty of his feelings of inadequacy as a lover...

Postnatal Marital Adaptation

Ratings reflect improvement in marital adaptation between the first and third trimesters. The impact of the child on the marriage in the early postnatal period is disruptive, however, and the six-month postnatal ratings reflect a lower level of marital adaptation.

In the follow-up groups women discuss their lack of privacy, that they can no longer pick up and go. "You have to pack the baby bag." "You're never sure when he is going to open his mouth and bellow." "You want to sit on your husband's lap and the baby climbs all over you." One woman resented her husband because he could sleep through the night.

Postnatal marital adaptation improves, however, in those cases where couples were helped prenatally to anticipate the negative impact of the child. When the results obtained using anticipatory guidance are compared with those of the control group by categorizing the data as shown in Table 1 below, it was found that differences were statistically significant, suggesting that this counseling method was effective in promoting marital adaptation.

TABLE 1. *Direction of change in ratings for marital adaptation: anticipatory guidance versus control cases**

	Down	Same	Up	Total
Postnatal marital adaptation as compared with prenatal marital adaptation				
Control	15	11	0	26
Anticipatory guidance	1	5	3	9
Total	16	16	3	35

*Based on comparison of ratings in Schedule B (seven months prenatal) and Schedule H (six months postnatal).

Chi-square computed for the above table showed a significant difference at the 0.01 level, although the results must be taken with caution because of the small theoretical frequencies in some cells. When the frequencies in the "same" and "up" categories were compared, a one-tailed *t*-test showed significance at the 0.005 "same" and "up" categories, resulting in a significant difference at the 0.02 level.

Table 1 also shows that fully one-third of the anticipatory guidance cases showed high ratings when evaluated six months postnatally, compared to none in the control group.

Anxiety and Fears Related to Pregnancy

Regressive forces stimulated by some of the physical changes in the woman are reminiscent of earlier concerns. Preoccupied with constipation and diet, she views herself with almost a parental concern. The involuntary processes, vaginal discharge, nipple discharge, urinary pressure, recall episodes of bedwetting and early adolescent concerns. "I change my underclothes several times a day, take many showers, but I still don't feel clean." Some of the play between husband and wife, examining the navel and feeling the baby, has an early "doctor game" quality.

Occasionally the woman's conversation reflects "primary process" thinking.

> Mrs. J. was hurt because a neighbor thought she was too flighty to settle down to motherhood. She complained of a hollow feeling in her ears. After a few moments of silence she said she had not felt life yet, revealing that the hollowness belonged to another part of her body.
>
> She digressed then to talk about food, and explained that although she enjoys eating and can understand the craving, when she sees the end result she would not do it, no matter what.
>
> "If you like something or desire something—even if you see a baby—you love that baby; or if you have certain desires for something, the inside of your stomach turns red. It does actually, physically, and the feeling you get is one of liking something and wanting to eat it. In other words, you want part of your own body, and so if you figure that you know, I don't know if it's people or things, if you want something you want to eat them. Your stomach conditions itself to become part of your body."

Actually this is a woman who fluctuates between overeating and severe dieting. The symbolic meaning of oral incorporation was not pursued. The counselor listened attentively, reassured her that she had checked with the obstetrician herself and he had confirmed that with a first baby one might not feel quickening as early as with subsequent children.

The reaction to quickening was indicative of the woman's object relations.

> Mrs. E. was very frightened by sudden pain. She discussed her pain with the doctor and they decided she was feeling life.

When the psychological meaning of quickening was negative, we attempted to help the woman view the fetal movements differently in an effort to condition her feeling toward the coming child.

> Mr. M. said what worried him most was the pain his wife felt. It is very hard for him to think of her suffering. Mrs. M. explained to the counselor that the movement of the baby was very painful to her. She knew it was not supposed to be, but nevertheless it did seem to roll around and push against her so that it was very hard for her to take. The counselor acknowledged that the contractions and muscle pain might be uncomfortable but wondered whether her husband might be imagining pain far beyond what she was acutally experiencing. She readily agreed that this was so. The pain was certainly bearable, but unexpected...

Rarely do the women verbalize a fear of injury or death, but as the delivery draws near their restlessness becomes more pronounced. There is an expressed eagerness to have the baby, but a feeling of panic that it will come too soon.

> Mrs. F. is irritated by her relatives who tell her that she looks ready to deliver when she is still several weeks from her due date. She imagines that passengers on the bus are afraid she will deliver on the bus. She begs the obstetrician for reassurance that it is still not time.
> Another woman who is obsessional and phobic talks about ESP and her occult powers with respect to predicting death, her attempt to gain control through childish omnipotence.

"This knowledge of an event that will happen on a certain date, upon which one depends, and which nevertheless one cannot influence, this mixture of power and submission, has something fatal and inevitable about it, like death" (Deutsch, 1945, p. 321).

The fear of loss of control is expressed by the women in their concern about how they will behave during labor and delivery. The influence of suggestion plays an important part during this period.[7]

Mrs. H. talked about women who had been in labor for two or three days and her fear of injury during delivery. Her husband listened anxiously. An extremely anxious and immature man, Mr. H. has a long history of illness and has grave doubts about his capacity to be a parent.

The counselor accepted Mrs. H.'s concerns as normal worries but went on to discuss the delivery realistically and mentioned the feeling of accomplishment and exhilaration that most women experience during labor and delivery. Mrs. H. contemplated this positive suggestion with interest. It was reassuring for Mr. H., who was frightened of his aggressive impulses, to hear that his wife would not be torn apart in the delivery.

Anticipatory Guidance

In prenatal therapy the therapist deals not only with the immediate concerns of the patient but with those aspects of her personality which the therapist surmises may interfere with good mothering. Considerable resourcefulness is required to enable the patient to explore issues which she may regard as irrelevant. Although anticipatory guidance was used to some extent with all the counseled patients, it was the primary approach with one group of women in an effort to modify the experience of delivery and the early period of infancy.

The main concepts which underly anticipatory guidance are elucidated by Gerald Caplan (1959) who regards psychological preparation for future stress as a strengthening procedure for the individual not unlike physical training. Anticipatory guidance with the project patients was directed toward (1) preparing couples for the reactions they would experience in each stage of pregnancy, labor, and delivery; (2) preparing them for the stresses of parenthood; and (3) discussing ways of coping with the expected and unexpected problems of the infant. This approach hypothesizes that if a woman can be helped to see the difficulties inherent in parenthood ahead of time, their impact will be lessened when she becomes a mother.

Anticipatory guidance made use of the woman's current life experience as well as past events in her life in helping her to foresee the time ahead. For example, the infant's dependency needs could not be overemphasized. Occasionally a woman would acknowledge that a mother might have feelings of resentment toward a baby, but for the most part the women were silent and it was difficult to know how much they were hearing. It did have the effect of making the child more an object, however. Deutsch (1945, p. 153) suggests that this is an important part of the psychic hygiene of pregnancy. Several women during these discussions shielded their abdomens as if to reassure themselves that child and mother were still one.

In the following illustrations the counselor addressed both husband and wife.

> I talked with them about the impact of a baby's dependence in these first months, that the baby's needs were so enormous that parents could feel the infant's crying as willful behavior. I stressed that an infant could not be regarded as a mature person and they, like most parents, would be feeling resentful and overwhelmed from time to time. Undoubtedly they would express some of this anger; this was human. They must try not to be too harsh with themselves and each other when they did make mistakes. I emphasized how important the father's support was during the early postnatal period. Any mother, even one with Mrs. Y.'s experience, feels uneasy and unsure from time to time, and it is helpful when she can lean on her husband.

The O.'s planned to sail and to water ski with the baby. The counselor attempted to make the child more real to them.

> The counselor emphasized the infant's need to be held and comforted and mentioned that some parents are afraid to hold the baby for fear of spoiling him. Mr. O. said that a baby could cry just to be crying, just as a dog barks just to be barking. Mrs. O. said she did not intend to give in to temper tantrums. The counselor explained that a tiny infant could not really be said to have temper tantrums. . . .

Mrs. F. is helped to anticipate problems with breastfeeding.

> Overworked nurses could not always be helpful in assisting the mother with breastfeeding, the counselor said. Mrs. F. would have to be assertive about having the baby brought in to her even if she were told she had no milk. Mrs. F.

said it was much easier for her to be aggressive than it used to be.

Anticipatory Guidance and Maternal Adaptation

In the nine cases in which anticipatory guidance was the primary approach, four were rated as above average in maternal adaptation. None was below average. In the twelve cases in which dynamic and genetic interpretation was the predominant technique, seven of the women were rated below average in maternal adaptation. Two were above average. Of the eight cases in which the treatment approach was the clarification of feelings and object relationships, none was rated below average in maternal adaptation. One case was rated above average. The results of the three techniques are summarized in Table 2 below.

TABLE 2. *Maternal adaptation ratings for three counseling techniques*

Counseling Technique	Number of cases				Per cent		
	Below	Average	Above	Total	Below	Average	Above
Clarification	0	7	1	8	0	87.5	12.5
Interpretation	7	3	2	12	58.3	25.0	16.7
Anticipatory guidance	0	5	4	9	0	55.6	44.4
Total	7	15	7	29	24.1	51.7	24.1

This table is based on maternal adaptation ratings at six months postnatally. A *chi*-square test showed the differences to be significant at the 0.01 level, but because of the small cell frequencies this result cannot be taken as conclusive. The table was condensed into a 2 × 2 table by pooled frequencies for the clarification and anticipatory guidance groups and for the average and above-average categories. Then a *chi*-square test showed statistical significance at the 0.01 level. Thus, marked differences were found in the ratings for maternal adaptation, at least between clarification and anticipatory guidance on the one hand and interpretation on the other.

A further attempt was made to test for possible differences between clarification and anticipatory guidance with regard to the observed frequencies in the average and above-average categories. For clarification, 12.5 per cent of the cases were in the above-average category compared to 44 per cent for anticipatory guidance. However, the significance of this difference was at the 0.10 level, not sufficient to warrant a high degree of confidence in the observed difference between the two methods. But given the small number of frequencies involved, the results strongly suggest that anticipatory guidance was more effective in promoting a higher level of maternal adaptation.

The distribution of frequencies is quite different among the three counseling techniques. Both clarification and anticipatory guidance registered no below-average cases, whereas interpretation yielded a majority of cases in that category. The highest per cent of cases in the above-average category was found for the anticipatory guidance technique.

Termination

The woman's delivery marked the termination of the counseling. The counselor visited the new mother in the hospital but her role now shifted from therapist to observer.[8] In the research design the birth of the child marked the ending of the counselor-patient relationship. However, most of the women felt deserted at a time when they most needed support. They suffered the simultaneous separation from the fetus and the good mother.

The women who had had particular difficulty in seeing the child as a reality object were the very deprived women described earlier. The termination was experienced by them as a betrayal and in some cases seemed to nullify the counseling gains in the early prenatal period. The counselor's present neutrality was a negation of the earlier therapeutic involvement and redolent of the inconsistent mothering some women had experienced during childhood. The therapist rarely reviewed the treatment process in the final interview. The patient seldom verbalized her feeling of loss. Several women had a depressive reaction. The baby lost its special significance in relation to pregenital narcissistic entitlement for these women (Blitzer and Murray, 1964, p. 89). The separation from the therapist may also bring about a depressive reaction (Deutsch, 1965, p. 340). A number of women maintained contact with the counselor through phone calls or visits. In these instances the patient was able to integrate the therapy with her ongoing life.

The counselor's efforts at helping the woman to anticipate her feelings about ending were not successful, perhaps because of the counselor's own conviction that the woman needed her most on becoming a mother.

> I said that I did not know how many times I would see them after today and that made me feel bad because at the point where I might be more useful to them our contact would be cut off. There was only silence. Then they asked questions about the mechanics of processing data....

Even when the counselor discusses termination during the first trimester she meets with denial.

> I told Mrs. G. that during this counseling period we would get to know each other very well and that it would be very hard when we had to end. She flew instantly to a story of a deaf woman she had met, also how delighted she was with her new church. Her old minister used to deliver negative sermons. She wants to hear only positive sermons.

Mrs. Z. accepted termination passively. She promised the counselor a picture of the baby but it never was sent. Two years later she told group members:

> I think the counseling should have continued, maybe, four to six weeks afterwards. The social worker really helped me and my husband. A lot of things that we would be discussing we would talk about afterwards. I'd come to pick him up or he'd come to pick me up and he'd usually ask me, "What did you talk about?" and then I'd tell him things that I wouldn't have said to him ordinarily. Things came out that otherwise would have stayed inside, and afterwards when we didn't have this, there were still some things that we could have discussed that we didn't discuss. It would have helped.

With an interval in time and group support the women can reveal the extent of their dependency.

> After I had the baby and I knew my social worker was coming to the hospital, I just couldn't wait. I said, "Oh

boy, now she can see my baby," you know, right away. I thought about it because I had been talking to her all along, about the baby and everything. We had been discussing back and forth and about how I felt and about the baby, and I just wanted so badly for her to come and see it.

Value of Prenatal Counseling

We have been presented with an enormous amount of material in this project about the women's lives and their adaptation to pregnancy. The assessment of the prenatal therapy is still elusive, but it is clear that in most instances the woman gained a sense of worth and value.

> Mrs. X., in her eighth month of pregnancy, is a far less constricted woman than she was. She wears bright colors, bemoans her loss of a waistline but makes no effort to close her coat. She is more sensual, her posture is more relaxed and she laughs more freely. She has been able to relate to her neighbors more easily and enjoys the easy, gossipy exchange. She is frightened that her dreams will mark the baby. She could discuss and at least partially resolve the fear of being cut (episiotomy) as well as her superstition in not preparing for the child. I have attempted little interpretation but have reassured her by accepting easily some of the feelings and behavior she describes as being part of her pregnancy. I laugh with her about the desserts she craves, explain her pregnant girl friend's misconceptions. It is easier for her to talk about her worries in the guise of her friend. My approach is at all times empathic and direct. The relationship between husband and wife is much closer.

There is no quantitative evidence that the counseling promoted self-understanding. Murphy (1965, p. 530) reminds us, however, that a great deal of working through of newly acquired insights must be left up to time and the patient. He points out that the effects of therapy extend outside the therapist's office and continue to operate long after therapy has come to an end.

At six months postnatally the women were asked by both the counselor and the psychiatrist to assess the value of the project. These responses were sometimes dissimilar.

> Mrs. H. continues to visit the clinic to see and talk with the counselor who "is almost one of the family." However, to the psychiatrist she said she would think twice before getting into the project again.
>
> Mrs. D., who expressed only scientific interest in her initial interview, remains uncommunicative in her final interview with the psychiatrist. "As far as the project is concerned, she is curious to find out what has been proved, if anything. I asked her if she thought that the project had any value for her and she replied that there was none that she could see. I asked her if anything was made worse by the project, and she replied that there was not. She thinks studies of this type are interesting, but it seems pointless until all the data are in. She feels that there were no problems that she had which required any help. She spoke highly of Mrs. J. (counselor); she felt she was a very nice person."
>
> Mrs. R. reports that her counselor had been very helpful. Mrs. R. had worried about having a retarded child but talking with the counselor made her forget her worry.
>
> The F.'s write a note to their counselor: "This year has been one of newness and growth for us, so likewise we hope you find what you are looking for in the program. It's been exciting working with you and discovering the world of parenthood."

The patient's perception of the counseling process may be considerably affected when periods of stress are experienced. Some of the couples were facing job changes, financial problems, housing moves. They felt cut off from help at a crucial period. Mosak (1952, p. 8) points out also the need of some patients to placate, manipulate, or express hostility toward the therapist. A patient who feels worthless, he suggests, feels he does not deserve to improve and may conceal whatever personal benefits actually have accrued to him.

The staff tended to underestimate the value of counseling. Pfeffer (1959, pp. 440-441), reporting on a procedure for evaluating the results of psychoanalysis, states that both patient and analyst seem to focus on what remains undone and tend to forget or ignore what has been done.

Summary

Grete Bibring (1961, pp. 12, 13) suggests that the pregnant woman is more in need of supportive psychotherapy than intensive treatment. Our findings would confirm this suggestion. Zinberg (1964, pp. 6-8) states that for some people "any goal short of thorough insight into unconscious conflicts and the resulting reorganization of the personality is insufficient." We believe with Zinberg, however, that psychiatric knowledge and insight is not lessened by minimizing interpretation. Interpretation, when used with our prenatal patients, caused some regression and augmented depression in the last trimester of pregnancy. These women had greater difficulty in accepting motherhood and in re-establishing the marital relationship. Support and the clarification of feelings and behavior enabled the woman to accept her pregnancy fully but it did not sustain her sufficiently to cope with the stress of the early postnatal period.

We believe that psychic intervention which is aimed at maternal adaptation calls for psychological knowledge on the part of the therapist together with the implementation of anticipatory guidance methods. Personality material is important in predicting critical areas in the woman's maternal adjustment. When the woman is able to gain some perspective on her problems and is helped to recognize her strengths, she is then prepared to draw on them as a mother. When the counselor can also help her to anticipate regression, disharmony in the marriage, and rivalry with the infant, she is enabling her patient to mobilize herself in meeting the problems of parenthood.

COMPARISON OF COUNSELED AND NON-COUNSELED GROUPS
AND WITHIN-GROUP DIFFERENCES

Pauline M. Shereshefsky and Robert F. Lockman

Despite the increasing recognition in earlier studies of the significance of psychological factors during pregnancy, there have been few attempts to provide special services geared to the needs of the pregnant woman and her family. A major purpose of this project was to develop a social work counseling service for pregnant women and their families as an adjunct of the obstetrical services of the sponsoring agency, the Group Health Association, Inc. The need for this phase of the project—intervention through casework counseling—was based on research by Cyr (1957), Caplan (1957, 1959), Bibring (1959), and others, which, while focused on the psychodynamics of pregnancy, recognized the preventive mental hygiene potential in services directed to the emotional needs of pregnant women and their families. This section is concerned with the use of casework counseling as a method of providing special services for this sample of normal women and their husbands during a first pregnancy.

The project undertook to explore the question: To what extent is the counseling program effective (a) in reducing the degree of emotional disturbance associated with the stress of pregnancy, (b) in reducing physical complications and difficulties during pregnancy and during delivery, and (c) in helping to promote a satisfactory relationship between husband and wife during pregnancy and in facilitating their assumption of satisfactory parental roles. The effectiveness of counseling in relation to these objectives would be determined, we thought, by evaluating and comparing the counseled and control groups on the outcome variables.

Statistically Significant Differences Between Groups

Initial Differences, Three Months' Prenatal Study. The families who met the criteria for inclusion in the project were randomly assigned to the control and counseled groups. Of 43 items of a factual nature defining social characteristics, the two groups were comparable in all except seven items, none of which was relevant to the purposes of the study.

Although the subjects were randomly assigned to the control and counseled groups, our initial study of the two groups indicated that the groups differed on several variables of potential significance for the outcome of the counseling. The control group was superior on one life history variable—a better relationship of the woman to her mother prior to age twelve—and on two current background factors: the controls as a group had better marital relationships and a smaller number of external stresses. In one other aspect the control group seemed somewhat at an advantage: they had a significantly lower number of women in the psychiatric diagnostic classification, "normal, with tendency toward character or personality disorders."[9]

Significant Differences Between Groups Subsequent to Initial Study Period. At the seventh-month period, the pregnancy experience was re-evaluated by a two-member team, the psychiatrist and social worker. Differences between groups and within each group over time were analyzed against the initial, first trimester ratings.

In Chapter IV, the changes over time in a number of rating items dealing with the pregnancy experience strongly suggest that, from the first to the second trimester, the women in both groups were moving in the direction of a growing acceptance of the pregnancy.[10] The data indicate, further, that the control group continued the higher level of husband-wife adaptation that was noted in the initial study period, in that two of three higher mean differences in the second trimester deal with the husband-wife relationship. During the course of the pregnancy and counseling (which terminated at the time of the birth of the infant), the counseled group showed changes that were especially marked in two important areas: the woman's capacity in visualizing herself in the maternal role, and the husband-wife relationship as indicated in the woman's greater identification with her new family (both significant at the 0.001 level) and the better ratings for "fewer fears regarding her sexual role with her husband." Visualization of self as mother is predictive of pregnancy outcome and highly correlated with the other outcome variables, so that change in this area was clearly relevant to the purpose of the study. The items on family identification and reduced anxiety for the woman regarding the sexual role with her husband suggest that the counseling was in fact having some impact in marital adjustments in this group, in which the husband-wife adaptation was not initially as good as in the control group. In several items in which changes over time occurred for both groups, the degree of change was distinctly accentuated for the counseled group, suggesting that the counseling had had an effect in intensifying changes precipitated by the pregnancy.

The degree of change in the control group, compared to its own baseline, is generally lower than that of changes in the counseled group. However, the controls rated higher over time on adaptability to the changes of pregnancy. This may be a reflection of the personality characteristics that were initially rated more favorably for that group and that would be expected to persist. The higher rating may also reflect the same problems that make all comparisons difficult: the counseled women were more open in telling of their concerns and doubts and expressing anxieties and fears, and the counselors knew them better, so that such defensive maneuvers as denial or repression could be evaluated and somewhat corrected in the rating (generally resulting in lowered ratings).

Labor and Delivery

Significant differences were found which indicate that the women in the counseled group went through the labor and delivery experience with better adaptation than those in the control group. The findings are summarized in Table 3.

The significant differences between the two groups are particularly noteworthy, especially when considered with a group of items showing non-statistically significant differences that are in the same direction. When doing the ratings, the obstetricians involved in the project did not know whether the case was in the counseled or control group. Moreover, the stage of admission to the hospital was a specific factual item, and thus it was freed from the rater bias issue that arises in some of the ratings. Medical observations support an interpretation that patients coming into the hospital at a later stage of the labor process as here defined are generally more relaxed about labor and delivery. The narrative accounts of their reactions to the labor and delivery experience by the women, as related to members of the project team, supported this interpretation, with appreciably more of the counseled women viewing their experience as "easy" than the controls (34 per cent compared to 10 per cent). At the same time, 42 per cent of the control women felt that the labor experience was very

TABLE 3. *Medical staff observations: labor and delivery*

	Counseled			Control				Superior group
	Mean	S.D.	%	Mean	S.D.	%	p	
Labor—stage at which woman was admitted to hospital:								
Late (7 to 10 centimeters dilation)			16			0	0.01	Counseled
Early (1 to 3 centimeters dilation)			53			83	0.01	Counseled
Dilation in centimeters upon admission to hospital	4.2	2.3		2.9	1.0		0.01	Counseled
Sedation administered at late stage of labor			47			23	0.05	Counseled
Little reaction to procedures during labor*			25			7	0.05	Counseled
No complaints during postpartum hospital stay			88			63	0.05	Counseled

*Checked as: overreacted, normal degree of reaction, or little reaction.

hard, compared to only 14 per cent of the counseled women. We conclude that the counseling relationship, by helping the woman in her preparation for labor and delivery, enabled her to cope better with the childbearing experience.

Husband-Wife Adaptation—Comparison Of Groups Over Time

Both groups showed improvements in husband-wife relationship during the prenatal period. The first postnatal ratings showed a trend downward, for the control group especially, doubtless reflecting the strains introduced in the relationship by the arrival of the infant. By the time of the overall six-month rating (Schedule H), the counseled group was found to have held the level of adaptation of the early prenatal period, while the controls were significantly less well adapted as compared to their initial level ($p = 0.025$). This movement in the ratings suggests an impact from counseling on this strategic aspect of family adaptation.

Summary Of Findings

The counseled group was found superior to the control group on these criteria:

1. Pregnancy-related adaptations in:
   a. Visualization of self as a mother—the counseled group made marked gains ($p = 0.001$) between the first and second trimesters of the pregnancy on clarity in visualizing self as mother and substantial gains in confidence in visualization of self as mother.
   b. Evidence of growth towards new-family identification—the counseled women showed an intensified movement ($p = 0.001$) towards identification with the new family (as against childhood family identification).
2. Labor and delivery—the counseled women showed more adequate coping with the labor and delivery experience, as determined by a number of factual criteria.
3. Husband-wife adaptation—whereas the control group, postnatally, had difficulty in maintaining the level of marital adaptation represented by the initial ratings in the prenatal period, thus showing the strain and disruptive impact of the birth of the infant, the counseled group were apparently better able to maintain themselves under that impact.

TABLE 4. *Superfactor scale means for control and counseled groups by counseling techniques*

Superfactor scale	Counseled group					p Anticipatory Guidance vs. Interpret.	p Clarification vs. Interpret.
	Interpretation	Clarification	Anticipatory guidance	Total Counseled	Total Control		
I. Feminine identification	66	80	87	76	78	0.01 Anticipatory Guidance	0.025 Clarification
II. Infant adjustment	81	78	82	80	83		
III. Woman's intelligence	113	119	108	113	115		
IV. Infant alertness (1 month)	176	161	170	170	172		
VI. Maternal responsiveness	117	139	139	130	129	0.025 Anticipatory Guidance	0.025 Clarification
VIII. Woman's self-confidence	52	61	64	58	63	0.025 Anticipatory Guidance	
IX. Husband-wife adaptation	46	53	49	48	52		
XI. Husband's responsiveness to paternal role	35	36	37	36	35		
N = 57	12	8	9	29	28		

No p values for counseling vs. control.

A fourth major finding deals with the counseling technique of anticipatory guidance, presented in the preceding section, Techniques in Prenatal Counseling.

Within-Group Differences, Based on Counseling Techniques

In the pioneering work of Gerald Caplan (1961) in preventive psychiatry, the technique which he calls "anticipatory guidance" holds a prominent place as a method recommended for short-term, therapeutic intervention during crises. This is one of three techniques used in providing counseling in this project.

The preceding section identified the different techniques as: (1) Interpretation, directed to major reorganization of the personality and involving uncovering of conflicts and interpretive interventions; (2) Clarification, which placed emphasis on a supportive relationship focused on feeling and stresses during pregnancy, and involving therapeutic collaboration in dealing with whatever interpersonal problems the family presented; and (3) Anticipatory Guidance, which, while utilizing psychoanalytic understanding, kept clearly in view limitations of time and goals and was closely focused on psychological preparation for the stresses of pregnancy, delivery, and parenthood.

In the overall view of the project, some eight major components or dimensions emerged, referred to as superfactor scales. With this reduced number of factors, the process of evaluating the varied techniques of counseling was facilitated. The differences among the three major techniques (interpretation, clarification, and anticipatory guidance) were tested for the superfactor scales; the results appear in Table 4. In comparing each pair (counseled and control) in each of the three caseloads, significant differences beyond those expected by chance arose. There was a significant counselor effect which probably masked differences in the comparisons of the total counseled and control groups.

Since the techniques used were found to have varying outcomes, evaluation of the counseling required a consideration of differences *within* the counseled group to supplement our analysis of differences between counseled and control groups:

1. There was no significant difference on any superfactor scale between counseled and control groups.
2. Comparing the two techniques, clarification and anticipatory guidance, the means were not significantly different on any superfactor scale.
3. The means for anticipatory guidance and clarification are both significantly higher than for interpretation on some of the most pertinent factor scales, as follows:

	Anticipatory guidance compared with interpretation	Clarification compared with interpretation
	p	p
Feminine identification	< 0.01	0.025
Maternal responsiveness	0.025	0.025
Woman's self-confidence	0.025	

These data, in summary, point to anticipatory guidance as the most effective of the three methods used with families undergoing a first pregnancy. On the superfactor scales, the cases in the anticipatory guidance subgroup were significantly higher than cases in the interpretation subgroup on three important scales. Comparing the subgroups, clarification and interpretation, the cases in the clarification subgroup were higher on two of these superfactors only, and anticipatory guidance exceeds in degree the differences noted with respect to the most inclusive factor, feminine identification.

Observations on Differences Between Groups Based on Follow-up Group Sessions

Further data on differences between groups were obtained in a series of group sessions led and reported by a member of the research team (Liebenberg, 1966):

> Follow-up group sessions were initiated as an additional approach in ascertaining the usefulness of psychotherapeutic intervention during pregnancy. The group session proved to be a more valuable procedure than we had anticipated, in that it yielded significant clinical data and opened up important areas in our own thinking....
>
> The content of these meetings covered the predominant themes of the pregnancy period as well as current problems relating to the child. Thus a typical meeting might deal with anxieties experienced during pregnancy, post-partum moods of depression, the emotional reaction to labor and delivery, lack of maternal fulfillment, the impact of the pregnancy on the marriage....
>
> Tentatively we can state that among the counseled women there does seem to be a difference in the woman's satisfaction in her role as mother....
>
> The competition between husband and wife in the control groups seems greater; the husbands tend to feed into their wives' lowered self-esteem by devaluing the mother's role with the child. In contrast, the counseled fathers talked more appreciatively about their wives' competence. It may be that the emphasis during the counseling period on meeting the husband's needs and affirming his ability to give support to his wife accounts for her greater satisfaction as a mother.
>
> The difference that emerges most clearly between the two groups is in the quality and quantity of group interaction. The counseled group is characterized by a lively free-flowing exchange of emotional viewpoints. The control patients are more defensive, tend to deny and intellectualize feeling. There is more warmth and approval in the response of experimental members toward each other. It does point to the possibility that therapeutic intervention during pregnancy enabled these women to ventilate anxiety more easily and to acknowledge and clarify their feelings.

Problems in Designing Research Involving Evaluation of Therapeutic Outcome

We recognize the crucial importance of enabling women to cope better with labor and delivery. The finding that counseling had this effect has special meaning in view of data from other research which show a similar trend (Grimm, 1961; Chertok, 1969). The statistically significant findings with respect to effectiveness of counseling in other facets of the study were, however, less definitive. The question of the relation of counseling to the goals set forth at the beginning of the study could not be answered unequivocally—again, with the important exception regarding reduction of anxiety during labor and delivery.

In attempting to understand why the positive results were few, we saw in retrospect that selected aspects of the program complicated the task of counseling and evaluating therapeutic outcomes. The problems of major proportions are discussed below.

Self-selection Aspect in Accepting Project Participation. Families with recognized need—the more problem-ridden families—tended to accept participation, when offered opportunity to come into the counseled group, more consistently than those with less need. The statistically significant greater incidence of stress found in the counseled group, especially serious marital disharmony, can probably be understood in these terms, despite the random assignment of cases to the counseled and control groups. Dependent on the group, the project had to be presented differently to candidates for each group. Some couples, knowing they were in difficulty, accepted the offer of project participation for the very reason that it held out the promise of counseling; this was explicitly stated by a few participants. Thus an element of self-selection may have characterized the counseled group especially.

Incidental Therapeutic Effects of the Study Process. The incidental therapeutic effects of psychological study is a familiar problem in clinical research (Stechler, 1961). The whole sample, control and counseled cases, were subjected to the same study process during the first phase of collaboration and later, in the postnatal period. Exposed to questioning and tests by the psychiatric team, the participants were stimulated to introspection and many drew on the experience for an increase in self-understanding and the achievement of some perspective on their interpersonal problems.

The more sensitive, self-aware, and introspective gained more from this study process than those who were heavily defended. Of many examples, the following is typical:

> In the seventh month interview, a woman of the control group states that she feels greater closeness in the relationship to her husband. She is not sure what the difference is, but she knows the relationship is not the same and that it is better. She then volunteers the observation that she and her husband found it had been helpful to talk to the counselor a few months ago because they have been more free to talk things over with each other ever since.

Similar statements and more clearly observable shifts in relationship or attitude occurred in a number of the control cases. Since incidental therapeutic effects of the psychiatric study had an impact on the non-counseled as well as the counseled group to some degree, counseling effects were obscured for purposes of comparison and evaluation.

Variations in Receptivity to Intervention. The degree of involvement with us varied greatly. Among the counseled group, some used the help available to them to work seriously on emotional needs and relationships, with full investment of themselves in the process. At the other extreme, some of the women and some of the men (not always those in the same family) were largely uninvolved, lending themselves to the counseling in form only and persisting in maintaining the role of research subjects in relation to us.

Differences in Theories of Psychotherapeutic Intervention. The divergence of theoretical viewpoints in the research counselors was not fully appreciated until the project was well under way, and differences were never fully reconciled. A consistent, integrated approach could not be achieved within the life-span of the project. It was finally recognized that the setting forth of issues was in itself a contribution in this still unclarified area of research on outcomes in psychotherapy.

SUMMARY OBSERVATIONS

Evaluated in terms of its effect on maternal functioning and infant adaptation, the project has not established an unequivocal role for counseling as a method of intervention for normal couples during a first pregnancy. It has established the fact that the counseled group as a whole coped better with labor and delivery than the non-counseled women. The counseled group as a whole also managed to ward off the disruptive effects in the marital relationship of the first postnatal period, which were seen in the control group. A substantial proportion of this population went through pregnancy and the early postpartum months with significantly better ways of adapting and coping, especially in the families that were counseled by the technique of anticipatory guidance.

The distinctive nature of this service aspect of the program is that a "normal" group, for the most part not consciously seeking help with psychological problems, was engaged in an experience of taking help. Theoretical and technical problems arising from this circumstance range from those specific to the participants (motivation, "stayability,"[11] involvement) to those specific to the therapist (theoretical orientation, sensitivity to patients' varying areas of "readiness," capacity to adapt skills) (Ripple, 1964).

Further studies of therapeutic intervention in pregnancy management would need to find solutions to these theoretical and technical problems. Possibly the most urgent need in therapeutic intervention studies, consistent with the provocative findings of Truax and Carkhuff (1967), is to structure research to take into account basic differences in personal qualities and theoretical approaches of individual therapists. In any case, the problem of evaluation of psychotherapeutic outcomes still largely eludes a precise quantitative approach.

[1]See Chapter VI, The Dreams of Pregnant Women and Maternal Adaptation.

[2]The appeal of one doctor for women who had enrolled in a health service using multiple doctors reveals the particular anxiety related to pregnancy.

[3]Schedule A, permitting the quantification of life history data, was rated by the project investigators for each woman during the first trimester of pregnancy. See Appendix B for Schedules.

[4]"Interpretation" as used here follows Edward Bibring's (1964, pp. 55-62) definition and refers exclusively to unconscious material. Insight gained through interpretation is dynamically different from that obtained through clarification.

[5]Patients who had completed the project study were invited to participate in small group discussions on pregnancy. These sessions were initiated as an additional method of ascertaining the usefulness of psychotherapeutic intervention during pregnancy. (Reported at Workshop on Psychology of Pregnancy, American Orthopsychiatric Association Conference, San Francisco, 1966.)

[6]Ferreira (1960) points out that the fear of harming the baby corresponds to greater unconscious hostility toward the baby-to-come.

[7]The medical findings in this study point to the value of preparation for the experience of labor and delivery. The counseled women had less fear and concern about childbirth than the control patients. See later section on Comparison of Counseled and Non-Counseled Groups.

[8]This was recognized as an impediment to the research design but dictated by practical necessity.

[9]Appendix B, Schedule A, contains the diagnostic classifications developed for our purposes, and this is discussed briefly in Chapter III, section on Psychological Study of the Woman.

[10]Chapter IV lists the items showing statistically significant changes for the total group from the first to the second trimester.

[11]This term is borrowed from Stieper and Wiener (1965) to differentiate people who remain in therapy from "dropouts;" a significant dropout between three and four sessions was reported as a characteristic problem in therapy.

REFERENCES

Bellak, L. (1952) The Emergency Psychotherapy of Depression. In: *Special Techniques in Psychotherapy*, edited by G. Bychowski and J.L. Despert. New York: Basic Books.

Bibring, E. (1964) Psychoanalysis and the Dynamic Psychotherapies. In: *Psychiatry and Medical Practice in a General Hospital*, edited by N.E. Zinberg. New York: International Universities Press.

Bibring, G.L. (1959) Some Considerations of the Psychological Processes in Pregnancy. *The Psychoanalytic Study of the Child*, Vol. XIV. New York: International Universities Press.

Bibring, G.L., Dwyer, T.F., Huntington, D.S., and Valenstein, A.F. (1961) A Study of the Psychological Processes in Pregnancy and of the Earliest Mother-Child Relationship. In: *The Psychoanalytic Study of the Child*, Vol. XVI. New York: International Universities Press.

Blitzer, J.R., and Murray, J.M. (1964) On the Transformation of Early Narcissism during Pregnancy. *International Journal of Psychoanalysis*, 45:89-97.

Caplan, G. (1957) Psychological Aspects of Maternity Care. *American Journal of Public Health*, 47:25-31.

Caplan, G. (1959) Concepts of Mental Health and Consultation. U.S. Department of Health, Education and Welfare, Children's Bureau. Washington, D.C.: Government Printing Office.

Chertok, L. (1969) *Motherhood and Personality*. Philadelphia: J.P. Lippincott.

Cyr, F.E., and Wattenberg, S.H. (1957) Social Work in a Preventive Program of Maternal and Child Health. *Social Work*, 3:32-39.

Deutsch, H. (1945) *The Psychology of Women: Motherhood*, Vol. II. New York: Grune and Stratton.

Deutsch, H. (1965) *Neuroses and Character Types*. New York: International Universities Press.

Fenichel, O. (1945) *The Psychoanalytic Theory of Neurosis*. New York: W.W. Norton and Co.

Ferreira, A.F. (1960) The Pregnant Woman's Emotional Attitude and Its Reflection on the Newborn. *American Journal of Orthopsychiatry*, 30:553-561.

Gillman, R. (1968) Manifest Dreams of Pregnant Women. *American Journal of Orthopsychiatry*, 38:688-692.

Grimm, E.R. (1961) Psychological Tension in Pregnancy. *Psychosomatic Medicine*, 23:520-527.

Jessner, L. (1964) Pregnancy as a Stress in Marriage. In: *Marriage Counseling in Medical Practice*. Chapel Hill: The University of North Carolina Press.

Knight, R. (ed.) (1954) *Psychoanalytic Psychiatry and Psychology*, Vol. I. New York: International Universities Press.

Liebenberg, B. (1966) First Pregnancy in Retrospect: A Follow-up Using Group Technique. An unpublished paper. Presented at Annual Meeting, American Orthopsychiatric Association.

Mosak, H.H. (1952) Problems in the Definition and Measurement of Success in Psychotherapy. In: *Success in Psychotherapy*, edited by W. Wolff and J.A. Precker. New York: Grune and Stratton.

Murphy, W.F. (1965) *The Tactics of Psychotherapy*. New York: International Universities Press.

Pfeffer, A.Z. (1959) A Procedure for Evaluating the Results of Psychoanalysis. *Journal of the American Psychoanalytic Association*, 7:418-444.

Ripple, L. (1964) Studies in Casework Theory and Practice. *Social Service Monographs*, 2nd Series, School of Social Service Administration, University of Chicago.

Stechler, G., and Geller, H. (1961) Psychological Evaluation of Pregnancy. A Follow-up Comparison. Presented at the American Psychological Association, New York City.

Stieper, D.R., and Wiener, D.N. (1965) *Dimensions of Psychotherapy.* Chicago: Aldine Publishing Co.

Sullivan, H.S. (1954) *The Psychiatric Interview.* New York: W.W. Norton and Co.

Truax, C.B., and Carkhuff, R.R. (1967) *Toward Effective Counseling and Psychotherapy.* Chicago: Aldine Publishing Co.

Zinberg, N.E. (ed.) (1964) *Psychiatry and Medical Practice in a General Hospital.* New York: International Universities Press.

Psychological Aspects of a First Pregnancy and Early Postnatal Adaptation.
Raven Press, New York © 1974

Chapter VIII
Maternal Adaptation

Pauline M. Shereshefsky, Beatrice Liebenberg, and Robert F. Lockman

INTRODUCTION

To be a good mother, a woman must have sense, and that independence of mind which few women possess who are taught to depend entirely on their husbands. Meek wives are, in general, foolish mothers. Unless the understanding of woman be enlarged, and her character rendered more firm, by being allowed to govern her own conduct, she will never have sufficient sense or command of temper to govern her children properly.

> From "A Vindication of the Rights of Woman,"
> by Mary Wollstonecraft (quoted in Flexner, 1972)

In 1792 Mary Wollstonecraft, the author of this first manifesto of women's rights, forcefully stated the relationship between the personality characteristics of the woman and her capacity for good mothering. Nevertheless, even in recent decades, relatively few investigations have approached the study of mother-infant interaction through personality evaluation of the woman prior to the birth of the child.

Studies of early mother-infant interaction have expanded in number, time span covered, and depth of penetration in the past several decades. The early investigations by Levy (1928), the longitudinal Berkeley studies (Bayley, 1968), and the interdisciplinary conferences on infancy sponsored by the Josiah Macy, Jr. Foundation (Senn, 1947) represent initial developments in this study area. Despite these developments it should be kept in mind that: "The idea that infants need a continuous and emotionally satisfying relationship to one person has been explicit in the literature for only a short time. It gained notice as a result of observations of infants in adverse conditions—those affected by the last war in Great Britain and those living in institutions" (Brody, 1956, p. 84).

In this research we undertook to study the personality of the woman partly at least with the purpose of evaluating its relation to the woman's adaptation to maternity, particularly her interaction with the infant in the first six months postpartum. This chapter will focus on the woman's response to her new role as mother; Chapter XI, on mother-infant adaptation.

The woman's postnatal adaptation was evaluated and rated at one, three, and six months, as outlined in Chapter II. The ratings were made by the interdisciplinary team consisting of social worker, infant observer, and pediatrician; the first two members of the team based their judgments on interviews and observations in the home setting, and the pediatrician on interviews, examinations, and observations in the clinic setting. At the end of project participation, the entire research team made an overall evaluation, which included maternal adaptation. The 29 items in the Maternal Adaptation schedule[1] were grouped as follows:

(1) the mother in relation to the infant—mother-infant adaptations;
(2) the woman's adaptation to her new role—her feelings, predominant mood, and sense of adequacy in coping with physical and psychological needs of the infant;
(3) the woman in relation to her husband—more comprehensively, the level of satisfying interaction in the family, with emphasis on the effect of the infant on family homeostasis.

As in the preceding chapters, the statistical findings will be presented as the basis for further discussion.

STATISTICAL FINDINGS REGARDING MATERNAL ADAPTATION

Factors Comprising the Outcome Variable, Maternal Adaptation

As in the analysis of pregnancy adaptation, a set of factors extracted from the individual rated items were used as comprising the outcome variable, Maternal Adaptation. Twelve factor scales derived from ratings at one, three, and six months postnatally comprise the outcome variable, Maternal Adaptation, as follows:

Factor scale no.	Name of factor[2]	Schedule and time period
26	Acceptance of maternal role	E-III, 1 month postnatal
27	Acceptance of infant	E-III, 1 month postnatal
28	Individualization of infant	E-III, 1 month postnatal
29	Reponsiveness to infant (amount and quality of physical contact, sensitivity and responsiveness, amount of stimulation)	E-III, 1 month postnatal
30	Responsiveness to infant (amount and quality of physical contact, degree of expression of affection)	F-III, 3 months postnatal
31	Acceptance of infant	F-III, 3 months postnatal
32	Confidence in maternal role	F-III, 3 months postnatal
33	Acceptance of maternal role	F-III, 3 months postnatal
34	Responsiveness to infant	G-III, 6 months postnatal
35	Acceptance of infant and maternal role	G-III, 6 months postnatal
36	Individualization of infant	G-III, 6 months postnatal
46	Mother-infant adaptation (infant feeding adjustment, infant's functioning—overall rating; mother's adequacy in coping with physical needs of infant; mother's adequacy in coping with emotional needs of infant)	H, 6 months postnatal

Predictors of Maternal Adaptation

Table 1 presents those factors derived from data evaluating the prenatal period that correlated at a statistically significant level with at least five of the twelve maternal adaptation scales, and that are representative of all study periods in which maternal adaptation was rated. The factors that attain this degree of correlation are seen as *predictors* of maternal adaptation.

Of the life history factors—perception of own experience in being mothered, school and peer relationships, and interest in children and experience with them—the one factor that reaches the significance of a predictor of maternal adaptation is interest in children and experience with them. This variable, as indicated earlier,[3] was initially included in our study of the woman's life history because of the findings by Levy (1958) associating childhood attitudes toward babies with maternal behavior.

Of five predictor variables, three are factors which summarize the woman's acceptance of and adjustment to the pregnancy for each trimester.

TABLE 1. *Maternal adaptation factor scales—predictor factors statistically significant correlates (N = 57)*

Prenatal scales			Correlated with maternal adaptation scales	Correlation*
No.	Name			
2	Interest in children (3 months)	Scale 26	Acceptance of maternal role (E-III)	0.37
		30	Responsiveness to infant (F-III)	0.33
		32	Confidence in maternal role (F-III)	0.33
		34	Responsiveness to infant (G-III)	0.34
		35	Acceptance of infant and maternal role (G-III)	0.28
8	Adaptation to pregnancy experience (3 months)	26	Acceptance of maternal role (E-III)	0.27
		33	Acceptance of maternal role (F-III)	0.45
		34	Responsiveness to infant (G-III)	0.40
		35	Acceptance of infant and maternal role (G-III)	0.45
		36	Individualization of infant (G-III)	0.25
11	Adaptation to pregnancy experience (7 months)	27	Acceptance of infant (E-III)	0.39
		32	Confidence in maternal role (F-III)	0.39
		33	Acceptance of maternal role (F-III)	0.44
		34	Responsiveness to infant (G-III)	0.44
		35	Acceptance of infant and maternal role (G-III)	0.65
		36	Individualization of infant (G-III)	0.30
13	Reaction to pregnancy fears (7 months)	28	Individualization of infant (E-III)	0.26
		29	Responsiveness to infant (E-III)	0.25
		32	Confidence in maternal role (F-III)	0.39
		33	Acceptance of maternal role (F-III)	0.30
		35	Acceptance of infant and maternal role (G-III)	0.31
		36	Individualization of infant (G-III)	0.25
16	Overall reaction to pregnancy experience (9 months)	27	Acceptance of infant (E-III)	0.28
		32	Confidence in maternal role (F-III)	0.40
		33	Acceptance of maternal role (F-III)	0.42
		34	Responsiveness to infant (G-III)	0.45
		35	Acceptance of infant and maternal role (G-III)	0.63

*$r = 0.25$ ($p = 0.05$); $r = 0.34$ ($p = 0.01$)

The scales from the first two trimester ratings, called adaptation to pregnancy experience, were comprised of the following items initially rated individually: predominant attitude or mood of the woman; her level of anxiety and fear regarding physical aspects of pregnancy;

the effect of the pregnancy on her feeling of well-being, and a more general item on adaptability to changes precipitated by the pregnancy.

The factor, reaction to pregnancy fears, which was another of the predictor variables, includes four items from the pregnancy experience ratings, three dealing with anxieties and fears specific to pregnancy and one with the mother-daughter relationship during pregnancy. The implication of this factor as a predictor of maternal adaptation is that a supportive mother-daughter relationship during pregnancy tends to be accompanied by little anxiety regarding various aspects of the pregnancy and to eventuate in a good maternal adaptation. This factor has the special significance that it is one of the few points at which statistical evidence clearly indicates the importance of maternal support during pregnancy.

The last of the predictor factors, entitled overall reaction to pregnancy experience, was rated at nine months, just after the birth of the infant. The items that loaded on this factor in a real sense measure overall reaction to the pregnancy: subjective reaction of woman to physical aspects of the pregnancy; medical evaluation of the pregnancy (by the obstetrician); subjective reaction to the emotional experience of the pregnancy; and objective evaluation of total pregnancy experience (physical and emotional), this last representing a consensus evaluation of the obstetrician and the psychiatric team.

Thus a good maternal adaptation in the early period of mothering her first-born child could be predicted for the woman who had had an early interest in children and who adapted well at each stage of the pregnancy, as indicated by: her predominant mood, relatively little anxiety regarding the physical aspects of the pregnancy and delivery or regarding the unborn child, and adaptability to physiological and other changes precipitated by the pregnancy. Since pregnancy adaptation was clearly predictive of maternal adaptation for this group, one of the hypotheses of the study was confirmed.

Feminine Identification and Maternal Behavior and Attitudes

Some of the less inclusive correlations between factor scales derived from the prenatal period and Maternal Adaptation scales lend support to the predictor variables and at the same time add some new dimensions (Table 2), establishing an expected close relationship between maternal adjustments and factors specific to feminine identity. The factors, interest in children, visualization of self as mother, confirmation of sexual identity, and the personality factor, nurturance,

TABLE 2. *Prenatal scales closely associated with maternal adaptation—statistically significant correlates (N = 57)*

Prenatal scales No.	Name		Correlated with		Postnatal schedule	r*
	Full Scale I.Q.	Scale 33	Acceptance of maternal role		F-III (3 months)	0.25
		34	Responsiveness to infant		G-III (6 months)	0.30
		35	Acceptance of infant and maternal role		G-III (6 months)	0.33
1	Perception of own mothering experience (3 months)	Scale 28	Individualization of infant		E-III (1 month)	0.29
3	School and peer relationships (3 months)	Scale 33	Acceptance of maternal role		F-III (3 months)	0.26
4	Ego strength (3 months)	Scale 33	Acceptance of maternal role		F-III (3 months)	0.41
		35	Acceptance of infant and maternal role		G-III (6 months)	0.39
		36	Individualization of infant		G-III (6 months)	0.26
5	Nurturance (3 months)	Scale 26	Acceptance of maternal role		E-III (1 month)	0.30
		34	Responsiveness to infant		G-III (6 months)	0.25
		35	Acceptance of infant and maternal role		G-III (6 months)	0.34
6	Husband's responsiveness to wife (3 months)	Scale 27	Acceptance of infant		E-III (1 month)	0.29
9	Visualization of self as mother (3 months)	Scale 26	Acceptance of maternal role		E-III (1 month)	0.34
		33	Acceptance of maternal role		F-III (3 months)	0.39
		34	Responsiveness to infant		G-III (6 months)	0.31
		35	Acceptance of infant and maternal role		G-III (6 months)	0.34
10	Reaction to characteristic fears of pregnancy (3 months)	Scale 29	Responsiveness to infant		E-III (1 month)	0.26
		36	Individualization of infant		G-III (6 months)	0.32
12	Pregnancy as confirmation of sexual identity (7 months)	Scale 26	Acceptance of maternal role		E-III (1 month)	0.34
		27	Acceptance of infant		E-III (1 month)	0.34
		33	Acceptance of maternal role		F-III (3 months)	0.46
		34	Responsiveness to infant		G-III (6 months)	0.34
14	Visualization of self as mother (7 months)	Scale 29	Responsiveness to infant		E-III (1 month)	0.25
		35	Acceptance of infant and maternal role		G-III (6 months)	0.26
15	Response to project experience (9 months)	Scale 26	Acceptance of maternal role		E-III (1 month)	0.25

*r = 0.25 (p = 0.05); r = 0.34 (p = 0.01)

all correlated significantly with Maternal Adaptation scales of varied time periods. The same interrelationship is indicated in the superfactor, feminine identification (described in Chapter II, Research Design and Methodology), which is especially representative of the woman in her roles as wife and mother.

Postnatal Factors Closely Associated with Maternal Adaptation (Concurrent Ratings)

Marital Adjustment and Maternal Adaptation. The statistical findings show a striking correspondence between postnatal marital adjustment and maternal functioning, as we indicated in reviewing background variables (Chapter III, section on Marital Adaptation). Factors concerned with husband-wife relationship were significantly related to eight to ten of twelve Maternal Adaptation scales at every study period. The superfactor scale entitled husband's responsiveness to the paternal role correlated with the two superfactor scales, maternal responsiveness and woman's self-confidence.

This statistical evidence from factor analysis at varied periods supports conclusions drawn from interviews with the husband and wife and observations in the home. In families in which the husband was responsive to his newborn infant and his wife and helpfully involved with, and accepting of, the new household routines, the mood and self-confidence of the woman and the level of mother-infant interaction were almost invariably good. Mother and infant had distinctly more problems in working out their early relationship on a mutually satisfying basis in families in which the husband did not undertake added functions at this time for his wife or the infant, or was unable to tolerate disruption to established routines, or, in more subtle terms, competed with the infant for nurturant care from his wife, or with his wife in proving his superior capacity in caring for the infant.

Earlier, in reviewing the statistical data regarding Pregnancy Adaptation as an outcome variable, some questions arose about the fact that the measures regarding the marital relationship in the prenatal period did not correlate significantly with pregnancy adaptation. If during pregnancy some tendency on the part of the woman toward excluding the husband was evident, in the postnatal period the women were, on the whole, eager for help, dependent on husbands and others to supplement in practical ways and to advise, reassure, and sustain them psychologically.

Personality Characteristics and Maternal Adaptation. The statistical findings on the personality variables and Maternal Adaptation have also appeared earlier (Chapter III, section on Psychological Study of the Woman). As Table 2 indicates, the variables delineating the personality of the woman as evaluated in the initial *prenatal* study were closely related to Maternal Adaptation.

The personality factors as evaluated *postnatally* show an even greater correspondence to Maternal Adaptation. The nurturance factor which is derived from the six months' restudy of the woman correlated highly with ten of the twelve Maternal Adaptation scales, at 0.01 significance level or better for six scales. The ego strength scale (postnatal score) correlated at the 0.01 significance level with five Maternal Adaptation scales (Chapter III, Table 3, presents these data in detail).

Maternal Behavior and Infant Adaptation. We developed two separate sets of data on the infant, one from the pediatrician's evaluations in clinic visits and the other from the infant observer's tests, observations, and interviews in the home. As indicated earlier, the statistical findings on the mother in relation to the infant are presented in Chapter XI. In the original analyses of items and factors dealing with maternal responsiveness to the infant, no differentiation with regard to the sex of the infant was made. Subsequently, a selective analysis was made of items dealing with maternal responsiveness and infant emotional equilibrium differentiated by the sex of the infant. The report of that study is contained in Chapter XII, Infant Temperament and Sex of Infant: Effects on Maternal Behavior.

Evidence of Maturation as Related to Pregnancy and Maternity

Two facets of the study, not included in the correlations, are suggestive of personality development apparently related to the experiences of pregnancy and early mothering activities. The nurturance factor, as measured at the three months' prenatal period and then at six months postnatally, shows a statistically significant increase ($p = 0.01$) over this one-year period for the total group under study. An item, level of personality integration (defined as "effectiveness of coping, feelings about self, relationships") was rated at one time only, at the six-month postnatal overall evaluation by the entire research team. Ratings on level of personality integration revealed change in both directions: 5 per cent were evaluated as having deteriorated, 39 per cent as having improved, during the year.

The increase in the nurturance factor scores during the year and the sizable group rated as improved in level of personality integration provide some evidence that processes of developmental change are set in motion or accentuated by pregnancy and maternity. It is recognized that many of these young women had only recently married; this fact, and other environmental circumstances, as well as intrapsychic developments, would have to be studied to achieve full understanding of these data. In general, the psychiatric team inclined to the view that only in the perspective of a longer span of time is it likely that developmental changes can be identified and assessed. Certainly it was seen clinically that some women in the sample who maintained contact with the research team over a three- to five-year period appeared to have had a time lag in integrating the impact of the pregnancy and the mothering experience, as well as the effects of counseling.

These findings suggest that childbearing and the early months of mothering an infant have some developmental impact for a substantial proportion of women. It is clear that many of the women, the majority in fact, tend to remain at approximately the same level of personality development (whether high or low or in between). A further sobering consideration, as we know from the follow-up study of postpartum psychiatric disorders, is that a few of the women suffered serious deterioration or disorganization in the next few years after the period of collaboration in the project, as reported in Chapter IX.

THE EARLY PHASE OF MOTHERING A FIRST CHILD

On homecoming with their first-born, some of the women were fully engrossed in, and in harmony with, an intricately interdependent and highly confining existence with the infant. Many adapted to this circumstance easily, some with delight. For many others, the situation was difficult; for a few, it was all but intolerable.

If one were to try to capture with some realism the varying moods and characteristic reactions of the first weeks and months after becoming a mother, one would have to deal with the impact on the women of the need for new concepts of time, a different organization of self, and a changed coordination of routine. Women accustomed to office or classroom routines have first of all to unlearn the virtues of adherence to time schedules and become attuned to a new kind of demand, one that emanates either from the infant or from within the self. Keeping one's self ready for feeding on demand, or awakening from sound sleep to determine the basis for an infant's discomfort (or of one's own discomfort, from too-full breasts), trying to take advantage of the infant's hours of sleep either to gain much-needed rest, meet other obligations, or undertake a cherished outing—all this requires a new organization of one's time and energies, and the women reacted with greatly varying capacity for flexibility and readiness to find satisfaction in their different rhythm.

One relatively unvarying personal circumstance was the fact of persistent pervasive fatigue. Affecting most of the women with a first baby was a certain degree of uncertainty and anxiety about the infant's cues and their meaning. Any tendency towards a depressed state (which did not always occur or was not recognized as such by many of the women) was doubtless exacerbated by fatigue and by the lag in being fully restored in physical strength.

The help that the woman had on homecoming with the infant was important, both in relieving some of her anxieties about her adequacy in caring for the baby and in making it possible for her to have some outside stimulation and freedom of movement when desired. In the first two weeks after coming home from the hospital with the infant, over half of the women had help from their mothers. As to the amount of help the women had during this two-week period, one-third had full-time help, over one-half had half-time help, and approximately 10 per cent had no outside help. Following the first two weeks, only two women had full-time help for a time, one-fourth had half-time help, and nearly three-fourths had no help.

An abridged, taped recording of a group session with women who had completed participation in the project is included in an unpublished paper, entitled, "First Pregnancy in Retrospect: A Follow-up Using Group Technique" (Liebenberg, 1966). There the women speak for themselves in describing initial adjustment to the role of mother and to the infant's demands.

"Almost all of the women indicated that they had not anticipated their fatigue, their disorganization, the physical complications following delivery, and their feeling of inadequacy in the face of the infant's demands and the demands of their husbands. To listen to the taped sessions is painfully moving. A young mother describes her first day home from the hospital almost three years ago:

> "It was really scary because the day I brought him home
> he slept all day and then that night I gave him his bottle
> for the 10 o'clock feeding, he started to cry and he wouldn't

stop crying. I rocked him and I held him. He cried steadily until his 2 o'clock feeding, and I thought that this will surely put him to sleep. He cried all night long until 8:30 the next morning. I thought he was going to die, to have something so small cry for almost nine hours. He turned all kinds of funny colors and was gasping. I could give him a bottle, rock him or anything you could think of....I didn't want to call him (the pediatrician) in the middle of the night. I don't know—I was embarrassed because I was so stupid that I couldn't take care of it myself. My husband sleeps like a rock and the next morning when he got up he said, 'Gee, that baby is amazing, he slept right through the night.' I said, 'Yes, he is, yes he is'...I could hardly move I was so exhausted."

And at a later point in the session when the women discuss help, she says, "I had to do it all myself. I don't have any sisters and no grandmothers and no anybody."

"With the realization that other women have forbidden negative feelings, the women become less guarded. Thus in discussing the resentment one can feel towards the infant, Yetta says:

I don't think I was prepared at all because you read in books and you talk with people and you think that all of a sudden there is going to be this motherly surge of love which is not true. In my case it wasn't. I had this colicky baby that spit up and we had to stay home. It took me a long time....I don't think motherly love is automatic as a lot of times you are led to believe. I think you should be prepared for this because you think you're unusual. There is a lot of guilt.

"Another mother joins in:

How can someone prepare you for this feeling? You're going to have a baby and everyone knows that a parent loves a child. It's something that all of a sudden they wake you up out of this sleep, shove this thing....I was so tired ....I didn't even want to touch him. I just wanted to sleep. They were shaking me and telling me that I have to give this baby a bottle. Now how much love can you have at that particular moment when I ache from my head to my toe and wanted to sleep....

"In another group Susan echoes the same feeling:

I guess it was after maybe the first two or three weeks and the baby would get up in the middle of the night, rattle the crib and I would try to satisfy her, nurse her, burp her, she'd be washed and cleaned and she still kept on crying and couldn't get back to sleep. I got to the point where I thought I would slam her against the wall. Oh, and then I started thinking what's happening to me? What am I doing? There's something wrong. I need help. It doesn't happen at nearly the same intensity any more but still occasionally there are times when there doesn't seem to be anything wrong—that's when it gets the worst and I still want to throw her....

"Kitty:

The first few nights at home, especially since I was breast-feeding and I cound never tell my husband, 'Go get her,' I started resenting him because he was able to sleep. If you want an honest answer here is the whole story. I resented my husband because he was able to sleep; I hated the baby because she was not a child who could do with just one feeding; until she was several months old she had the 10 o'clock and the 2 o'clock and sometimes the 4 o'clock. So I resented the baby for being so darn big and hungry and I would get one big mood of depression and warn my husband in advance, 'If I suddenly burst into tears, just ignore me,' I did, once....

"Sylvia:

When I was in the hospital I guess I felt like a mother but it was just like playing house and the least little thing she did, I said, 'Gee, what an exceptional baby!' and it was just so much fun there. But the first couple of weeks I was home I don't think I felt like a mother. I didn't feel much like anything for the first month. I was just tired and I was just glad to see that baby sleep. (There is much sympathetic laughter and mingling of voices.) I think when the baby started to be more or less on her own, and now that she calls me 'Mommy,' then it makes me feel like a mother.

Approximately one-third (30 per cent) of the women experienced difficulty beyond those characteristic of the transitional period of adjustment for all the group, some of the difficulty different only in degree and some in kind. Despite much denial, several women gave evidence of resentment of the demands of the infant, anxiety regarding the totality of his dependency, or insensitivity to his needs. The insensitivity took the form of overreaction to real problems, such as exaggerated concern over feeding adjustments, spitting up, or bowel movements. The occasional more serious problem was one of underreaction, such as ignoring signs of hunger or illness, and especially symptoms that might be particularly hard to face—hyperactivity, for example.

In one instance involving illness of the infant, necessitating his hospitalization for a time, a rather obvious withdrawal of emotional investment on the part of the mother took place, apparently out of her need to defend herself against the contingency of total loss. It was not clear, by the end of her participation in the project, whether the initial degree of involvement had been re-established.

It may be relevant to refer to incidents that were possibly predictive of future problems in the individual case, though not representative of the whole sample. An occasional instance of hostile, even punitive action was reported in this sample, such as episodes of slapping the baby, walking out of the house because he was screaming and leaving him alone for an unspecified period of time; and, in one instance, literally throwing the child back and forth between two immature quarreling parents. Discovering punitive action toward infants under six months of age in this relatively favored, knowledgeable group of families is important in terms of social planning. Clearly such developments are by no means limited to one segment of the population; practical help for the new mother and legislation for the protection of young children need to be directed to the community as a whole.

SUMMARY

1. The pregnancy adaptation was found to be predictive of maternal adaptation. Of five factors derived from the prenatal period that were identified as predictors, four are factors summarizing the woman's level of adaptation to the pregnancy.

2. The early history of the woman as expressed in her interest in children and experience with them was also found to be predictive of maternal adaptation. This variable is probably closely related, in terms of meaningfulness for the purpose of this study, to other variables—notably visualization of self as mother and nurturance —which, in correlating significantly with Maternal Adaptation scales, emphasize the close relationship between the woman's clarity about her feminine identity and her satisfaction and competence in mothering a young infant.

3. In the current, postnatal circumstance, the most significant single aspect or grouping of factors that correlated with Maternal Adaptation scales of each study period was the husband-wife adaptation as evaluated in the postnatal period. The nature of the woman's accommodation to the infant and her acceptance of the maternal role was found highly interrelated with the quality of the relationship with her husband.

4. The personality factor, nurturance, as measured at the postnatal rating period, also correlated significantly with almost all of the scales measuring maternal adaptation as an outcome variable. At a somewhat less inclusive level, the factor scale, ego strength, as measured at the six-month period also, is found to be highly correlated with maternal adaptation as an outcome variable.

5. The rating on the single item, level of personality integration, evaluated at the end of the year's collaboration, indicated that a substantial proportion of the women (two-fifths) were evaluated as having achieved a somewhat improved level of integration. A small proportion (5 per cent) were found to have a lowered level of integration at this point. The finding that a substantial proportion achieved an improved level of personality integration, when taken in conjunction with the statistically significant increase of the nurturance factor between the pre- and postnatal periods, suggests that the experience of a first pregnancy and of the first months of mothering an infant may accentuate developmental changes for a substantial proportion of women.

These findings emphasize attitudes of acceptance and adaptability to the pregnancy as predictive of the woman's maternal adaptation, indicate the relationship between her clarity as to feminine identity and her mothering capacities, recognize the husband's role (confidence-building, sustaining) as highly correlated with the woman's maternal functioning, and view the woman's personality characteristics (ego strength, including self-confidence, and her nurturant qualities) as basically determinative of her capacities as a mother.

In the sample, approximately one-third of the women were found to have special difficulty in the early period of undertaking maternal care of their first-born infant. The difficulty was exhibited in such varied ways as: intense, sometimes disruptive, anxiety about the care of the infant or about adequacy in the mothering role; overreaction to realistic problems (notably feeding adjustment); depressed states for varying periods of time; and hostile, punitive attitudes toward the infant.

The problem that presents itself, especially in view of similarity of the findings to those of studies[4] of different populations and even different socio-economic and cultural strata, is to find ways of converting poor mothering attitudes and methods to good ones, so that a child of an unhappy marriage and a not-very-nurturant mother is given opportunity for a more nearly equal start in life with children born into better psychological circumstances.

[1]The Schedule, Maternal Adaptation (E-III at one month and F-III and G-III at three and six months) is contained in the set of Schedules, Appendix B. The compendium of factor scales, Appendix C, indicates the items that were grouped together for each scale.

[2]While the items that were found to group together at each rating period differed somewhat, the factors were given the same title at separate periods because the nature of the factor was determined by the higher loadings within each grouping. Specific items have been listed under a few factors above to suggest the nature of the groupings.

[3]Chapter I, Premises and Assumptions.

[4]See especially Fearing, 1966; Goshen-Gottstein, 1966; Gordon, 1967; Heinstein, 1967; Larsen, 1967; and Wenner and Cohen, 1968.

REFERENCES

Bayley, N. (1968) Behavioral Correlates of Mental Growth: Birth to Thirty-six Years. *American Psychologist,* 23:1-17.

Brody, S. (1956) *Patterns of Mothering.* New York: International Universities Press.

Fearing, J.M. (1966) Anxiety: How, Not Why. *Medical Opinion and Review,* 2.

Flexner, E. (1972) *Mary Wollstonecraft*. New York: Coward, McCann and Geoghegan, p. 153.

Gordon, R.E., and Gordon, K.K. (1967) Factors in Postpartum Emotional Adjustment. Presented at the American Orthopsychiatric Association Annual Meeting.

Goshen-Gottstein, E.R. (1966) Marriage and First Pregnancy: Cultural Influences on Attitudes of Israeli Women. *Mind and Medicine Monographs*. Philadelphia: J.B. Lippincott.

Heinstein, M.I. (1967) Expressed Attitudes and Feelings of Pregnant Women and Their Relations to Physical Complications of Pregnancy. *Merrill-Palmer Quarterly of Behavior and Development*, 13:217-236.

Larsen, V.L., Evans, T., and Martin, L. (1967) Differences Between New Mothers: Psychiatric Admissions vs. Normals. *Journal of the American Medical Women's Association*, 22:995-998.

Levy, D.M. (1958) *Behavioral Analysis*. Springfield, Ill.: Charles C. Thomas.

Levy, D.M. (1928) Fingersucking and Accessory Movements in Early Infancy: An Etiological Study. *American Journal of Psychology*, 7:881-918.

Liebenberg, B. (1966) First Pregnancy in Retrospect: A Follow-Up Using Group Technique. Presented at the Annual Conference of the American Orthopsychiatric Association in San Francisco (unpublished).

Senn, J.M.E. (ed.) (1947) Problems of Early Infancy. Transactions of the First (1947) Conference. New York: Josiah Macy, Jr. Foundation.

Wenner, N.K., and Cohen, M.B. (eds.) (1968) Emotional Aspects of Pregnancy. Final Report of Washington School of Psychiatry Project, Washington, D.C.

Psychological Aspects of a First Pregnancy
and Early Postnatal Adaptation.
Raven Press, New York © 1974

Chapter IX
Seven Women: A Prospective Study
of Postpartum Psychiatric Disorders*

Walter A. Brown and Pauline M. Shereshefsky

INTRODUCTION

Mental disturbances in women occurring soon after childbirth have been noted and described since the Fourth Century B. C. (Hamilton, 1962). Data from recent studies utilizing adequate controls suggest that women have an increased vulnerability to psychological decompensation in the first three postpartum months and particularly in the early postpartum weeks (Pugh et al., 1963; Melges, 1968; Reich and Winokur, 1970). This requires an explanation. Hippocrates speculated that suppressed lochial discharge could be carried toward the head "and result in agitation, delirium, and attacks of mania" (Hamilton, 1962, p. 126). Today, we are not much closer to understanding the interaction between experience, physiology, and psychopathology in the postpartum period.

The conceptual framework into which the postpartum disorders have been placed has varied over the centuries with the changing emphases and theories in psychiatry. The early notion of postpartum disorders

*This article is reproduced with slight adaptation from *Psychiatry,* Vol. 35, May 1972, pp. 139-159, with permission of the Editor. Copyright is held by the William Alanson White Psychiatric Foundation.

Mr. David Heppel helped evaluate and present the quantitative data and Mrs. Linda Brown provided editorial assistance. Beatrice Liebenberg, ACSW, E. James Lieberman, M.D., Harold Plotsky, M.D., and Sara Saltzman, M.A., read and commented on the manuscript. Leon Yarrow, Ph.D., contributed thoughtful suggestions during every phase of this endeavor, and Mrs. Joanne Mechler provided technical assistance.

as unique syndromes with specific organic etiologies gave way in the late 19th and 20th Centuries to the notion that these disorders are phenomenologically identical to the standard psychiatric diseases. The most recent diagnostic and statistical manual of the American Psychiatric Association reflects the conceptual ambiguity surrounding postpartum psychiatric disorders today. It lists "psychosis with childbirth" under the organic syndromes, with an appended note stating that this diagnosis should be used only if no other diagnostic categories are appropriate. The prevalent thinking in this country seems to be that the psychiatric syndromes which occur in the postpartum period do not differ phenomenologically from those occurring at other time periods and that childbirth, if it plays any etiological role at all, functions as a nonspecific stress. Critical evaluation of the recent and past literature indicates that this prevailing belief is not grounded in clinical investigation. Important questions remain unanswered:

1. Are there one or more unique psychiatric syndromes for which childbirth is a necessary precipitant? Careful scrutiny of studies which utilize broad nosological categories and a recent study which includes patient observation suggest that it is often difficult to place the postpartum patient in one of the standard nosological categories (Strecker and Ebaugh, 1926; Hamilton, 1962; Melges, 1968; Reich and Winokur, 1970). Emotional lability and mild confusion have been found as frequent symptoms regardless of diagnosis (Hamilton, 1962; Melges, 1968).

2. What is the nature of the relationship between parturition and a contiguous psychiatric disorder? The psychological impact of the rapid hormonal changes during the puerperium is unclear. Equally unclear in the genesis of these disorders are the roles of labor, delivery, and awareness of motherhood, as specific or nonspecific psychological stresses.

3. Can the woman who is prone to a severe postpartum disturbance be identified during pregnancy? There have been no prospective studies utilizing psychological or physiological variables. Prospective data on the "postpartum" patient have been limited to the demographic and medical information available from obstetrical records after a woman has developed a psychiatric disorder. These patients when compared to normal postpartum controls have been found to have shorter gestation, greater age, and a longer interval between the last two pregnancies (Paffenbarger, 1961). The woman with one postpartum hospitalization has a greatly increased probability of having another, and there is a suggestion that "postpartum blues" may presage a more severe disorder in a subsequent postpartum period (Paffenbarger,

1961; Melges, 1968). Retrospective data regarding premorbid history and personality have been inconclusive. An overly close mother-daughter relationship has been described (Markham, 1961; Daniels and Lessow, 1964), and the non-supportive husband, chronic frigidity, and a schizoid personality have been considered predictive (Zilboorg, 1928, 1957; Boyd, 1942; Daniels and Lessow, 1964; Kaplan and Blackman, 1969).

Some of the ambiguity in this area can be attributed to the great variety of psychiatric syndromes, precipitating circumstances, and times of onset which previous investigators have included under the rubric "postpartum." In some studies, women who are hospitalized for a psychiatric condition either during or following pregnancy are included in the "postpartum" sample (Martin, 1958; Paffenbarger, 1961; Pugh et al., 1963; Kaplan and Blackman, 1969). Other investigators include only those women who are hospitalized or have the onset of illness within a specified postpartum period such as two, three, or six months (Madden et al., 1958; Thomas and Gordon, 1959; Seager, 1960; Daniels and Lessow, 1964; Reich and Winokur, 1970). Broad diagnostic labels have been utilized without specifying the criteria for inclusion in each category (Strecker and Ebaugh, 1926; Madden et al., 1958; Paffenbarger, 1961). Some of the widely quoted studies employ the diagnoses from mental hospital records as the sole source of psychiatric information (Fondeur et al., 1957; Paffenbarger, 1961). Conclusions about phenomenology, prognosis, and pre-morbid status have been derived from studies which compare hospitalized postpartum patients with other hospitalized patients, without further differentiation within each group (Tetlow, 1955; Fondeur et al., 1957; Seager, 1960).

It is difficult to generate knowledge about prediction, etiology, and phenomenology without stringent, meaningful criteria for defining postpartum disorder and for differentiating one postpartum disorder from another. This study is addressed to the issue of developing these criteria.

In the study population of this research, seven of the women developed severe psychiatric disorders within the six months following their first or second pregnancy. Three of them were hospitalized. The psychiatric disorders of these women represent the broad spectrum of mental disturbances which have been described in the postpartum period.

The fact that each of these women was sufficiently disturbed to warrant psychiatric attention within six months of childbirth would have justified their inclusion in several previous investigations of postpartum disorders, and there is no question that the three hospitalized women met the usual criteria for inclusion in a postpartum sample. The data on each woman were sufficiently comprehensive to provide a basis for evaluating the significance of parturition in the development of her symptoms.

Through this evaluation we attempt to distinguish the postpartum disorder which is critically related to parturition from that which is incidental to it, and to identify the variables—prenatal, perinatal and postnatal—which are important to the development of symptoms in each situation.

METHODS

We defined postpartum psychiatric disorder as any psychiatric disturbance occurring up to six months postpartum for which a woman sought or was referred for psychiatric treatment. Three women were referred for psychiatric treatment following their first pregnancy. One was hospitalized. During the six years following the initial study, four additional women were referred for psychiatric treatment after second pregnancies. Two of these women were hospitalized. As far as we can determine from Group Health Association records and informal contact with the research subjects over the years, none of the others have been identified or have identified themselves as having a mental disturbance in the postpartum period requiring intervention.

Prospective data on the seven "postpartum" subjects were obtained from the research files of the project on prenatal and early postnatal adaptation. Included in this material were the comprehensive case studies by psychiatrists and social workers, reports of psychological testing, obstetrical records, and the item and factor scores used in the project data analysis. Psychiatric hospital records and case records were obtained for each woman. In addition, the psychiatrists who treated the women were personally contacted for information regarding the subject's precipitating circumstances, symptomatic picture, and subsequent course. In the spring of 1970 the authors saw each of the four women who had suffered a severe psychiatric disorder conjointly for a one-hour open-ended interview focused on detailed recollection of the psychiatric episode and present adjustment.

Chapter II on Research Design and Methodology reported that factor analysis using the principal components method with varimax rotation reduced the data on the final project sample to 46 prenatal and postnatal factors (Tables 1 and 2). All but one of the postpartum subjects were included in the final data analysis by the project staff.

Initial inspection of these data indicated wide variance within the postpartum group. For this reason and because we were interested

TABLE 1. *Prenatal factors*

Factor	Time measured (months)
Perception of experience being mothered	3
Interest in children	3
School and peer relationships	3
Husband's responsiveness to wife	3
Husband's responsiveness to pregnancy	3
Ego strength	3
Nurturance	3
Visualization of self as mother	3 and 7
Adaptation to pregnancy experience	3 and 7
Reaction to pregnancy fears*	3 and 7
Confirmation of sexual identity*	7
Response to project experiences*	9
Overall reaction to pregnancy experiences*	9

*These factors did not differentiate any of our subjects from the large group and were excluded from the final analysis.

TABLE 2. *Postnatal factors**

Factor	Time measured (months)
Acceptance of maternal role	1 and 3
Acceptance of infant	1 and 3
Responsiveness to infant	1, 3, and 6
Acceptance of infant and maternal role	6
Mother-infant adaptation	6
Family adaptation	6
Husband-wife adaptation	1, 3, and 6
Reaction to paternal role	1, 3, and 6
Ego strength	6
Nurturance	6
Confidence in maternal role	3
Individualization of infant	1 and 6
Infant adjustment	1, 3, and 6
Infant alertness	1, 3, and 6
Infant functioning	1, 3, and 6

*Because of the consistency of our subjects between 1- and 3-month scores, the 3-month scores were not utilized in the final comparisons. Husband-father factor scores showed consistency over time, and final comparisons included just the 6-month scores. "Individualization of infant" was not included in the final analysis.

in investigating the relationship between each postpartum psychiatric syndrome and the premorbid data, we decided to compare each postpartum subject with the total group of 57 subjects rather than the entire group of postpartum subjects with the larger group. In order to do this, we standardized the scores for the 46 prenatal and postnatal factors, using as the standardization group the total group of 57. Further comparisons between each "postpartum" woman and the total group were made for the number of prenatal stresses (specified external events, such as illness or death in the family), number of physical complaints during pregnancy, length of labor, and infant weight.

RESULTS

Based on the personality and adaptation data gathered during the prenatal period, each of the seven women seemed to fall into one of three premorbid categories: (1) well adapted and functioning well, (2) considerable neurotic symptomatology and character problems but functioning adequately, (3) severe long-standing characterological problems with recurrent disruptive anxiety or dysfunctional behavior. For clarity of presentation the case material and quantitative data will be presented in three sections corresponding to the three premorbid groupings.

The Healthy Woman Decompensates

Case 1—Mrs. Smith, age 21, an attractive, vivacious young woman, seemed delighted to be having a baby. Observers noted her contentment with marriage and the pregnancy and concluded that she had a tendency toward the development of psychosomatic symptoms but was generally a "healthy, positive, and forward-looking young lady."

Throughout her pregnancy Mrs. Smith demonstrated her strong attachment to her mother, whom she saw several times weekly. When Mrs. Smith was 15 years old, her mother's sixth child had been born, an infant with multiple congenital defects who died within three years. Mrs. Smith had been that child's godmother. Although she never expressed explicit concern over having a deformed infant herself, she spoke often during her pregnancy about the birth of her deformed sister and on several occasions about other tragedies involving young children.

Mrs. Smith experienced little physical discomfort during her pregnancy and had an uncomplicated labor and delivery. The project social worker who visited her 48 hours after delivery noted that she expressed pleasure in her infant and seemed at ease. One week later, after being home for several days, Mrs. Smith called the obstetrics department and was noted to be in "an upset state." Her obstetrician saw her the next week (two weeks postpartum) and reported that she seemed to be in the midst of a psychotic reaction marked by excessive activity and talking. This impression was confirmed by a social worker and a psychiatrist who saw her during the ensuing week. They noted her disorganized speech, hyperactivity, and bizarre behavior. She was diagnosed as having a schizophrenic reaction, and was given chlorpromazine. Two weeks later her condition had worsened. At eight weeks postpartum she was admitted to the psychiatric service of a general hospital. Her agitated, at times violent behavior did not respond to chlorpromazine and she was given electroshock therapy to control her agitation. Within two weeks her disorganization and agitation had cleared considerably and she was discharged. Over the following week she became increasingly erratic and irrational and was rehospitalized for three and a half weeks during which she received a second course of electroshock therapy.

At six months postpartum Mrs. Smith was reevaluated by the project staff. Particularly noticeable were her good-humored remarks to the effect that at times she wasn't sure whether she or her mother was the mother of the baby. The project psychiatrist felt that her thought processes were perhaps somewhat slow but that her thinking was organized, and there was no gross evidence of psychosis. Projective tests showed no evidence of psychotic disorder.

Mrs. Smith continued in outpatient supportive therapy and remained on a low dose of chlorpromazine. One year after her first delivery she gave birth to a second son. Pregnancy, labor, and delivery went smoothly, as did her postpartum course. Nine months after the birth of the second son she relapsed in a setting of several upsetting events— including a visit from her father-in-law, the illness of her two children, and a fall in which she sustained a concussion. She was rehospitalized for six weeks in an agitated, labile, paranoid state, and she was treated with electroshock therapy and chlorpromazine. Since then she has been feeling well and functioning effectively as a mother, homemaker, and wife. In April of 1968 she gave birth to a third boy without complication.

At the time of our interview, Mrs. Smith's youngest child was 14 months old. There was no evidence of disturbance in her mood, behavior, or thinking. She was seeing her psychiatrist about every six weeks for evaluation and was on 50 mg of chlorpromazine. In reviewing her psychiatric episodes four and six years previously, she stated that her "mind just snapped." She spoke in an amused way of some of the uncharacteristic things she had done, such as throwing a glass at her mother and not recognizing people. She reported that things have been going well for the past few years. Her marital adjustment continues to be unusually good, and she is involved and satisfied with her role as homemaker.

Case 2—In the third month of her first pregnancy, Mrs. Allen was an attractive, bouncy, gregarious young woman. Psychiatric and social work interviews throughout her pregnancy lent weight to the initial impression of "normality." She had a lively, diverse social life, was deeply involved with her husband of two years, and was delighted that she was pregnant. Labor and delivery were uncomplicated and at six months postpartum she seemed delighted with her infant and was adapting well to her change in routine.

Mrs. Allen became pregnant for the second time when her first child was one and a half. She was overdue this time, labor was induced, and she remembers it in contrast to the previous labor as being "very painful." She gave birth to a girl who had multiple congenital anomalies including heart defects unamenable to surgery, and abnormalities of the hands and face. The infant required specialized care, was institutionalized, and died within three months.

The night that Mrs. Allen returned from the hospital the Allens received a phone call informing them that Mr. Allen's father had died suddenly of a heart attack. Two days later Mrs. Allen's mother, who had come to help out, started hearing voices and behaving in a bizarre manner. Within days she made a suicide attempt, and Mrs. Allen had to drag her, naked and unconscious, from the bath tub. Over the ensuing week Mrs. Allen became restless and agitated and was unable to sleep or eat. Her thoughts began to race, she developed pressured speech, and was unable to remember what she had just done or said. Particularly upsetting were uncontrollable persistent thoughts about her husband's premarital sexual activites. She remembers feeling that what was happening to her was "paralleling" what had happened to her mother and that she didn't want it to continue. Six days after her mother's breakdown, she found herself unable to prepare a meal and called one of the project social workers. The psychiatrist who saw her the next day felt that she was having an acute dissociative reaction with marked elements of depression. She was hospitalized immediately and treated with phenothiazines and psychotherapy. Her symptoms began to abate within a week and she was discharged after a 17-day stay with a hospital diagnosis of "psychoneurotic depressive reaction."

Mrs. Allen was in outpatient treatment for several months following discharge. During this time she readjusted to her home situation and was able to cope with child and husband. Six months later she sought psychiatric consultation for feelings of anxiety and depression. It was recommended that Mrs. Allen go into therapy, and she and her husband were in family therapy for six months.

The authors interviewed Mrs. Allen four and a half years after her initial contact with the pregnancy project and one year after her psychiatric hospitalization. She spoke happily about her son and was tentatively planning a pregnancy for some time in the next year. There were only glimmers of her old verve and enthusiasm.

Comparisons with the Total Sample

Standard scores for Mrs. Smith and Mrs. Allen on the prenatal personality and adaptation factors are shown in Fig. 1. It is immediately apparent that those scores which deviated more than one standard deviation from the group mean were for the most part in the direction of unusually good health or adjustment.

Seven external events were designated as prenatal stresses.[1] The average number of "stresses" for all project participants was 1.4 with a range of 0.4. Mrs. Allen had one "stress" and Mrs. Smith had

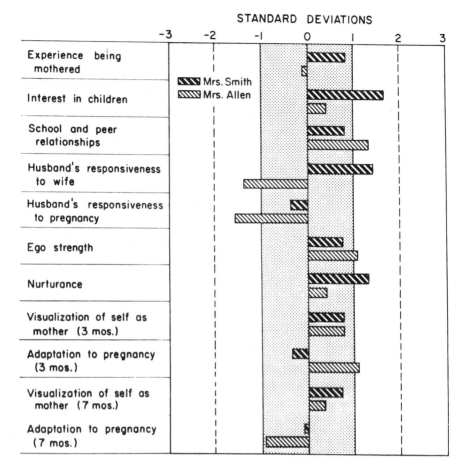

FIG. 1. Standard scores on prenatal factors (first pregnancy) for Mrs. Smith and Mrs. Allen.

none. Both of these women, in addition, reported less than the average number of physical complaints to their obstetricians. They were rated as having minimal anxiety during labor, and like the majority of the women, they were considered to have normal reactions to pain. Mrs. Allen's mood state in the hospital was characterized as euphoric, Mrs. Smith's as contented.

The maternal adaptation factor scores for Mrs. Smith and Mrs. Allen are shown in Fig. 2. Not surprisingly, Mrs. Smith's scores were extremely low for the first month (psychotic episode), but by the sixth postpartum month her maternal adaptation was close to the group mean. Neither infant was unusual in his overall adjustment or functioning during the first six months.

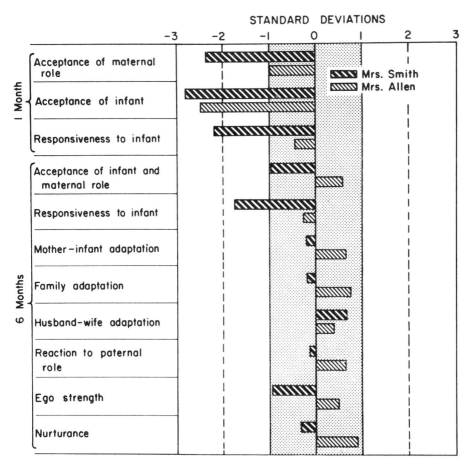

FIG. 2. Standard scores on postnatal factors (first pregnancy) for Mrs. Smith and Mrs. Allen.

Comment

The panic and personality disorganization which both of these women experienced within days of childbirth suggest the temporary psychological disintegration which occurs in some healthy individuals faced with an overwhelming threat. Mrs. Allen was faced with a series of external stresses associated with childbirth which might well have produced some degree of strain in most people. Mrs. Smith developed her symptoms in the context of an objectively unremarkable labor, delivery, and early puerperium. Her history of a congenitally deformed sibling seems worthy of note, particularly in view of the extremely close mother-daughter relationship and the gross identity diffusion which Mrs. Smith experienced postpartum. These data suggest that childbirth had idiosyncratic associations for this woman which made the inner reality of childbirth unusually threatening. The fact that Mrs. Smith did not have recurrences with two subsequent pregnancies is subject to a variety of interpretations. Possibly the experience of bearing a normal child neutralized the threat of congenital deformity.

The role of physiological changes of the early puerperium in the development of these disturbances cannot be determined from our data. The ego vulnerability common in the early puerperium is probably related in part to the direct effects of multisystem physiological changes on brain functioning (Yalom et al., 1968). We can hypothesize that the psychological defensive capacity of these women was limited by these baseline changes, and that the affective lability common in the early puerperium colored their symptomatology.

The Neurotic Faces Motherhood

Case 3—In the third month of her first pregnancy Mrs. Forbes, age 21, was seen by the project staff as an immature, passive young woman suffering from a strong sense of guilt. She was found to be inhibited, guarded, and given to occasional impulsive outbursts. Both Mrs. Forbes and her husband made frequent references to the fact that prior to marriage she had been subject to periods of moodiness and depression.

Mrs. Forbes' early childhood was marred by frequent parental dissension and her father's alcoholism. At age 12 her father had a stroke when she was alone with him. Some months later he died, and Mrs. Forbes felt guilty for having failed to go to the hospital the night before her father's death. Mrs. Forbes' relationship with her mother was consistently unhappy and guilt-ridden. She saw her mother as manipulative, intrusive, and oppressively vigilant to slights and rejections, and she experienced considerable guilt over the fact that she had little affection for her. Mrs. Forbes also expressed guilt over the fact that she and her husband had had premarital sex relations, and she spoke often of her fears of death and of dying while still in a state of sin.

Throughout her pregnancy Mrs. Forbes complained of

nausea and of constipation which had been a lifelong problem for her. Labor was induced two and a half weeks beyond her due date but the birth of her son was otherwise uncomplicated. The social worker who visited Mrs. Forbes in the hospital noted that she seemed concerned about her physical well-being, as she had been during her pregnancy, but the social worker did not notice any disturbance in mood or behavior.

At one month postpartum Mrs. Forbes reported to the social worker that she had been depressed during the last day in the hospital and the first two weeks at home. She said that she had cried quite a bit and although very tired, had been unable to unwind and get to sleep. She remembered wanting to leave home and go off by herself and being inundated with remorse for having such thoughts.

At six months postpartum Mrs. Forbes reported that she had been depressed for the first three months, crying frequently during this period and having recurrent suicidal thoughts. At times she had been about ready to commit herself. The project psychiatrist felt that by the sixth postpartum month she had come out of her depression but was still vulnerable.

Mrs. Forbes was most anxious to avoid having similar postpartum difficulties following her next pregnancy. Two years after the birth of her first child she started planning for the second and undertook to do everything differently this time. The Forbeses moved into a large apartment and decided that they would have help when the baby came. Pregnancy, labor, and delivery were uncomplicated, and she was happy to have a girl. Mrs. Forbes felt that her second depressive episode came on in the same manner as the first. Immediately after the birth of each child she was fine. Then on the fourth day the depression came on suddenly and severely—"like a black cloud," "a sinking sensation." Mrs. Forbes wanted to go home but feared that she would be unable to cope. Upon returning home from the hospital she felt like escaping and was preoccupied with feelings of guilt. She had difficulty sleeping, poor appetite, and extremely bothersome headaches. Mrs. Forbes felt that the second episode was more severe than the first. "It felt more like a trap." This time Mrs. Forbes sought help. She first consulted her obstetrician, who felt that she was having a depressive reaction with anxiety and prescribed a tranquilizer. This was not helpful and at five weeks postpartum she sought psychiatric help. She reported her numerous somatic complaints to the psychiatrist, spoke of her persistent thoughts of death and auto accidents, and at one point begged to be put in a hospital. Many of Mrs. Forbes' symptoms cleared on a regimen of mild tranquilizer and twice-weekly psychotherapy. After two months of treatment she was essentially asymptomatic and therapy was discontinued.

Mrs. Forbes has not required any psychiatric treatment during the past four years. She is somewhat more nervous now than she was before her first pregnancy, tends to become "depressed" from time to time, and still has periods during which she is preoccupied with thoughts of death.

Although Mrs. Forbes dislikes "being on the pill for the next 25 years," she finds this choice clearly preferable to that of risking another period of postpartum depression. These episodes were "the worst things that had ever happened" to her. She states that she is happy with her current situation but that the two depressions "left scars."

Case 4—At the time of her first pregnancy Mrs. Gordon was 28 years old and had been married one year. During the initial months of prenatal evaluation she demonstrated an unusual amount of concern over her physical well-being but in general seemed to be a fairly competent woman. With further evaluation during her pregnancy and early postpartum months, her neurotic character style, dysfunctional marriage, and marked tendency to somatization became quite apparent.

Mrs. Gordon complained of constipation and evening nausea throughout her pregnancy. She went ten days past her due date, became quite anxious, and labor was electively induced. She complained bitterly about her hospital experience, cried throughout her hospital stay, and expressed much concern about the baby's size and the problems of breast-feeding.

At one month postpartum Mrs. Gordon was obviously having more than the usual degree of difficulty adjusting to her new role. She reported a good deal of physical discomfort, was irritable, and cried easily. Her resentment of the infant and anger at its demands were clear. The social worker concluded that "the childbirth experience seems thus far to have accentuated Mrs. Gordon's infantilism, dependency and preoccupation with her physical self." Neither Mr. nor Mrs. Gordon found the experience of parenthood pleasurable or in any way gratifying.

At six months postpartum the project psychologist saw Mrs. Gordon as a repressed, constricted, compulsive woman who was immature and "very much identified with and tied to her baby." By this time she was handling the infant and household in a competent manner but was still resentful of the baby's demands and anxious to escape from her.

A year and a half after the birth of her first child Mrs. Gordon became pregnant for the second time. She felt well during this pregnancy and again labor was induced (for convenience) but was otherwise uncomplicated. During the early postpartum months she had a number of situational problems. The Gordons had just moved into a new house, a recently hired maid was not working out well, and the infant had persistent projectile vomiting. Mrs. Gordon remembers becoming "depressed" and losing ten pounds during the first three postpartum months. Toward the end of this period, just as these situational problems were resolving, Mrs. Gordon "got worse." She felt driven to engage in numerous social activites, keeping her calendar full night and day. "I was sort of running—I felt safer that way." At about this time she also had an exacerbation of a chronic ear infection, was plagued with dizziness, and developed a urinary tract infection. Her internist suggested that she consider the possibility of psychiatric help. After spending a week of lying in bed doing nothing and feeling that she was not living, Mrs. Gordon began to see a psychiatrist. She was noted to be overactive and agitated. After three months Mrs. Gordon discontinued therapy. During the ensuing two-month period she made increasing demands on her husband and friends for attention and care. Her husband gradually assumed more of the household responsibilities. At the urging of husband and friends she sought psychiatric care again, and, in an agitated state, she was admitted to a private psychiatric hospital. At this time she was quite

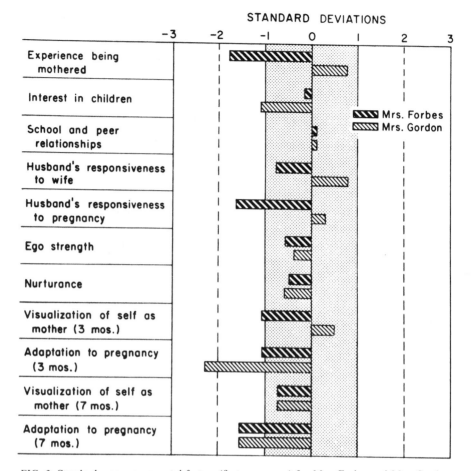

FIG. 3. Standard scores on prenatal factors (first pregnancy) for Mrs. Forbes and Mrs. Gordon.

anxious. Her behavior was described as clinging and demanding, and her speech was rapid and digressive but without a truly dissociative quality. Mrs. Gordon's diagnosis was borderline personality. She had group therapy and upon her discharge continued in individual therapy and in couples therapy with her husband.

We interviewed Mrs. Gordon one year after her psychiatric hospitalization. She said that she was finding out about herself in therapy, particularly about her guilt in regard to her lack of maternal feelings, and that she and her husband were improving their relationship as a result of couples therapy. Mrs. Gordon was making plans to do part-time rehabilitation work in a local hospital. She felt that her "breakdown" resulted from a piling up of responsibilities that she couldn't cope with.

Comparisons with Total Sample

The prenatal personality and adaptation factor scores for Mrs. Forbes and Mrs. Gordon are shown in Fig. 3. It is of particular interest that they had extreme scores not on dimensions of personality but on their adaptation to the experience of pregnancy. Both women had less than the average number of external stresses during pregnancy and both expressed less than the average number of physical complaints to their obstetricians.

Mrs. Gordon was among the minority (28%) of the women who were rated as overreactive to pain but she was not noted to be unusually anxious during labor. During her hospital stay her mood state was rated as temporarily depressed. This placed her among the small number (12%) of women who after uncomplicated deliveries were notably dysphoric. Mrs. Forbes, like Mrs. Gordon, was not unusually anxious during labor but was noted to be temporarily depressed during her hospital stay.

The postnatal factor scores in Fig. 4 reflect the unusual amount of difficulty which Mrs. Gordon experienced in handling her infant and in adjusting to the demands and restrictions of motherhood. The considerable distress which Mrs. Forbes experienced during her postpartum period is somewhat reflected in the factor scores. Unlike Mrs. Gordon, by the sixth postpartum month, most of her scores for maternal adaptation did not deviate appreciably from the group mean. Neither infant was unusual in his overall adjustment during the first six months.

Mr. Gordon's unusually poor adjustment to the paternal role is notable as is the poor husband-wife adaptation in both families during the postpartum period.

Comment

Neither of these women received or actively sought psychiatric treatment until after a second pregnancy. It is abundantly clear, however, that the postpartum difficulties which landed them in treatment were not appreciably different from those which they experienced after a first pregnancy. The similarity is more striking in Mrs. Forbes. Her depressive episode came on each time in the first postpartum

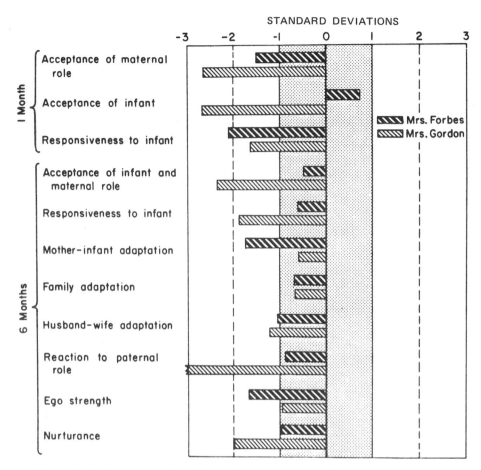

FIG. 4. Standard scores on postnatal factors (first pregnancy) for Mrs. Forbes and Mrs. Gordon.

week and persisted for about three months. Her overwhelming feeling was that she could not cope with the new demands imposed on her by childbirth. Feelings of entrapment, fear of falling apart, and profound guilt characterized each depression, as did frequent crying, restlessness, and insomnia. Her depressive disorder seemed to have an almost autonomous quality.

This guilt-ridden, hysterical woman was certainly vulnerable to periods of depression and for many years had experienced transient periods of depressed mood. The two depressive episodes following childbirth, however, were strikingly different from the transient mood changes that she had experienced in the years before and which she experienced after these episodes. The contiguity between childbirth and the acute onset of her profound mental changes certainly suggest that childbirth was in some sense a precipitant of these changes. The replication of the syndrome after her second parturition and the fact that each had its onset four days postpartum invite speculation about the effect of the perinatal fall in progesterone on her depressive illness. Progesterone has been demonstrated to reduce the excitability (raise seizure threshold) of the central nervous system (Hamburg, 1966). Correlative studies indicate that the rapid drop in progesterone and estrogen secretion in the premenstrual period is accompanied in some women by anxiety, depression, and irritability (Benedek, 1950; Hamburg, 1966). More direct evidence for a mood-stabilizing effect of progesterone comes from studies which demonstrate the efficacy of large doses of progesterone in the prevention of the premenstrual recurrence of postpartum disorders and a recent study in which psychiatric patients on oral contraceptives were found to show symptomatic improvement (Hamilton, 1962; Kane et al., 1969).

In Mrs. Forbes the possibilities for interaction between character structure, the physiological changes of parturition, and the psychological impact of parturition are highlighted. The relative contribution of each to her depressive illness is indeterminable from this data. It does seem, however, that the total experience of parturition was both a necessary and a sufficient cause of her depressive illness.

Mrs. Gordon, on the other hand, developed her difficulties gradually and seemingly in response to the demands of motherhood. Following her first pregnancy she was unusually rejecting of her infant and her new role. Her difficulties following a second pregnancy had their onset not immediately after delivery but after several months of caring for an infant. Childbirth *per se* was not a precipitant of her symptoms. With a character structure ill-suited to mothering, she gradually decompensated in what was for her an untenable situation.

Three Vulnerable Women

Case 5—Mrs. Norton married at age 19. The pregnancy which occurred within the first month of marriage caught her by surprise: "It never entered my head that I would be pregnant; it doesn't feel real to me."

Her father was an alcoholic who frequently beat her, and at age 17 Mrs. Norton was ejected from home. An older man took her in to live with him and soon became abusive, and she attempted suicide by cutting her wrists. Shortly thereafter she found a job, made different living arrangements, and entered into the relationship with Mr. Norton which culminated in marriage.

Mrs. Norton found pregnancy distasteful. She resented the nausea and ungainliness, and the fact that she was no longer able to sing, dance and "act wild." The project team saw Mrs. Norton as schizoid—shy, inarticulate and withdrawn—and noted her failure at impulse control and her feelings of emotions getting out of hand. Throughout pregnancy she suffered from intense disruptive anxiety, and she remained anxious and frightened throughout the six-month postpartum period. All observers noted her depressive affect during this time. At four months postpartum she made two suicide attempts, apparently precipitated by marital crises.

Mrs. Norton's second infant was born when the first child was approximately a year and a half old, and again Mrs. Norton was extremely anxious during the pregnancy and dysphoric following parturition. Five or six months postpartum she withdrew to bed for a week, responding neither to husband nor to children.

When her second child was a year and a half of age, Mrs. Norton discovered that she was pregnant for the third time. She was evaluated by three psychiatrists at this time, all of whom recommended therapeutic abortion. Each psychiatrist noted her immaturity, history of recurrent depression with childbirth, and suicidal potential. Following termination of the pregnancy, the family situation deteriorated further. Mrs. Norton became addicted to narcotics, the four-year marriage ended in separation, and not long thereafter she again attempted suicide. She is currently in a mental hospital.

Case 6—Mrs. London, age 21 and married for a year and a half, experienced the first few months of pregnancy as difficult and unpleasant. She was seen as restrained, blocked, depressed, and fixated in adolescence.

Mrs. London characterized her childhood as happy and uneventful. In early adolescence she began quarreling frequently with her parents, having increased difficulty in school, and fainting during examinations. Her school grades went from superior to poor. At age 13 Mrs. London took a bottle of aspirin in a suicide attempt. These problems were related to thyroid disease, and she was treated by an internist for three years and briefly by a psychiatrist. During her first year of marriage Mrs. London made two suicide attempts in the context of quarrels with her husband. Her husband's plans to get psychiatric treatment for her subsequent to these events bogged down, presumably for financial reasons.

In the last months of her pregnancy Mrs. London seemed to be taking considerable pride in the experience and began to feel "a greater sense of personal worth" in being able to have a child.

Labor and delivery went well, and from the first she was proud of her infant and devoted to her. In spite of this, Mrs. London spent the first two postpartum months crying a great deal, feeling lonely and sad, and at times contemplating suicide. At six months postpartum, however, she seemed considerably more content and confident than she ever had before.

Two years after the birth of her first child, Mrs. London gave birth to a second, and during the early postpartum months again experienced an intensification of her chronic feelings of depression, inertia, and anxiety. When a third pregnancy occurred six months after the birth of the second child, Mrs. London, feeling that she could not tolerate another pregnancy, obtained an illegal abortion. Following this she was referred for intensive psychotherapy. The psychiatrist who saw her at this time commented: "I get the feeling that I'm talking to a 15-year-old rather than a 24-year-old."

Case 7—Mrs. Jenkins was age 28 and in the fifth year of her marriage when she became pregnant for the first time. She was quite aware of her ambivalence about the pregnancy and her lifelong pattern of "nervousness."

When after a one-year courtship she had become engaged, her characteristic shyness and nervousness were accentuated and she stopped working because her nervous mannerisms, such as trembling hands, had become increasingly obvious. When after two years of marriage the couple moved to Washington, 400 miles from her childhood home, Mrs.

Jenkins had considerable difficulty. She felt more insecure than usual, was subject to crying jags, and considered getting psychiatric help but made no moves to do so.

Although Mrs. Jenkins had severe nausea and vomiting in the early months of pregnancy, had problems of weight gain and the realistic fears attached to being Rh negative, she reported that she felt more relaxed during pregnancy than she ever had felt before. Throughout her pregnancy, however, she expressed little confidence in her ability to take care of an infant. The psychologist felt that Mrs. Jenkins was childlike and very constricted.

The first two postpartum months were especially difficult for her. She felt depressed and was concerned with the fact that for the first time she felt as if she didn't love her husband. At three months postpartum Mrs. Jenkins was advised by the project social worker to obtain psychiatric help for the depression and anxiety which she was obviously experiencing. By six months postpartum Mrs. Jenkins decided to see a therapist and entered into a counseling relationship with a social worker which lasted for about a year and a half. A psychiatrist who evaluated her at the end of this period suggested that "her anxiety symptoms became more evidenced and troubling following the birth of her child." To date Mrs. Jenkins has had no further pregnancies.

Comparisons with Total Group

The prenatal scores for these women are shown in Fig. 5. Most striking are their deviantly low scores on ego strength and nurturance. Also of interest is the change from unusually poor adaptation to pregnancy at three months to fairly good adaptation at seven months.

Mrs. Norton underwent three external "stresses" during pregnancy, Mrs. London one "stress," and Mrs. Jenkins two "stresses." All three women reported fewer than the average number of physical complaints to their obstetricians.

Both Mrs. London and Mrs. Norton were rated by their obstetricians as overreactive to pain and unusually anxious during labor and delivery. Mrs. Jenkins, on the other hand, was rated as having little or no reaction to pain and as having little or no anxiety.

STANDARD DEVIATIONS

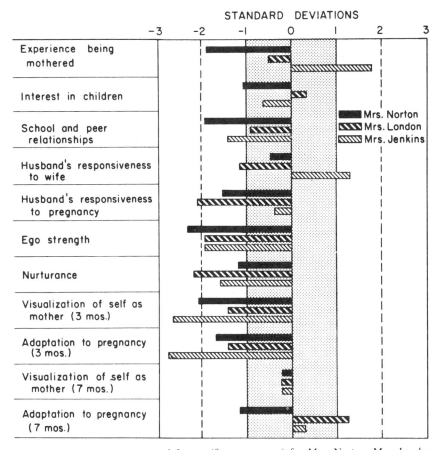

FIG. 5. Standard scores on prenatal factors (first pregnancy) for Mrs. Norton, Mrs. London, and Mrs. Jenkins.

Mrs. London and Mrs. Jenkins scored considerably higher on the Maternal Adaptation variables than did Mrs. Norton (Fig. 6). The differentiation between these women carried over into evaluation of the husband-wife adaptation. Also of note is the fact that at six months postpartum Mrs. London's ego strength score had risen considerably whereas the ego strength scores for the other two women remained low.

Comment

The prenatal evaluations of these women suggested that they were unusually vulnerable to stress, and one might have predicted that they would be likely to develop symptoms in association with the physical

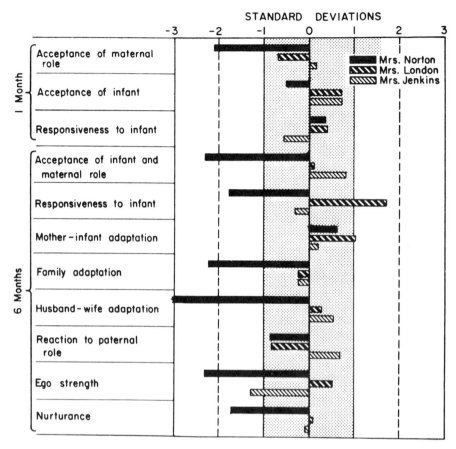

FIG. 6. Standard scores on postnatal factors (first pregnancy) for Mrs. Norton, Mrs. London, and Mrs. Jenkins.

and psychological stresses of parturition. Although these women did require psychiatric attention in what is often designated as the postpartum period, it is clear that parturition itself had little to do with the onset of their difficulties. Mrs. Norton made a suicide attempt four months postpartum in the context of a marital crisis; Mrs. London developed considerable anxiety when faced with a third pregnancy six months postpartum; and Mrs. Jenkins sought help six months following her first pregnancy for chronic recurrent dysphoria exacerbated by the responsibilities of infant care. These symptoms did not differ from those which they had experienced during periods of stress prior to pregnancy.

Each of these women responded to labor in a predictably frightened or constricted fashion, and each experienced periods of dysphoria in the early postpartum weeks. For two of them, however, the last months of pregnancy and early months of motherhood seemed to be ego-enhancing experiences. This ego enhancement or mood stabilization in the latter months of pregnancy has previously been noted in the chronically dysphoric woman and is subject to both endocrinologic and psychologic explanation (Benedek, 1950).

These data suggest that the woman with considerable ego deficits is likely to develop symptoms at some point in the "postpartum" period. Whether the disruptive stress will be pregnancy, childbirth, infant demands, or changes in the marital relationship can be determined only by close scrutiny of her environment and the meaning of these events to her.

Discussion

Childbirth is unique among expected life events in its physiological and psychological impact. Out of 1,000 women undergoing childbirth it is commonly estimated that one or two will develop a psychotic disorder in the postpartum period (Paffenbarger, 1961; Hamilton, 1962; Normand, 1967). An untold number of others suffer from incapacitating but less dramatic disturbances which often go unrecognized. The potential effects of these disorders on the woman and her infant pose an important problem in preventive mental health.

A first step in studying parturition as a disruptive stress is to limit consideration to those psychiatric disorders which are directly and critically related to parturition. Out of the seven women in our study who developed psychiatric symptoms within six month postpartum, only two, Mrs. Smith and Mrs. Forbes, had disorders which were directly related to parturition. These women had the onset of symptoms within days of parturition. One criterion, then, for a more rigorous definition of postpartum disorder both for diagnostic and research purposes might be the onset of symptoms in very close contiguity to childbirth. Since it is likely that different clusters of prenatal and parturition variables relate to different postpartum syndromes, it probably would be helpful for purposes of prediction and investigation of etiology to differentiate the depressive syndromes from those of profound personality disorganization. The complexity of intervening variables between parturition and psychiatric symptom guarantees the futility of investigating one variable—such as mother-daughter relationship or endocrine dysfunction—as predictor or etiologic agent. The data from this and other studies suggest that in the attempt to understand the development of symptoms following childbirth, premorbid character structure, sexual identity, the idiosyncratic meaning of childbirth, and the gradient of puerperal endocrine changes are among the variables worthy of study.

SUMMARY

Although mental disturbances occurring soon after childbirth have been noted and described since the Fourth Century, basic questions about the etiology and phenomenology of these disorders remain unanswered. This study is addressed to the development of meaningful criteria for designating a condition as postpartum and for differentiating one postpartum syndrome from another. Sixty women were investigated psychologically and medically from the first trimester of their first pregnancy through the sixth postpartum month. Seven of these women were referred for psychiatric treatment within the six months following their first or second pregnancy, with three requiring hospitalization. Childbirth was directly related to the onset of symptoms in only two cases. In the first a woman who had appeared well integrated during pregnancy developed a profound schizophrenic disorder in the week following delivery. In the second a woman who had a tendency toward depressive mood swings developed a severe depressive disorder four days postpartum after two consecutive pregnancies. Although each of the remaining five women had the onset of symptoms in what is usually designated as the postpartum period, it is clear that childbirth itself had little to do with the onset of symptoms. One woman decompensated ten days following her second pregnancy in a setting of multiple stresses which constituted an extreme situation. Another experienced unusual discomfort with the demands of infant care and at five months postpartum was referred for psychotherapy and soon hospitalized. None of the three women with premorbid histories suggesting marked ego deficits (multiple suicide attempts, recurrent disruptive anxiety) developed symptoms during the early puerperium; each of them did become symptomatic between four and six months postpartum—two in the context of situational crises. The data from this study indicate that the postpartum disorder which is precipitated by childbirth can be distinguished from a psychiatric disorder in the postpartum period which is not critically related to childbirth. It would be helpful for purposes of prediction and investigation of etiology to consider only those disorders with onset in close contiguity to childbirth as "postpartum" and to differentiate the depressive from the schizophrenic syndromes.

[^1](1) Illness or death in the extended family, (2) illness of husband or wife, (3) anxiety re: financial security, (4) crisis in or with extended family, (5) marital disharmony, (6) job dissatisfaction of husband, (7) geographical distances from extended family. (See Chapter III, Stresses.)

REFERENCES

American Psychiatric Assn. (1968) *Diagnostic and Statistical Manual of Mental Disorders* (3rd ed., DSM-II). Washington, D.C., APA.

Benedek, T. (1950) The Functions of the Sexual Apparatus and Their Disturbances. In: *Psychosomatic Medicine*, edited by Franz Alexander. New York: W.W. Norton and Co.

Boyd, D.A. (1942) Mental Disorders Associated with Childbearing. *American Journal of Obstetrics and Gynecology*, 43:148-163.

Daniels, R.S., and Lessow, H. (1964) Severe Postpartum Reactions. An Interpersonal View. *Psychosomatics*, 5:21-26.

Fondeur, M.M. et al. (1957) Postpartum Mental Illness. A Controlled Study. *AMA Archives of Neurology and Psychiatry*, 77:503-512.

Hamburg, D.A. (1966) Effects of Progesterone on Behavior. *Research Publications Assn. for Research in Nervous and Mental Disease*, 43:251-265.

Hamilton, J.A. (1962) *Postpartum Psychiatric Problems*. Mosby.

Kane, F.J., Treadway, R., and Ewing, J.A. (1969) Emotional Change Associated with Oral Contraceptives in Female Psychiatric Patients. *Comprehensive Psychiatry*, 10:16-30.

Kaplan, E.H., and Blackman, L.H. (1969) The Husband's Role in Psychiatric Illness Associated with Childbearing. *Psychiatric Quarterly*, 43:396-409.

Madden, J.J. et al. (1958) Characteristics of Post-Partum Mental Illness. *American Journal of Psychiatry*, 115:18-24.

Markham, S. (1961) A Comparative Evaluation of Psychotic and Nonpsychotic Reactions to Childbirth. *American Journal of Orthopsychiatry*, 31:565-578.

Martin, M.E. (1958) Puerperal Mental Illness. A Follow-up Study of 75 Cases. *British Medical Journal*, 2:773-777.

Melges, F.T. (1968) Postpartum Psychiatric Syndromes, *Psychosomatic Medicine*, 30:95-108.

Normand, W.C. (1967) Postpartum Disorders. In: *Comprehensive Textbook of Psychiatry*, edited by A.M. Friedman et al. Baltimore: Williams and Wilkins Co.

Paffenbarger, R.S. (1961) The Picture Puzzle of the Postpartum Psychoses. *Journal of Chronic Disease*, 13:161-173.

Pugh, T.F. et al (1963) Rates of Mental Disease Related to Childbearing. *New England Journal of Medicine*, 268:1224-1228.

Reich, T., and Winokur, G. (1970) Postpartum Psychoses in Patients with Manic Depressive Disease. *Journal of Nervous and Mental Disease*, 151:60-68.

Seager, C.P. (1960) A Controlled Study of Post-Partum Mental Illness. *Journal of Mental Science*, 106:214-230.

Strecker, E.A., and Ebaugh, F.G. (1926) Psychoses Occurring During the Puerperium. *Archives of Neurology and Psychiatry*, 15:239-252.

Tetlow, C. (1955) Psychoses of Childbearing. *Journal of Mental Science*, 101:629-639.

Thomas, C.L., and Gordon, J.E. (1959) Psychosis After Childbirth: Ecological Aspects of a Single Impact Stress. *American Journal of Medical Science*, 238:363-388.

Yalom, I.D. et al. (1968) "Postpartum Blues" Syndrome. *Archives of General Psychiatry*, 18:16-27.

Zilboorg, G. (1928) Malignant Psychosis Related to Childbirth. *American Journal of Obstetrics and Gynecology*, 15:145-158.

Zilboorg, G. (1957) The Clinical Issues of Postpartum Psychopathological Reactions. *American Journal of Obstetrics and Gynecology*, 73:305-312.

*Psychological Aspects of a First Pregnancy
and Early Postnatal Adaptation.*
Raven Press, New York © 1974

Chapter X
Maternal Personality and Early Adaptation as Related to Infantile Colic*

Benjamin A. Shaver

INTRODUCTION

Infantile colic is certainly one of the most common and distressing ordeals that confront young parents and their pediatricians. By colic, we refer to excessive night crying, usually beginning at about the third week of life and continuing until the infant is approximately three to four months of age. When infection and anomalies of the gastrointestinal and genitourinary tract have been ruled out medically, and the infant still continues to fuss excessively and cry through the evening hours, a diagnosis of colic is applied.

The cause of colic has been variously attributed to air swallowing, rapid feeding, improper burping, milk allergy (Wessel, 1954; Rambar, 1956), hyperirritability (Meyer, 1958) and progesterone dependence (Clark, 1963). In the older medical literature, we find colic attributed to the thymus (Barbour, 1933), that mysterious gland to which another generation of pediatricians attributed many poorly understood maladies of infancy and childhood. The most popular and time-honored theory concerning the etiology of colic attributes the symdrome to the reaction of the infant to an insecure, inexperienced, and perhaps inept mother,

---

*Adapted from a paper delivered at the American Orthopsychiatric Association Annual Meeting in Chicago, March 1968.

who is thought to transmit her feelings to her infant, who responds by being equally nervous and uncomfortable.

Alexander Schaffer (1966) writes concerning colic:

> We are convinced that no organic basis exists for the excessive crying of most newborns. Many of them choose a crying period, often between 6 and 10 p.m. during which they complain incessantly. We do not know why they select this particular period, but we suspect that the father's return from his daily labors has something to do with it. His presence may add a new bustle of activity, an added feeling of excitement or a superimposed feeling of apprehension to the environment....the sensitivity of the newborn to parental unsureness and jitteriness never ceases to amaze us.

Lakin (1957), on the basis of a psychologic study, and Wessel (1954) from a medical study both agree with Schaffer that colic is most often a reflection of the mother's mood and anxiety level.

We agree with these authors that babies are exceptionally sensitive to their mother's mood. However, colic rarely begins before the second or third week of life. If colic were due primarily to the mother's mood and level of anxiety, we would expect the symptom to begin in the first few days of life when the mother is the most anxious and unsure of herself, rather than later when she is more accustomed to mothering. Also, we would expect the first-born of several children to be the most colic prone. This is not the case, however, for ordinal position within the family does not appear to be correlated with development of colic (Clark, 1963).

METHODS

To test the validity of the hypothesis that infantile colic is etiologically related to the mother's mood, anxiety level, and maternal adaptation, we selected 54 items relevant to the mother's personality, maternal adaptation, and level of infant function. These items for the twelve cases (21 per cent of the total sample of 57 infants studied) in which colic was diagnosed were compared with the same items for the non-colic patient sample in order to discover differences in personality and level of functioning of the mother and her colicky infant. The items found to be statistically different between the colic and non-colic groups were obtained by correlation analysis.

TABLE 1. *Non-significant correlations between the occurrence of colic and mother-infant adaptation*

Mother's accommodation to the infant
    Amount of physical contact (holding the infant)
    Quality of physical contact (degree of physical involvement)
    Degree of expression of affection for infant
    Sensitivity and responsiveness to the infant's cues
    Amount of stimulation (social, visual, auditory, play)
Mother's psychological adaptation to the infant
    Feelings in regard to care of the physical needs of the infant
    Reaction to total dependency of the infant
    Anxiety regarding adequacy in her role as a mother
    Anxiety regarding the infant, his health, normality, development
    Prevailing mood since birth of baby
Mother's current personality
    Emotional adaptation—characteristic way of expressing feeling
      Hostile and explosive
      Impulsive
      Repressed
      Tender and affectionate
      Adapted
    Ease of fantasy production
    Responsiveness to others—giving and nurturant quality
    Flexibility
    Sense of humor
    Covert, underlying dependency pattern
    Ability to meet own needs, including pleasure
    Insight into self
    Sense of success as a wife
    Sense of success as a mother
    Sense of success as a homemaker
    Achievement of an adult role
    Capacity for closeness
    Ability to take help
    Overall evaluation of adaptive behavior
    Narcissism
Current stresses (such as: financial insecurity, illnesses or death in extended family, illness
    of husband or wife, problems with relatives, job dissatisfaction of husband)

RESULTS

In regard to the mother's accommodation to the infant (Table 1), the amount of physical contact between the mother and infant in periods of feeding, diapering, bathing, dressing, and play, was found to be the same for both the colic and non-colic groups. Similarly, the quality of physical contact and the mother's expression of affection for the infant both verbally and in demeanor were found to be comparable for both groups. The mothers of the colicky infants were no less sensitive and responsive to the infant's hunger, discomfort, and social needs, and the amount of visual, auditory, and social stimulation was comparable for both groups of infants.

The mother's psychological adaptation to the infant (Table 1) was not statistically different when the colic and non-colic groups were compared. The reaction of the colic mother to the dependency of her infant and his physical needs was the same as that of her non-colic counterpart, and she was no more anxious regarding her overall adequacy as a mother and concerning her infant's developmental status. A wide range of mood was found in the total group during the six months' postpartum study period, but, again, the two groups were comparable.

The current personality (Table 1) as reflected in her characteristic way of expressing feeling, ease of fantasy production, giving and nurturant quality, flexibility, sense of humor, dependency pattern, her ability to meet her own needs, her insight into self, and her sense of success as a wife, mother, and homemaker were comparable in both groups. Both groups of mothers had been equally successful in achieving an adult role, and both displayed a comparable capacity for closeness and ability to accept help when offered. The degree of narcissism was comparable for both groups. Stresses (Table 1) were comparable for both groups during the study period.

We do find significant differences when we examine infant adjustment and the mother-infant relationship. In the adjustment of the infant (Table 2) the "excessive crying" of the colicky infant is found to be significant at age six weeks and twelve weeks but not significant at 24 weeks. The colicky babies were judged by the infant observer and pediatrician to be more irritable and tense than the non-colic infants at age 24 weeks. Also at 24 weeks, the colic group of infants was judged to have a poorer feeding adjustment, whereas the feeding adjustment was comparable at the time of the six-week and three-month rating periods. We might postulate that by the time of the 24-week rating period, the problems of the colicky period may have contributed to an altered response to food and feeding on the part of the mother, her infant, or both. The problem of colic contributed to a lower overall evaluation of functioning of the infant at age six months.

At the twelve-week rating period (Table 2), the mother of the colicky infant was definitely less confident in coping with her infant. By the time the infant was 24 weeks old, two months after colic ceased to be a problem, the mother's confidence had returned and there appeared to be no significant difference between the two groups.

TABLE 2. *Statistically significant correlations between the occurrence of colic and mother-infant adaptation**

	Age of Infant		
	6 weeks	12 weeks	24 weeks
Infant adjustment			
Excessive crying	0.48	0.30	—
Low object responsiveness	—	0.26	—
Increased irritability	—	—	0.32
Increased tenseness	—	—	0.39
Less happy characteristic mood	—	0.34	—
Poor feeding adjustment	—	—	0.37
Lower overall evaluation of functioning of infant	—	—	0.31
Mother-infant relationship			
Mother less confident in coping with infant	—	0.36	—
Mother's reaction to infant as less accepting	0.30	0.27	—

*Correlations shown are significant at the 0.05 level of probability or better.

DISCUSSION

Contrary to the findings of Wessel (1954), Lakin (1957), Schaffer (1966), and those who have written on the subject in popular publications, we have found no statistical differences in current personality, current stresses, and maternal adaptation when these items for the mothers of the colic group were compared with the non-colic group of infants. This suggests that the mother's personality, anxiety level, and degree of success in adapting to the maternal role were not factors in the development of colic in the infants studied.

It is quite apparent from the data presented that infantile colic does have an appreciable impact on the mother. The mother of the colicky infant was quite significantly less confident in coping with her infant, and was significantly less accepting of her infant at age twelve weeks, than was the mother of the non-colicky infant. Women almost uniformly respond to a colicky infant with a sense of frustration and futility. Mrs. T., one of the mothers studied, said of her colicky baby, "It is so terrible to have him crying in such pain; nothing I do for him seems to help."

Much of the anguish suffered by parents and their colicky infants alike is the result of our not having effective treatment to offer. An occasional infant is quickly relieved by changing to a soybean formula, and undoubtedly milk allergy is an occasional etiologic factor in colic (Wessel, 1954). None of the infants in this series responded to a change of formula. Pediatricians often prescribe antispasmodics, sedatives, heat to the infant's abdomen, more frequent burping, changes in nipples and feeding technique, but often these measures are of little help. The use of drugs and changes in formulae and routine seem to assist the parents in tolerating the condition, because at least they are doing something for their baby. In our activist society, "doing something" is important, whether or not that which we do is helpful.

The most helpful "treatment" for colic, in our experience, is the reassurance that the symptoms will abate when the infant is three to four months of age. The fact that the condition is not interminable is often enough to keep the parents "holding on for a few weeks," as Mrs. M. expressed it.

The degree of reaction to the infant's colic varied enormously from one woman to another. Mrs. T., as we have already noted, was enormously distressed by her infant's difficulty, while in the case of Mrs. R's infant, the diagnosis of colic was made by the pediatrician after inquiring about the infant's sleeping, feeding, and crying pattern. Mrs. R., whose infant had moderately severe colic, accepted her infant's fussing and crying as "normal" for babies, and was not disturbed by it.

Though our data suggest that the mother's confidence in coping with her colicky infant returns by the 24th week of life (two months after colic has ceased to be a problem), the crying and sleepless nights are not easily forgotten. Under the stimulus of a subsequent pregnancy, the woman may voice her apprehension concerning the possibility of another colicky baby, or may comment after delivery that the new baby is "not colicky" as was her first infant.

The data presented here support the findings of Paradise who made a prospective study of the mothers of 146 normal newborns in which a diagnosis of colic was made in 23 per cent. Maternal personality factors were measured by the Minnesota Multiphasic Personality Inventory. No evidence was found to support the "frequently stated view that colic results from an unfavorable emotional climate created by an inexperienced, anxious, hostile, or unmotherly mother" (Paradise, 1966, p.191).

There has been a tendency on the part of the medical and paramedical professions to attribute all the ills of society to the neurotic, anxious mother. Our data suggest that infantile colic should be removed from the list.

SUMMARY

To test the validity of the traditional hypothesis that colic is often the result of interaction of the infant with a nervous and insecure mother, 57 women and their infants were studied from the second trimester of pregnancy through the six postpartum months. Twelve of these infants were diagnosed as having colic. The mothers of the colicky infants showed no statistically significant differences in personality and degree of success in adapting to the maternal role when compared with the non-colic sample, suggesting lack of etiologic relationship between infantile colic and maternal personality factors.

However, the infant's colic did appear to have a significant effect on the mother-infant relationship. The mothers of the colicky infants were less confident by the end of the first three months of the infant's life and somewhat less accepting of the infant at that time, suggesting that colic made it harder for the mother to cope with her infant. However, at six months postpartum (two months after the disappearance of colic in all the infants in this series), these mothers were no longer seen as less confident or less accepting when compared with the non-colic group.

ACKNOWLEDGMENTS

The author gratefully acknowledges the assistance of Robert F. Lockman, Ph.D., in the preparation of the statistical analysis.

REFERENCES

Barbour, O.E. (1933) Pylorospasm as a Manifestation of Thymic Disturbance. *Archives of Pediatrics,* 50:851.

Clark, R.L., Ganis, F.M., and Bradford, W.L. (1963) A Study of the Possible Relationship of Progesterone to Colic. *Pediatrics,* 31:65.

Lakin, M. (1957) Personality Factors in Mothers of Excessively Crying (Colicky) Infants. *Monographs of Society for Research in Child Development,* 23:No. 64.

Meyer, H.F. (1958) A Clinical Interpretation of the "Colicky" Infant. *Postgraduate Medicine,* 24:627.

Paradise, J.L. (1966) Maternal and Other Factors in the Etiology of Infantile Colic. *Journal of American Medical Association,* 197:191.

Rambar, A.C. (1956) Colic in Infants, General Considerations. *Pediatrics,* 18:829-832.

Schaffer, A.J. (1966) *Diseases of the Newborn* (2nd Ed.). Philadelphia: W.B. Saunders Co.

Wessel, M.A., Cobb, J.C., Jackson, E.B., Harris, G.S., and Detwiler, B.A. (1954) Paroxysmal Fussing in Infancy, Sometimes Called "Colic." *Pediatrics,* 14:421.

Psychological Aspects of a First Pregnancy and Early Postnatal Adaptation.
Raven Press, New York © 1974

Chapter XI
Dimensions of Infant Behavior in the First Half Year of Life*

Elaine F. Gerson

INTRODUCTION

Belief in the importance of early environment for the development of personality has been part of our recent cultural climate. Yet speculation about the effect of the emotions of the pregnant woman upon her unborn child goes back into antiquity. Elizabeth, wife of Zacharias, after her sixth month of pregnancy, ". . . heard the salutation of Mary, and the babe in her womb leaped for joy" (Luke 1:41).

The interaction between the state of the infant, his reactivity pattern, and maternal response has long been within the awareness of clinicians dealing with the mother-baby dyad. The ways in which maternal handling mediates the infant's capacity to respond to his environment have been studied by a number of researchers in recent times, including Yarrow (1963), Wolff (1965), Korner (1966), Fantz (1966), and others.

To record the complexity and richness of the infant's behavior repertoire, summary ratings were used. The central question of the study is: what prenatal and postnatal maternal variables are related to the infant's adjustment and functioning? The following section presents

---

*This chapter is adapted from a dissertation submitted in partial fulfillment of the requirements for the Ph.D. degree in Clinical Psychology at the Pennsylvania State University, 1968, excerpts from which were presented at the 77th Convention of The American Psychological Association, 1969, and published in the Proceedings of the Convention.

the study of the baby using scaled tests and ratings gathered from observations in the natural setting of the home and in the clinic during routine pediatric examinations.

DETAILED PROCEDURE FOR INFANT OBSERVATIONS

During a prenatal visit, the social worker explained the nature and purpose of the infant observer's visit. On telephoning the mother to arrange for the first interview, the observer briefly explained her role again. The infant observer had no knowledge of the woman's history.

Two home visits on consecutive days were made around the baby's one-, three- and six-month birthdays. One observation was made in the afternoon and one in the morning around feeding and bathing times. Occasionally, one situation was omitted or observed twice, depending on the infant's schedule. The infant observer watched ongoing routines (feeding, bathing, changing, and play) and tried to remain as neutral as possible. Behavior of baby and mother was recorded. Observations in the home totalled about four hours at each age period.

The Revised Bayley Scales of Infant Development (Bayley, 1965) were administered at the time of the home visit, usually at the baby's first content, wakeful period.

Following the second day's observation, the baby was rated on the Infant Characteristics Schedule.[1] A case summary was written by the infant observer about the baby's development after each age observation.

The development of the Infant Characteristics Rating Schedule evolved from scales developed by Yarrow (1963). Areas of interest included intellectual, motor, affective, social, and coping capacities.

The following items were rated on a five-point scale:

Object responsiveness (alertness, interest in objects)
Tension (how tense or relaxed baby is)
Characteristic mood (actively unhappy to actively happy)
Affective stability (variability in mood)
Level of social responsiveness (unresponsive to interested)
Appropriateness of social responsiveness (for age level)
Adaptability (capacity to handle change)
Irritability (ease of being upset)
Vulnerability to stress (ease of disintegration of functioning)

Ease of recovery (lengthy or rapid recovery from upset)
Goal directedness (low to high persistence)
Overall rating (poor to smooth overall functioning)

The pediatrician, concerned primarily with health aspects and age-appropriate neurological development, reported his observations on a separate schedule.[2] The areas of interest that were recorded included a number of factual items: (a) physical status (including such items as birthweight, physical condition, neurological status); (b) feeding behavior; (c) mother's reaction; and (d) the infant's overall adaptation (from poorly integrated with significant deviation in many areas of functioning to extremely well integrated, smoothly functioning). The pediatric examination differed slightly in timing from the observation periods of the infant observer in that the first pediatric observation period was at six weeks of age instead of one month; the others were at the same time periods, namely, three months and six months.

INFANT ADAPTATION AS AN OUTCOME VARIABLE

Factor Analysis: Infant Adjustment, Alertness, and Functioning

Factor analysis of the postnatal rating schedule, Infant Characteristics, resulted in the extraction of two significant factors: The first factor, *adjustment,* consists of these items: tension, characteristic mood, affective stability, adaptability, irritability, vulnerability to stress, ease of recovery (from upset), and overall rating. Thus the adjustment factor seems concerned with affective response. The second factor, *alertness,* consists of: object responsiveness, level of social responsiveness, and goal directedness. The factor alertness seems concerned with responsiveness to the environment.

Factor analysis of the pediatric evaluation schedule resulted in a factor called *infant functioning* which consists of: feeding behavior, adjustments to routines, and overall integration of the infant. This factor largely reflects the infant's physiological adaptation.

The three factors, adjustment, alertness, and functioning of the infant, were combined to obtain a score on the outcome variable, Infant Adaptation.

Infant Characteristics and the Woman's Adaptation to Pregnancy

A few prenatal factors were significantly related to infant adaptation in the first half year of life, although the correlations occur at one or two rating periods only. They are presented in Table 1.

TABLE 1. *Significant correlations of pregnancy factors and infant factors*

Time during pregnancy (months)	Prenatal factor scale	Corre-lation*	Infant factor scale	Time period in infancy (months)
3	Visualization of self	0.26	Alertness	1
	as mother	0.30	Alertness	6
7	Adaptation to pregnancy	0.32	Adjustment	6
	experience	0.29	Infant functioning	3
9	Overall reaction to	0.28	Adjustment	6
	pregnancy experience	0.25	Infant functioning	6

*$r = 0.25$ ($p = 0.05$)

The factor *visualization of self as mother* has already been identified in an earlier chapter as a sensitive indicator and predictor for two of the three outcome variables in this study. The ability of the woman to envision herself clearly and confidently in her forthcoming role as a mother may permit some rehearsal in fantasy of the things that she will do with her infant and enable her to be better prepared to offer the baby nurturant care and stimulation appropriate to his needs.

Significant Correlations Between the Woman's Adaptation to the Maternal Role and the Infant's Adjustment

The relationship between postnatal maternal factor scale findings and infant factor scale findings always assumes an interaction of effects. Generally, the accepting confident mother tends to be seen with an effectively coping infant. Significant correlations range from 0.26 to 0.53. The results are presented in Table 2.

A group of maternal factors (acceptance of maternal role, acceptance of infant, individualization of infant, and responsiveness to infant) rated at the one-month time, are related significantly to infant functioning based on the pediatrician's rating, at the six weeks' time. It is of interest to note that confidence in maternal role is correlated at each infant age period with the pediatrician's rating of infant functioning. The issues of interactive effects or the mother's differential reporting cannot be partialed out.

At six months the factor of mother-infant adaptation relates significantly to the factors, infant adjustment and functioning; earlier,

TABLE 2. *Significant correlations: postnatal maternal factors and infant factors (N = 57)*

Time post-natally (months)	Maternal factor scale	Correlation*	Infant factor scale	Time period in infancy
1	Acceptance of maternal role	0.30	Infant functioning	6 weeks
1	Acceptance of maternal role	0.29	Infant functioning	6 months
1	Acceptance of infant	0.26	Infant functioning	6 weeks
1	Acceptance of infant	0.26	Infant functioning	6 months
1	Individualization	0.33	Infant functioning	6 weeks
1	Individualization	0.36	Infant functioning	3 months
1	Response to infant	0.34	Infant functioning	6 weeks
3	Acceptance of infant	0.53	Infant functioning	3 months
3	Acceptance of infant	0.47	Adjustment	3 months
3	Acceptance of infant	0.48	Adjustment	6 months
3	Confidence in maternal role	0.28	Adjustment	3 months
3	Confidence in maternal role	0.34	Adjustment	6 months
3	Confidence in maternal role	0.44	Infant functioning	3 months
3	Confidence in maternal role	0.50	Infant functioning	6 months
6	Mother-infant adaptation	0.41	Infant functioning	6 months
6	Mother-infant adaptation	0.53	Adjustment	6 months
6	Acceptance of infant and maternal role	0.30	Infant functioning	6 months

*$r = 0.25$ ($p = 0.05$); $r = 0.34$ ($p = 0.01$)

at one and three months, the relationships are not statistically significant. The woman's confidence in her maternal role and acceptance of her infant at the age of three months correlates significantly with the infant adjustment factor at three and six months of age. It would be reasonable to assume that whatever would enhance the mother's confidence in herself as a mother and her acceptance of the infant would affect the infant's capacity to adjust. That the well-adjusted infant has the effect of supporting the mother's confidence and her acceptance of the baby appears validated in another phase of the project, the study of Maternal Personality and Early Adaptation as Related to Infantile Colic, reported in Chapter X.

The postnatal maternal factor scales are not generally significantly related to the alertness factor in the infant. It would seem that the alertness factor may be tapping more of the infant's own pattern of reactivity and so be less responsive to the mother's state, except as she mediates such stimulation as is essential and appropriate to the infant's evolving needs.

THE BAYLEY SCALES OF MENTAL AND
MOTOR DEVELOPMENT

The Bayley Scales of Mental and Motor Development were administered to the same infants at the three time periods of the postnatal assessments. Table 3 presents the results of the Bayley Scales testing for the 57 infants.

The trend over time for our group appears to be different for DIQ and DMQ. For the Bayley Scale of Mental Tests (DIQ), the mean of our total group remains constant at one and three months and rises at the six-month period. For the Bayley Scale of Motor Tests (DMQ), the mean of our total group remains constant at one and three months and drops at the six-month period.

To investigate the extent to which we can predict Bayley Scale Test results at one time period from an earlier test, the test results of the total group of 57 were correlated for paired age periods. The results show that for neither DIQ nor DMQ is it possible to predict the results of a test at three or at six months from a test at one or at three months.

TABLE 3. *Results of Bayley Scales Mental and Motor Tests*

Test	Age (months)	Mean	S.D.	S.E. Mean
DIQ	1	101.7	10.6	1.40
	3	101.2	10.3	1.37
	6	106.6	7.6	0.99
DMQ	1	118.0	11.6	1.55
	3	116.8	9.5	1.26
	6	107.4	12.1	1.60

INFANT OBSERVER RATINGS: ITEM CHANGES OVER TIME

The items of the infant observer ratings show interesting changes over time.

The ratings on object responsiveness, level of social responsiveness, and goal directedness show an increase with age from one to six months. These items constitute the factor *alertness,* which, in showing a consistent rise over time, reflects the infant's capacity to demonstrate behaviorally his widening interest in the world of objects. This finding is congruent with the common sense observation that infants become more responsive to the environment as they mature and that they direct their interest increasingly toward objects in the environment (Piaget, 1952).

Two items show no change over time, appropriateness of social response and ease of recovery. These behaviors were generally rated at midpoint, and therefore did not discriminate among the infants. Three "mood" items (tension, characteristic mood, and affective stability) are stable from one to three months, but rise significantly at the six-month time. Four items (adaptability, irritability, vulnerability to stress, and overall rating) show a significant decrement at three months of age. The observations of the infant and the mother's reporting of the infant's behavior result in the rating of the three-month period as less adaptable and more reactive to stress. This apparent change in mood might be seen as a reflection of the mother's differential reporting once the excitement of the infant's arrival is over, or as a more differentiated infant response reflecting more awareness of environment. The infant's irritability may be a function of neurological immaturity resulting in motoric inability to master retrieval of objects or body positioning. The six-month period, with increasing maturation, seems to result in better affective equilibrium.

The factor *adjustment,* composed of a more inclusive cluster of items concerned with affective response, does not reflect the lowered three-month ratings discussed above, but remains constant from one to three months of age and rises at the six-month period. The infant *functioning* factor shows a rise at each rating period, namely, six weeks, three months, and six months of age. In summary, alertness, adjustment, and functioning increase in the first half year of life to a peak at the six-month age.

SUMMARY

For our group of 57 infants born to middle-income parents, we have studied certain dimensions of infant behavior, ordered the many variables, reduced them to three factors—adjustment, alertness, and infant functioning—and related the findings to prenatal and postnatal characteristics of the woman. The Revised Bayley Scales of Infant Development were used to study the babies.

Factor analysis helped to reduce the dimensionality of the multiple ratings of the infant. While certain items remained invariant over time, broad factors such as adjustment, alertness, and functioning tend to go up during the first six months. Of the first half year of life, the six-month point seems to be characterized by the most adaptive functioning.

Prenatal factors (visualization of self as mother, adaptation to pregnancy experience, overall reaction to pregnancy experience) showed small but significant correlations with all three infant factors at some age period studied. Postnatal maternal factors show larger correlations with infant adjustment than prenatal factors.

The interaction between the mother and child seems well illustrated by the significant correlations between maternal acceptance of the infant and confidence in her role as a mother, and infant adjustment and functioning. Certain aspects of infant behavior, as measured by the alertness factor, seem less related to maternal factors and may be reflective of patterns of reactivity unique to each infant.

---

[1]See Appendix B for Postnatal Rating Schedule: Infant Characteristics. Schedules E-1, F-1, and G-1.

[2]See Appendix B for Rating Schedule: Pediatrician's Evaluation of Infant.

REFERENCES

Bayley, N. (1965) Comparisons of Mental and Motor Test Scores for Ages 1-15 Months by Sex, Birth, Order, Race, Geographical Location, and Education of Parents. *Child Development,* 36:379-411.

Fantz, R.L. (1966) The Crucial Early Influence: Mother Love or Environmental Stimulation? *American Journal of Orthopsychiatry,* 36:330-331.

Korner, A., and Grobstein, R. (1966) Visual Alertness as Related to Soothing in Neonates: Implications for Maternal Stimulation and Early Deprivation. *Child Development,* 37:867-876.

Piaget, J. (1952) *The Origins of Intelligence in Children.* New York: International Universities Press.

Wolff, P. (1965) The Causes, Controls, and Organization of Behavior in the Neonate. *Psychological Issues,* 5, No. 1, Monograph 17.

Yarrow, L.J. (1963) Research in Dimensions of Early Maternal Care. *Merrill-Palmer Quarterly of Behavior and Development,* 9:101-114.

Psychological Aspects of a First Pregnancy
and Early Postnatal Adaptation.
Raven Press, New York © 1974

Chapter XII
Infant Temperament and Sex of Infant:
Effects on Maternal Behavior

Gordon W. Keating and Tracey Manning*

INTRODUCTION

A number of researchers in child development have discussed the problem of direction of effects (Sears, 1951; Thomas et al., 1963; Korner, 1965, 1971; Bell, 1968, 1971) and have argued that the parent-child relationship should be viewed as a reciprocal interaction rather than a one-way influence of parent on child. The generally poor correlations between child-rearing attitudes and practices and later child characteristics (Caldwell, 1964) may stem in part from the failure to take into account the influence of child characteristics on parental attitudes and behavior. Relatively little research has considered the influence of child on parent. Undoubtedly this is partly due to the problem of developing suitable research designs.

One approach to the investigation of child effects is to study the influence of very early temperamental characteristics of infants on their caretakers. Characteristics studied during the neonatal period can be considered constitutional in origin rather than a result of interaction with the mother. Moreover, in early infancy the mother-infant relationship is actively developing, and thus both infant and mother characteristics probably have an especially immediate and critical impact on the newly emerging relationship. Of the many observational

*Dr. Keating is a Fellow in Child Psychiatry, Department of Psychiatry, University of Washington, Seattle. Mrs. Manning is completing her doctoral dissertation in the Psychology Department, Catholic University of America.

and experimental studies of individual differences in infancy, few have been concerned about the impact of these differences on maternal behavior towards the infant. One factor-analytic study of mother-infant dyads described the interaction in terms of nine factors along a continuum from child-centered to mother-centered (Stern et al., 1969). Both infant and mother characteristics loaded on all factors.

The effect of sex of child on parental behavior has perhaps received more attention in the literature than any other child characteristic (Rothbart and Maccoby, 1966; Goldberg and Lewis, 1969). The sex of an infant is a biological fact and is not subject to parental influence. In many cases, however, it may be difficult to distinguish the direct effect of child's sex on parental behavior via parental sex-typing from an indirect effect on the parent due to sex-related differences in infant behavior and temperament. Some evidence exists for behavioral sex differences in early infancy (Kagan and Moss, 1962; Kagan and Lewis, 1965; Garai and Scheinfeld, 1968; Watson, 1969; Korner, 1969).

In this paper we have looked at two issues: (1) the relationship of an infant characteristic, emotional equilibrium, to maternal behavior toward the infant; (2) the interactive influence of sex of infant and maternal personality on maternal behavior.

Although the study reported in this volume was not designed to investigate the effects of sex of infant or infant temperament on maternal behavior, some of the data collected in the process of the study are suitable for analyzing this problem. The data to be presented in this chapter were drawn from the research of the original study.

The final sample includes 30 mothers with male infants and 27 with female infants.

MEASURES

In the larger study a great many measures of personality and adaptation to pregnancy were obtained. Four measures were used in the analyses in this chapter: (1) maternal personality, (2) adaptation to pregnancy, (3) maternal behavior toward the infant, and (4) infant characteristics.

Maternal Personality

Clusters of variables were derived from the item ratings through correlational analyses, factor analyses, and conceptual considerations.[1]

The personality variables used in this chapter, ego strength and nurturance, represent a somewhat different cluster of items than those encompassed in the personality variables by the same name in other parts of the study, notably in Chapters III and IV.

The variable, ego strength, consists of the following items:

(1) Emotional adaptation: the degree to which the individual can release feelings, verbally or otherwise, and still be in consonance with her environment.

(2) Flexibility: the ability to accommodate to changes in the environment.

(3) Ability to meet own needs: the capacity to utilize activities and relationships for the satisfaction of emotional needs.

(4) Acceptance of identity: the acceptance of own sociocultural and personality characteristics.

(5) Achievement of adult role: the woman's self-confidence, personal satisfaction in her roles, and emotional integration.

(6) Adaptive behavior: the adequacy of the woman's defenses in dealing with both instinctual and super-ego demands.

The ratings of each of these items were added, using standard scores when indicated, to give a score for ego strength. The correlations of each item score with the combined score range from 0.70 and 0.90 for both prenatal and postnatal scores. Item intercorrelations range from 0.37 to 0.75.

The personality variable, nurturance, consists of the following items:

(1) Tender and affectionate feelings to family members.

(2) General responsiveness to others: awareness of the needs and demands of others, as opposed to strong dependency needs.

(3) Ability to give help and support: capacity to respond to the emotional and physical needs of husband, sibling, or other—especially in times of crisis.

The ratings on these items were added to give a nurturance score. The correlations of each item with the total score range between 0.76 and 0.90 for both prenatal and postnatal scores. Item intercorrelations range between 0.35 and 0.66.

Adaptation to Pregnancy

To evaluate the women's adaptation to pregnancy, the subjects were studied intensively at the third and seventh months of their pregnancies.

The variable, adaptation to pregnancy, consists of the following items:

(1) Feelings about pregnancy: from extremely rejecting to enthusiastic.

(2) Anxiety about physical aspects of pregnancy: from intense, disruptive anxiety to little or no anxiety.

(3) Effect of pregnancy on maternal well-being: from hypochondriasis to enhancement of well-being.

(4) Adaptability to changes of pregnancy: from resentment of changes to enthusiastic adaptation.

Maternal Behavior Toward the Infant

This group of variables represents an attempt to evaluate the quality of the mother's interaction with her infant. Each variable consists of a cluster of rating items which intercorrelated reasonably well at each time period. (The correlation coefficients ranged from 0.33 to 0.77.) The score on each variable at each time period is obtained by summing the item ratings. The variables, along with the items composing them, are listed below:

1. Affective Reaction to Maternal Role
    a. Feelings regarding physical care of infant: the extent to which the mother enjoyed, accepted, or rejected giving physical care to the infant.
    b. Reaction to total dependency of infant: the extent to which she enjoyed or rejected the infant's total dependency on her.
    c. Reaction to curtailment of freedom: the degree to which she accepted or resented the limitations in her activities resulting from the need to care for the infant.
    d. Prevailing mood since birth of baby: the general affective tone of the mother.
2. Physical and Affectionate Responsiveness to Baby

a. Amount of physical contact.
b. Quality of physical contact: the degree of physical involvement and closeness.
c. Degree of expression of affect: the degree of demonstrativeness in expressing affection.
3. Acceptance of Infant
a. Overall acceptance.
b. Acceptance of individual traits of infant.
4. Individualization: The extent to which the mother perceives infant as an individual and guides her behavior toward the infant by her awareness of his uniqueness.

Infant Behavior

The stability of the infant variables over the first six months is of importance, if indeed these variables do influence maternal behavior. Stability was explored by calculating correlation coefficients for each variable as rated at one and three, three and six, and one and six months. For the most part, these correlations were not very high. Variables relating to emotional behavior showed the highest stability. Furthermore, these variables were moderately to highly intercorrelated. Hence, a new summary variable called Emotional Equilibrium was obtained by summing the ratings of each component item.

Emotional equilibrium is composed of a summary rating of the following items:

1. Quality of crying under conditions of frustration: from very strong to little crying or protest.
2. Affective stability: from highly unstable to extremely stable.
3. Irritability or ease of being upset: from very low threshold to very high threshold.
4. Vulnerability to stress or ease of disintegration of functioning under stress: from low threshold to high threshold.
5. Ease of recovery from being upset: from prolonged to rapid recovery.

The stability of emotional equilibrium proved greater than that of its components but still is only moderate (Table 1). There are no sex differences in the stability of emotional equilibrium.

TABLE 1. *Individual stability across time of infant emotional equilibrium*

Time period	Males (n = 30)	Females (n = 27)
1 month to 3 months	$r = 0.66$	$r = 0.50$
3 months to 6 months	0.56	0.53
1 month to 6 months	0.41	0.36

RESULTS

The Relationship of Infant Characteristics to Maternal Behavior

The infant characteristic, emotional equilibrium, related significantly to some maternal behavior variables. There is a significant positive relationship between infant emotional equilibrium and maternal acceptance of infant for girls but not for boys (Table 2). The relationship for girls is significant both at three and six months.

TABLE 2. *Correlation of infant emotional equilibrium and maternal acceptance of infant, and significance of sex differences in correlation*

Time period	Boys (n = 30)	Girls (n = 27)	Sex difference
1 month	$r = 0.09$, NS	$r = 0.20$, NS	NS
3 months	0.28, NS	0.65, $p < 0.01$	$p < 0.10$
6 months	0.21, NS	0.37, $p < 0.05$	NS

The correlations of emotional equilibrium with individualization show quite a different pattern (Table 3). Emotional equilibrium at one and six months is negatively related to individualization of the baby boy by his mother. This relationship does not hold at any time for girls.

TABLE 3. *Correlation of infant emotional equilibrium and maternal individualization, and significance of sex differences in correlation*

Time period	Boys (n = 30)	Girls (n = 27)	Sex difference
1 month	$r = -0.57$, $p < 0.01$	$r = 0.01$, NS	$p < 0.05$
3 months	−0.21, NS	−0.24, NS	NS
6 months	−0.40, $p < 0.05$	−0.01, NS	NS

These results suggest that emotional equilibrium of the infant is related to maternal behavior in a sex-specific manner. Although at all three time periods the boys have a lower mean emotional equilibrium than the girls, at no time does this difference approach significance.

It might be argued that mothers tend to individualize boys more or less *because* they are boys or accept girls more or less *because* they are girls. If this were so, there should be consistent mean differences on individualization and acceptance for mothers of male and female infants. The only mean sex difference in acceptance is found at one month, with boys more accepted than girls ($p < 0.05$, *t*-test). This is not surprising in view of the greater preference for boys, especially among mothers of first-borns. This difference does not persist after one month. In short, although there are no sex differences in the means of either infant emotional equilibrium or maternal acceptance (except at one month) or individualization, sex of infant seems to mediate the relationship between infant emotional equilibrium and maternal acceptance and individualization of the infant.

Sex-specific Influences of Maternal Personality on Maternal Behavior Toward the Infant

In the previous section, a complex interaction was noted between sex of infant, emotional equilibrium, and maternal acceptance and individualization of the infant. Further analysis of the data reveals a sizable number of correlations between certain maternal personality characteristics and maternal behavior toward the infant. These correlations differ dramatically depending on sex of infant. For example, nurturance, a maternal personality measure, is highly positively related to several dimensions of maternal behavior toward girls but not toward boys.

The data on the relationship of nurturance and maternal behavior toward the infant are shown in Tables 4-6.[2] These data show that for mothers of female infants, nurturance is positively related to affective reaction to maternal role, acceptance of infant, and physical and emotional responsiveness to baby. For mothers of male infants, these relationships do not hold.

Another dimension of personality which relates to maternal behavior is ego strength. Tables 7-9 show the data relating ego strength to maternal behavior. The correlations of ego strength with various

TABLE 4. *Correlation of nurturance (postnatal) with affective reaction to maternal role (1, 3, and 6 months postnatal), and significance of sex differences in correlation*

Time period	Boys (n = 30)	Girls (n = 27)	Sex difference
1 month	r = 0.25, NS	r = 0.52, p < 0.01	NS
3 months	0.00, NS	0.57, p < 0.01	p < 0.05
6 months	0.17, NS	0.75, p < 0.001	p < 0.005

TABLE 5. *Correlation of nurturance (postnatal) with physical and affectionate responsiveness to baby (1, 3, and 6 months postnatal), and significance of sex differences in correlation*

Time period	Boys (n = 30)	Girls (n = 27)	Sex difference
1 month	r = 0.25, NS	r = 0.58, p < 0.01	NS
3 months	0.31, NS	0.52, p < 0.01	NS
6 months	0.13, NS	0.70, p < 0.001	p < 0.01

TABLE 6. *Correlation of nurturance (postnatal) with acceptance of infant (1, 3, and 6 months postnatal), and significance of sex differences in correlation*

Time period	Boys (n = 30)	Girls (n = 27)	Sex difference
1 month	r = 0.14, NS	r = 0.57, p < 0.01	p < 0.10
3 months	−0.15, NS	0.39, p < 0.05	p < 0.05
6 months	−0.30, NS	0.65, p < 0.001	p < 0.001

maternal behaviors toward the infant reveal a similar but less dramatic sex-specific pattern than those with nurturance. For mothers of girls the correlations are mostly positive and significant. For mothers of boys the correlations are positive and significant for affective reaction to maternal role only.

The mothers in this study were followed rather closely throughout their pregnancies. Their adaptation during pregnancy was highly positively related to the personality variables, ego strength and nurturance. Thus, it seemed likely that the measure, adaptation to pregnancy, as defined in this chapter, might also be related to later maternal behavior measures. Adaptation to pregnancy was measured in the first and third trimesters of pregnancy. The relationship of the scores for the two time periods was much greater for mothers of girls (r = 0.58) than for mothers of boys (r = 0.33).

Adaptation to pregnancy measured during the third trimester was found to be positively related to affective reaction to maternal role for mothers of boys and girls. Table 9 shows that for mothers of girls, but not for mothers of boys, adaptation to pregnancy and physical and affectionate response to baby are positively and significantly related at all times. The data suggest that the better adapted a mother is during pregnancy, the more she will accept her maternal role and the baby—whether boy or girl. However, adaptation to pregnancy relates positively to responsiveness to baby only for mothers of girls.

TABLE 7. *Correlation of ego strength (postnatal) with affective reaction to maternal role (1, 3, and 6 months postnatal), and significance of sex differences in correlation*

Time period	Boys (n = 30)	Girls (n = 27)	Sex difference
1 month	$r = 0.38, p < 0.05$	$r = 0.50, p < 0.01$	NS
3 months	$0.43, p < 0.05$	$0.64, p < 0.001$	NS
6 months	$0.40, p < 0.05$	$0.74, p < 0.001$	$p < 0.10$

TABLE 8. *Correlation of ego strength (postnatal) with physical and affectionate responsiveness to baby (1, 3, and 6 months postnatal), and significance of sex differences in correlation*

Time period	Boys (n = 30)	Girls (n = 27)	Sex difference
1 month	$r = 0.24$, NS	$r = 0.42, p < 0.05$	NS
3 months	0.10, NS	$0.59, p < 0.001$	$p < 0.05$
6 months	0.18, NS	$0.68, p < 0.001$	$p < 0.05$

TABLE 9. *Correlations of adaptation to pregnancy (third trimester) with physical and affectionate responsiveness to baby (1, 3, and 6 months postnatal), and significance of sex differences in correlation*

Time period	Boys (n = 30)	Girls (n = 27)	Sex difference
1 month	$r = -0.24$, NS	$r = 0.45, p < 0.05$	$p < 0.005$
3 months	-0.04, NS	$0.43, p < 0.05$	$p < 0.05$
6 months	-0.22, NS	$0.63, p < 0.01$	$p < 0.001$

DISCUSSION

There are several findings which might be interpreted as supporting the notion that maternal behavior can be influenced by some infant characteristics: for example, emotional equilibrium of infant boys is related negatively to maternal individualization. This negative correlation of emotional equilibrium with individualization seems meaningful. The irritable, unstable, easily stressed baby would essentially demand more individualization from his mother. But why should the relationship hold only for boys? This study provides no satisfactory answers to this question.

The above discussion has implied that the infant characteristic influences maternal behavior, but the direction of effects, whether from infant to mother or mother to infant, cannot be deduced from correlational studies. We cannot interpret these findings too simply, i.e., as a unidirectional infant influence on the mother. Rather, there is a complex interaction between the personality characteristics of the mother, the sex of the infant, and the infant's characteristics. Sex of the infant appears to influence the relationships observed between infant characteristics and maternal behavior, but it is not at all clear if this influence is mediated by sex-specific maternal behavior or sex-specific infant behavior, or both. What is needed is research which clarifies what both mother and infant contribute to the dyadic interaction of mother and son and mother and daughter.

Much of the data reported in this chapter concerns the relationship of certain maternal personality dimensions to dimensions of maternal behavior toward the infant. The results indicate that some maternal behaviors are highly related to maternal ego strength and nurturance and to adaptation to pregnancy for mothers of girls but not for mothers of boys. We can only speculate on the meaning of these sex differences.

A baby girl may elicit certain maternal feelings, attitudes, and behavioral propensities having to do with the mother's feminine identity which in turn may affect her acceptance and responsiveness to her baby girl. Logically, these feelings and attitudes would also be related to her acceptance of her maternal role. These feelings and attitudes relating to feminine identity may be of less significance for a mother interacting with a baby boy. We speculate that a woman learns how to be a mother to a baby girl by her own experience of being mothered. The experience of learning to mother while being mothered can be called complementary role learning. It may lead a mother to feel that she knows intuitively how to interact with her baby girl. This may be reflected in the stronger relationships we observed between maternal personality and maternal behavior for mothers of baby girls. Perhaps maternal interaction with a male infant is more strongly influenced by the infant's behavior or situational factors.

Although little research has been done on the effect of sex of infant on the determinants of maternal behavior toward the infant, some data reported by Moss and Robson (1968) are relevant. They found that attitudes about mothering measured during pregnancy were positively related to the amount of eye-to-eye contact between mother and infant at one and three months. At one month this relationship was significant for male and female infants, but by three months it was even stronger for females and not significant for males. Furthermore, one measure of maternal attitude was positively correlated with a laboratory measure of total time of fixation on a social stimulus. Moss and Robson found it of interest that "maternal attitudes were predictive of maternal behavior toward girls and that this behavior had a bearing on the social learning of girls."

While the notion that sex of infant might serve to link certain dimensions of maternal personality (e.g., feminine identity) to maternal behavior toward the infant or to mediate the influence of infant characteristics on maternal behavior is an appealing idea, it remains highly speculative. Hopefully, future studies will investigate sex of infant as an intermediate variable affecting the motivational and attitudinal bases of maternal behavior toward the infant. Clearly, all studies of infant effects on parents or of parent-infant interaction should take into account sex of infant.

SUMMARY

Mothers of 27 female and 30 male first-born infants were studied by interview and psychological testing during their pregnancies and postnatally for six months. Measures obtained included: (1) personality characteristics—ego strength and nurturance; (2) adaptation to pregnancy; and (3) maternal behaviors—acceptance of maternal role, acceptance and individualization of baby, and responsiveness to baby. A measure of infant temperament, based on observations of the infant in the home, related positively to acceptance of the baby for mother-daughter pairs, and negatively to individualization of the baby for mother-son pairs. The measures of maternal personality and adaptation to pregnancy correlated positively with many of the measures of maternal behavior for mothers of girls but not for mothers of boys. It is suggested that sex of infant may act as an important variable mediating the relationship of infant temperamental and maternal personality characteristics to maternal behavior toward the infant.

[1]In the original study the items were grouped by principal components factor analyses. Often the same factor was defined by different items at different time periods. For conceptual reasons the factors were altered in this analysis so that they were composed of the same items at each time period. No new items were added to any factor.

[2]For reasons of economy, correlations with prenatal measures of maternal personality will not be presented. In general, these show very similar though less dramatic trends than the postnatal data. One would expect somewhat lower correlations in view of the greater time period separating the measures being correlated. The important point, however, is that the sex differences in correlations are still evident.

REFERENCES

Bell, R.Q. (1968) A Reinterpretation of the Direction of Effects in Studies of Socialization. *Psychological Review*, 75:81-95.

Bell, R.Q. (1971) Stimulus Control of Parent or Caretaker Behavior by Offspring. *Developmental Psychology*, 4:63-72.

Caldwell, B. (1964) The Effects of Infant Care. In: *Review of Child Development Research*, Vol. 1, edited by M.L. Hoffman and L.W. Hoffman. New York: Russell Sage Foundation.

Garai, J.E., and Scheinfeld, A. (1968) Sex Differences in Mental and Behavioral Traits. *Genetic Psychology Monographs*, 77:191-193.

Goldberg, S., and Lewis, M. (1969) Play Behavior in the Year Old Infant: Early Sex Differences. *Child Development*, 40:21-32.

Kagan, J., and Lewis, M. (1965) Studies of Attention in the Human Infant. *Merrill-Palmer Quarterly*, 11:95-127.

Kagan, J., and Moss, H.A. (1962) Birth to Maturity. New York: John Wiley and Sons.

Korner, A.F. (1965) Mother-Child Interaction: One or Two Way Street. *Social Work*, 10:47-51.

Korner, A.F. (1969) Neonatal Startles, Smiles, Erections and Reflex Sucks as Related to State, Sex and Individuality. *Child Development*, 40:1039-1053.

Korner, A.F. (1971) Individual Differences at Birth: Implications for Early Experience and Later Development. *American Journal Of Orthopsychiatry*, 4:608-619.

Moss, H.A., and Robson, K.S. (1968) Maternal Influences in Early Social Visual Behavior. *Child Development*, 39:401-408.

Rothbart, M.K., and Maccoby, E.E. (1966) Parents' Differential Reactions to Sons and Daughters. *Journal of Personality and Social Psychology*, 4:237-243.

Sears, R.R. (1951) A Theoretical Framework for Personality and Social Behavior. *American Psychologist*, 6:476-483.

Stern, G.G., Caldwell, B.M., Hersher, E.L., Lipton, E.L., and Richmond, J.B. (1969) A Factor Analytic Study of the Mother-Infant Dyad. *Child Development*, 40:163-181.

Thomas, A. et al. (1963) *Behavioral Individuality in Early Childhood*. New York: New York University Press.

Watson, J.S. (1969) Operant Conditioning of Visual Fixation in Infants Under Visual and Auditory Reinforcement. *Developmental Psychology*, 1:508-516.

*Psychological Aspects of a First Pregnancy
and Early Postnatal Adaptation.*
Raven Press, New York © 1974

Chapter XIII
Summary and Integration of Findings

Pauline M. Shereshefsky

During an important year in their lives, some 60 young, normal, middle-class, married couples involved themselves in a collaborative undertaking with a multidisciplinary research team concerned with an investigation into psychological aspects of pregnancy and early mother-infant adaptation. It was a year in which, in each family, the woman experienced a pregnancy and childbirth for the first time, and husband and wife assumed their new roles as father and mother. Each family involved themselves in exploring with the research team the psychological facts and meaning of their experiences during this year. When the infant was six months old, the formal collaboration ceased. Of the final sample of 57 families, 29 were engaged in casework counseling during pregnancy, and 28 participated in the research on a non-counseling basis. The families were all members of a comprehensive prepaid medical plan, and each woman had her own obstetrician throughout pregnancy and confinement. For three of the families the pregnancy ended with a reproductive casualty: a miscarriage, a stillbirth, and a premature birth resulting in death of the infant. Seven women of the group suffered postpartum psychiatric disorder following birth of the first child or within a six months' period after a second childbirth.

What we learned from the encounter with this study population is presented in terms of the two major areas of inquiry to which the study addressed itself: exploration of the psychodynamics associated with individual differences in adjustment to pregnancy and in early mother-infant adaptation; and evaluation of the effects of social work counseling on the course of pregnancy and on maternal adaptation.

SUMMARY OF FINDINGS

Adaptation to Pregnancy

Most predictive of the women's adaptation to a first pregnancy were several personality characteristics. Women high in nurturance and ego strength adapted well to the experience. The women who handled the pregnancy well also showed the capacity to visualize themselves as mothers both early in the pregnancy (the first trimester) and again during the second trimester. Concurrent with poor psychological adjustment during pregnancy was a high incidence of physiological disturbances.

A number of background variables, in addition to the personality variables, were explored in some depth: life history, which included the woman's perception of her own experience in being mothered, family adaptation, and external stresses (not pregnancy-engendered). Data on the woman's perception in being mothered yielded few correlations; these suggested a relationship between retrospective recall of her mother as being warm, empathic, close, and happy in her own mothering role, and current self-confidence and reduced anxiety about the physical aspects of the pregnancy, delivery, and unborn child.

The project showed that both external stresses and psychological needs (not pregnancy-engendered) are to be found in varied combinations in a large proportion of the families, even in a segment of the population in which a first pregnancy is experienced under relatively good socio-economic circumstances. Families burdened with more stresses had greater difficulty in accepting and adapting to the pregnancy and later in meeting the demands of the early period of adjustment to the newborn infant. Families already involved in serious marital disharmony at the time of the pregnancy (one-fifth of the sample) tended to have more stresses per family than others in the sample, implying special vulnerability and problem in coping preventively with potentially stressful conditions.

The psychological study of the woman (during the third or fourth month of the pregnancy) revealed no psychotic-like tendencies in the majority of women, unlike some of the researches of recent decades (Caplan, 1961; Bibring et al., 1961). Early in the pregnancy, many of the women (nearly three-fourths) gave anxious responses on psychological tests, and a number showed depressive feelings. Less than half gave responses indicating a happy, positive mood.

Most of the women were found to experience some heightening of emotional sensitivity and more lability than usual, especially in the first period of pregnancy. While many reported diminished vitality in the first trimester, by the seventh month approximately half of the group reported enhancement of a feeling of well-being.

There were fluctuations in reported anxiety; it was high in the first trimester, tended to subside in the second trimester, and then to rise again towards the end of the pregnancy when labor and delivery was imminent.

From the first to the third trimesters, marked changes occurred in several variables. The women showed increased clarity and confidence in visualizing themselves as mothers, and there was a concomitant reduction of anxiety regarding infant care, indicating movement in psychological preparation for maternity. There was also an improvement in husband-wife adaptation.

The woman's constant accommodations, throughout pregnancy, to bodily changes and alterations in her body image is most acute at the time of delivery. The opportunity to watch the delivery was found to have varying impact on the women, several women reacting with some feeling of anatomical assault and intensified fears about body intactness, and others with a sense of completion and discovery.

Our impressions from the interviews and test data were that a first pregnancy is a time of intensified psychological activity directed toward preparing for the culmination in labor and delivery and for the new tasks and commitment thereafter. It is an intrapsychic experience in which the woman tends to be primarily engrossed in immediate physiological changes and emotional developments in response to all aspects of the pregnancy.

Expectant Fathers

The expectant fathers also react to the pregnancy with considerable anxiety, a reactivation of parent-child conflicts, and intensified feelings about separation. We noted a marked increase in physical symptoms among the men; 65 per cent of the expectant fathers developed physical complaints similar to pregnancy symptoms (nausea, backache, gastrointestinal discomforts, etc.). Almost half of our sample reported a sharp decrease in sexual activity during the pregnancy; with the beginning of fetal movement, the husband is often disinclined to engage in sexual activity because of a fear of harming the baby. Fears for wife and baby are common. Many men expressed their envy of the pregnancy, either by denying its significance or, at the other extreme, almost fusing with the wife in an attempt to experience the pregnancy biologically. Overwork, auto accidents, drinking, and general restlessness gave indication of the degree of anxiety engendered by the pregnancy or the early period of fatherhood. We concluded that pregnancy and parenthood are crucial for the male as well as for the female.

Dreams During Pregnancy

The manifest dreams of these normal pregnant women clearly reflect the impact of pregnancy; almost half of the reported dreams were about the baby, and almost half of the dreams represented misfortune, harm, or environmental threat to the baby or mother. In this study the absence of masochism in dreams correlated with ratings signifying greater ego strength.

Maternal Adaptation

To what extent can we predict prenatally the woman's adaptation to motherhood? We found that acceptance of, and adaptation to, the pregnancy was significantly related to maternal adaptation. In addition, interest in and experience with children was significantly related. Of five predictors, four are variables summarizing the woman's level of adaptation during pregnancy. The pregnancy adaptation was thus clearly predictive of maternal adaptation. This important finding may, however, require some qualification as a result of a further study, which will be summarized briefly below, on the relation between maternal behavior and sex of the infant.

At all postnatal study periods (one, three, and six months), the personality variables measured postnatally, especially nurturance qualities of the woman, were highly related to maternal adaptation. Perhaps more striking is the close correspondence between the husband-wife adaptation and maternal adaptation; the woman's accommodation to the infant and her acceptance of the maternal role was found highly related to the quality of the relationship with her husband at this time.

A number of the women (39 per cent) were seen as somewhat better integrated following pregnancy and childbirth, and there was a statistically significant increase in the nurturant quality as between the prenatal and postnatal personality studies. These findings suggest that childbearing and the first months of mothering an infant facilitate positive developmental change for a substantial proportion of women.

Infantile Colic and Maternal Personality

Twelve of the 57 infants were diagnosed as having colic. There has been much speculation about the possible psychogenic origins of colic, with pediatricians and psychiatrists feeling that it may be related to the mother's personality. To test this hypothesis, we compared the mothers of colicky and non-colicky infants on a number of personality variables, and we found no significant differences. There were also no differences in adaptation to the maternal role.

Infant Adaptation

Maternal attitudes of acceptance of the maternal role and confidence in the maternal role were significantly related to several aspects of the infant's adaptation: his psychological adjustment and his physiological functioning (which included neurological status). The factor, infant alertness, was less related to maternal factors than were the infant adjustment and infant functioning factors, suggesting that the alertness variable may reflect patterns of reactivity that are at least partly constitutional.

Sex of Infant and Maternal Behavior

Subsequent to the initial analyses of maternal adaptation, in which no differentiation was made with regard to the sex of the infant, a selective analysis was made of items dealing with maternal responsiveness and the emotional equilibrium of the infant, differentiated by sex. The selected measures of maternal personality and adaptation to pregnancy were found to correlate positively with maternal behavior for mothers of girls but not for mothers of boys. Findings from this analysis suggest that sex of the infant may act as an important variable mediating the relationship of maternal behavior towards the infant.

Postpartum Psychiatric Disorders

Seven women in the study population were referred for psychiatric treatment within the six months following their first or second pregnancy; three were hospitalized. Each of the women fell into one of three premorbid categories: (1) well adapted and functioning well; (2) considerable neurotic symptomatology and character problems but functioning adequately; (3) severe long-standing characterological problems with recurrent disruptive anxiety or dysfunctional behavior. Three of the seven women had premorbid histories suggesting marked ego deficits, and two more had considerable neurotic symptomatology and character problems. The special study of these seven women, conducted a few years following completion of the initial study, led to the conclusion that the woman with considerable ego deficits is likely to develop symptoms at some point in the postpartum period, with childbirth itself not necessarily the disruptive stress. The data from this study indicate that the postpartum disorder which is precipitated by childbirth can be distinguished from a psychiatric disorder in the postpartum period which is not critically related to childbirth. We concluded that, for purposes of prediction and investigation of etiology, it would be helpful to consider only those disorders with onset in close contiguity to childbirth as "postpartum" and to differentiate the depressive from the schizophrenic syndromes.

Effects of Counseling

As a method of intervention aimed at reducing anxiety and facilitating maternal functioning, casework counseling was found useful and effective in some important phases of pregnancy adaptation. The women in the counseled group went through the labor and delivery experience with better adaptation than those in the control group. This finding, based on detailed obstetrical recording, was supported by subjective reports that the counseled women gave of their reactions to the labor and delivery experience (less fearful, less painful, more satisfying) as compared with reactions of the non-counseled group. We concluded that by helping the woman in her preparation for labor and delivery, the counseling relationship enabled her to cope better with the childbearing experience. Further findings from the prenatal period indicate that counseling served to accentuate changes precipitated by the pregnancy, such as in the woman's confidence and clarity in visualizing herself in the role of mother and in becoming more fully identified with her husband in the new family configuration.

There were no significant effects of the counseling on maternal adaptation nor were there any significant differences in the adaptation of the infants from the counseled and control groups. However, a comparison of the level of marital adjustment at six months postpartum and at the beginning of the pregnancy (first trimester) showed that the marital relationship of the non-counseled group had significantly deteriorated, while the counseled group was found to have held to the initial level. After the period of formal project participation, there were group sessions of project patients which revealed other differences between the counseled and control groups. It was our impression from these sessions that the counseled women were more content in the role of mother. They were clearly more open in acknowledging and discussing emotional reactions and psychological needs.

In the analysis of prenatal counseling, we identified three counseling approaches: Interpretation, Clarification, and Anticipatory Guidance. These were found to show substantial differences in outcome. Of the three approaches used, anticipatory guidance was the most effective in terms of promoting a higher level of maternal adaptation. It is probable that there were significant counselor effects which may have obscured evaluation of the impact of the counseling.

REVIEW AND INTEGRATION OF FINDINGS

The first chapter of this volume includes the major assumptions and premises which guided the development of this research design. Since a decade has elapsed between the time of planning the project and the task of preparing this report on it for a larger audience, it is appropriate to indicate where our further experience has led us.

The Mother's Psychological State and Infant Development

The hypothesis that the mother's psychological state is a crucial influence affecting infant development is certainly implicit in the findings of this research, even though it is not explicit. The woman's psychological state during pregnancy was clearly predictive of her adaptation to maternal functioning, and maternal behavior and infant adaptation were closely associated, except for one factor, infant alertness. An interesting complicating element was introduced into our perspectives on maternal adaptation by the finding that maternal behavior was predictable but only for mothers of girl infants, not for mothers of male infants; in other words, women react to the maternal role with more variation if the newborn infant is a boy.

Our results on the mother's psychological state during pregnancy indicate that adjustment to the circumstance of childbirth can be identified fairly early in pregnancy. Since the woman's personality characteristics of ego strength and nurturance, and her confidence and clarity in visualizing herself as mother, as assessed early in the pregnancy, were all *predictors* of pregnancy adaptation, the early assessment can be used to anticipate the woman's adaptive and coping capacity. The results also emphasize the close relationship between the woman's physical well-being and her predominant mood and emotional adaptations during pregnancy; the women with more pregnancy-related medical symptoms can be expected to suffer greater psychological strain (although this does not establish a cause-and-effect relationship between these variables). If women with special adaptive problems can indeed be identified early in the pregnancy, it then may be possible to bring psychotherapeutic measures to bear in selected cases determined to be especially vulnerable, so that maladaptive attitudes are less likely to become fixed and damaging to mother, child, or family as a whole.

The Concept of a First Pregnancy as Crisis

"Neither birth nor death has ever, anywhere, been regarded entirely as a 'natural' phenomenon. On the contrary, birth provides an ideal opportunity for understanding the way in which culture enmeshes the crucial facts of nature in a symbolic network.... The attribution of cultural significance blocks but also awakens anxiety, conceals but also expresses the human situation" (Chertok, 1969, p. 37). This statement, in the context of referring to the anthropological approach to conception and pregnancy by Mead and Newton (1935, 1965), leads into the issue of whether pregnancy, or at least a first pregnancy, is a "natural" phenomenon or is indeed a "crisis."

In the course of our study, we came to see that pregnancy-as-crisis may connote different meanings. If the term "pregnancy-as-crisis" is used to mean a stress involving threat or loss and requiring resources beyond the ordinary, then our data suggest that a first pregnancy is not, generally, a crisis in these terms. It is true that some of the families were especially susceptible to crisis and involved in crises in this meaning of the term, but under special circumstances. These were families either already burdened with stresses of various degrees of seriousness when the pregnancy occurred or they suffered some loss or threat which in combination with the pregnancy made the period one of major anxiety and distress.

However, in the use of the term crisis in the sense of a transitional phase or its dictionary definition of a "turning point," our young women and their husbands were indeed involved in a crisis. In all cases in our sample the first pregnancy made substantial demands for change in current routines of living and, obviously, in issues and decisions involving the future—demands which were sometimes onerous and resisted in different ways and degrees, and sometimes anticipated and met with an investment of positive feelings that varied from little to all-out involvement. Pregnancy was also a turning point in terms of inner reality in that it allowed or even forced the woman to become aware of her intrapsychic self—of her body image and her feeling responses especially. The impact on the man's self-concepts was often of equal force.

We think a distinction in use of the term is indicated to remove any lingering tendency to view pregnancy as illness and to differentiate and specify those circumstances that indicate clear need for psychological help. Perhaps we need new and different terms to carry the meaning of transitional or rites-of-passage experiences (van Gennep, 1960).

Receptivity of Pregnant Women to Psychological Study and Intervention

Several researchers report on the readiness of pregnant women to participate in programs of psychological study and their relative openness to psychotherapeutic intervention at this time (Caplan, 1961; Bibring, 1961; Wenner and Cohen, 1968; Grimm, 1969). Data from our study only partially confirm these findings. It is true that the women in our study, as in the others cited, quite readily volunteered to participate as research subjects, and those who were found to meet our criteria were entirely responsible in lending themselves to the procedures involved and faithful in remaining throughout the year designated for participation with us.

We recognized, however, that the nature of the collaboration varied greatly, from those situations in which the families invested themselves fully and worked seriously on their psychological problems, to those in which they participated in the counseling in form only and maintained the role of information-giving, research subjects throughout. Not all women in our sample found the pregnancy a time of major stress, in fact, and some couples seemed well able to sustain themselves and support each other in the more anxiety-laden aspects, drawing on varied resources within themselves and in the environment to make the transition to parenthood an essentially positive experience. Not all families wanted intervention during the period of the first pregnancy, as a few of the women indicated in our follow-up group sessions, and this was true for a variety of reasons, some healthful and sound, some questionable by any criterion of mental health.

It should be kept in mind that in our study the central criterion by which success or failure of counseling efforts was judged was the quality of the infant's environment created by the parents, the mother especially, in the first six months of life. While our study disclosed some areas in the adaptation to pregnancy, especially the aspect of coping with labor and delivery, in which counseling was clearly effective, on the basis of comparison of the counseled and non-counseled groups, neither maternal adaptation nor infant behavior showed effects of the counseling in quantitatively identifiable terms.

It was peculiarly difficult to tie to the brief engagement in counseling so subtle and pervasive a quality as maternal environment. In any case, we are inclined to the view that the pattern of mothering that comes into being with the infant has its origins in layers of emotional, familial, and cultural experience that a brief exposure to counseling or psychotherapy can scarcely influence appreciably. Moreover, the data from infant development studies increasingly point to the central unpredictable factor that may greatly affect the mothering response: the characteristics of the particular infant (Yarrow, 1963, 1968; Bell, 1968). In respect to the counseling phase of the project we ended with a sense of smaller gains than expected and concern that in a few instances the effect of the engagement may have been more nega-tive than positive.

Of the few other studies involving intervention during pregnancy, not all report complete satisfaction with their results from intervention. In reporting on the clearly positive findings from his study of the effectiveness of psychoprophylactic measures (PPM) in preparing a group of French married women, also primigravidae, for labor and delivery, Chertok notes, "Preparation essentially furnishes a model of behavior to which the women try to adhere." He indicates that a woman's behavior but not her subjective response to pain can be modified by this method of intervention. He concludes, "On the whole, our results suggest that the benefits derived from PPM, although unde-niable, nevertheless remain at a relatively superficial level and are accompanied only to a limited extent by the reduction of anxiety that one might expect to find" (Chertok, 1969, pp. 115-117).

That women with a defined problem around pregnancy and with

motivation for engagement in treatment—like the women suffering from habitual abortion, reported by Grimm (1967)—are clearly responsive to psychological help during pregnancy, while our sample were less universally responsive, suggests questions about the particular kinds of intervention that might be needed and useful. Are psychological services that are geared to psychopathology appropriate for the relatively healthy sector of the population?

The question of appropriate services may in part be answered by the fact that anticipatory guidance, as one of the three major techniques used in our project, was the one that was found to be most effective. As a technique that is not directed to curative ends but, rather, to facilitating the movement to a changed situation under circumstances that are both anxiety-provoking and challenging, anticipatory guidance may well result in allaying anxiety while freeing the woman and the man to respond to the dynamics of change, ushered in by childbirth and the infant, in its releasing, invigorating impact.

A Selective Approach to Intervention During Pregnancy

We have been at pains to explore and reconsider pregnancy-as-crisis and the view that women during a first pregnancy are more responsive to intervention than at other times. While this project did not, as indicated earlier, entirely substantiate these assumptions, it did indicate that, under special circumstances, many families can make effective use of even brief encounters with psychologically oriented professional people. The project also revealed important areas of need for psychological help during pregnancy.

Possibly the most burdensome and most pervasively disruptive stress was the circumstance of marital disharmony because of its portent for the future of the newborn infant as well as because of its effect in diverting energies of husband and wife at a time when support from the spouse might have been most needed and appropriate. The one-fifth of the couples who were already involved in serious marital disharmony at the time of the first pregnancy disclosed this drain on psychological resources that occurred in the conflict over the marriage.

Three of the seven women from this sample who developed postpartum psychiatric disorder either with the first or a second pregnancy, as described earlier in the report, had been found to be unusually fragile when tested and interviewed at the three months' prenatal study; they revealed recurrent, intense, disruptive anxiety and maladaptive functioning. Two others revealed neurotic symptomatology. From the follow-up study several years later, we came to the recognition that the woman with substantial ego deficits is likely to develop symptoms at some point in the postpartum period.

Both the families with serious marital problems and the women with considerable ego deficits were readily identifiable early in pregnancy through the study procedures outlined here.

Two groups have thus been singled out as particularly vulnerable during pregnancy: (1) those with non-pregnancy-related stresses to which they are reacting with a sense of marked difficulty in coping (most prominent among this group are families with serious marital disharmony at the time of the pregnancy), and (2) women with a chronic maladaptive pattern of response to new maturational tasks. We see these two groups as representing psychosocial hazards during pregnancy, in the sense that their current dysfunction and their vulnerability to stress represent threats to the adequacy and continuity of their mothering behavior and to family life.

It appears appropriate to suggest that diagnostic services should be offered during pregnancy in order to identify women and families in these two groups as a "population at risk" that cuts across socio-economic class lines, and to make psychotherapeutic services available to this group in the effort to prevent personality deterioration of the new parent and distortions in personality development of the young infant.

In Chapter I we set forth the fact that lower-class socio-economic populations have constituted a "population at risk" in the sense that reproductive difficulty of many kinds (stillbirth, neonatal death, congenital malformations of the central nervous system, prematurity, etc.) is closely correlated with lower socio-economic status and that there is a generational chain effect of lower-class economic conditions:

> Women begin their preparation for childbearing early in life—indeed, they begin it at the time of their own conception. Adult health, which has so strong a bearing on reproductive functioning, is the end result of a series of social and physical experiences which begin with fetal health or injury and continue throughout childhood and adolescence. The forces that determine childhood growth and adult health are interwoven with social processes which influence value systems and have significant effects on courtship, ages at marriage and conception, attitudes towards

...pregnancy, health and illness, and toward behavior concerning birth control and child spacing (Illsley, 1967), p. 76).

These observations with respect to the population at risk because of poverty are equally relevant to the population at risk because of the psychosocial factors that were identified in the study under consideration. Problems of screening and case finding are more difficult in cases of psychosocial issues but should not prove insurmountable, given adequate motivation to safeguard early infant development and the family environment.

Psychological and Physiological Realities

To the extent that there has been a single theme throughout this exploration of the psychodynamics of the maternity cycle, it has centered around the close interrelation of physiological and psychological developments. Each woman had to make accommodation to the physical aspects of pregnancy, childbirth, and lactation. For some this accommodation was made with relative ease; for others it came hard indeed.

Those women who had special difficulty with the accommodation responded to the physiological and other changes of this period as burdens superimposed on them, the whole development an occurrence controlled by some inexorable fate. Their womanhood itself became burdensome as they found themselves engaged in encounter with an alien, outside force.

For the essential adaptation, always in process but most keenly and unavoidably realized at this point in time, is to the fact of being a woman. That reality was now experienced in relation to a build-up of bodily discomforts, inconveniences, intermittent periods of marked fatigue, and some degree of pain—all of this, and the end to which it was directed, necessarily affecting body image and total self-concept.

The woman who, by the time of her first pregnancy, has accepted as her own the choice to have a child and, even more, the commitment of responsibility for another implicit in that choice, has achieved a sense of wholeness and self-acceptance—as a woman and as a person. With self-acceptance as a woman and recognition of her own part in this choice to have a child, she has, for the time at least, subordinated more individual self-expression to her generic role. Responding to pregnancy, childbirth, and maternity as self-willed, she is able to cope with, accept, and internalize the physiological processes as necessary and life-giving. It is this harmony of psychological involvement with the realities of childbearing and motherhood that makes discomfort and pain bearable and robs childbirth of a sense of threat or terror, freeing the woman's energies for moving into the role of mother with anticipation and excitement over her expanding capacities.

The preceding chapters have presented facts about the study sample, statistical correlations, case illustrations, taped sessions in which the study population speak for themselves, observations and interpretations in which the researchers attempt to fit the separate parts into general-izations of wider meaning and usefulness. It may be appropriate to leave the last word to the woman herself. Here is a woman in fiction in 14th Century Norway, who comes through a prolonged, tortured childbirth and sees that her infant lives and breathes: "It was as though she grew awake right into her inmost heart—this was her son, and he had striven for his life even as had she" (Undset, 1965, p. 344). And, from one of our 20th Century project women, a comment about childbirth close in feeling to the woman of fiction of another era and setting: "I felt alive in every part of me."

REFERENCES

Bell, R.Q. (1968) A Reinterpretation of the Direction of Effects in Studies of Socialization. *Psychological Review,* 75:81-95.

Bibring, C.S., Dwyer, T.F., Huntington, D.S., Valenstein, A.F. (1961) A Study of the Psychologi-cal Processes in Pregnancy and the Earliest Mother-Child Relationship. *The Psychoanalytic Study of the Child,* Vol. XVI. New York: International Universities Press.

Caplan, G. (1961) *An Approach to Community Mental Health.* New York: Grune and Stratton.

Chertok, L. (1969) *Motherhood and Personality. Psychosomatic Aspects of Childbirth.* Philadelphia: J.P. Lippincott.

Grimm, E.R. (1967) Psychological and Social Factors in Pregnancy, Delivery and Outcome. In: *Childbearing—Its Social and Psychological Aspects,* edited by S.A. Richardson and A.F. Guttmacher. Baltimore: Williams and Wilkins Co.

Grimm, E.R. (1969) Women's Attitudes and Reactions to Childbearing. In: *Modern Woman,* edited by G.D. Goldman and D.S. Milman. Springfield, Ill.: Charles C. Thomas.

Illsley, R. (1967) The Sociological Study of Reproduction and Its Outcome. In: *Childbearing—Its Social and Psychological Aspects,* edited by S.A. Richardson and A.F. Guttmacher. Baltimore: Williams and Wilkins Co.

Mead, M. (1935) *Sex and Temperament in Three Primitive Societies.* London: Routledge.

Mead, M., and Newton, N. (1965) Conception, Pregnancy, Labor and Puerperium in Cultural Perspective. In: *Proceedings of the First International Congress of Psychosomatic Medicine and Childbirth.* Paris: Gauthier-Villars.

Undset, S. (1965) *Kristin Lavransdatter.* New York: Alfred Knopf.

van Gennep, A. (1960) *The Rites of Passage.* London: Routledge and Kegan Paul.

Wenner, N.K., and Cohen, M.B. (eds.) (1968) Emotional Aspects of Pregnancy. Final Report of Washington School of Psychiatry Project. Washington, D.C.

Yarrow. L.J. (1963) Research in Dimensions of Early Maternal Care. *Merrill-Palmer Quarterly,* 9:101-114.

Yarrow, L.J. (1968) Conceptualizing the Early Environment. In: *Early Child Care,* edited by Laura Dittmann. New York: Atherton Press.

APPENDICES

TABLE OF CONTENTS

Appendix A
Some Facts About
Group Health Association

During the Fall of 1972, GHA marked its 35th year as a pioneering medical care organization. It was the first urban, prepaid group medical practice plan in the United States. The founders of GHA were a group of employees of the Home Loan Bank Board and the Home Owners Loan Corporation who wanted to provide for themselves and their families the best possible medical care at reasonable cost. After lengthy planning and study, this pioneer group laid down the basic principles upon which GHA was founded. They visualized a member-owned health plan that would provide both preventive and curative, prepaid, comprehensive medical care on a group practice basis.

With these simple principles as guidelines, and with the help of a loan from the Home Loan Bank Board, GHA opened its first medical center on November 1, 1937. Available at first only to employees of the Home Owners Loan Corporation, the Association soon opened its membership to a number of other government agencies. Shortly thereafter, the right to enrollment was extended to all employees in the executive branch of Government, and then to all civilian Federal employees. By 1947, the Association had opened membership to all residents of the Washington area, regardless of employment.

Responsiblity for managing the affairs and property of GHA rests with GHA's nine-member Board of Trustees. Members elect this Board to represent them. They serve on a voluntary basis without pay. The Board has the ultimate responsibility and authority to establish guidelines as to the scope of health services, subscription rates, group enrollment contracts, and capital requirements. It is also charged with reviewing and adopting an annual budget, and prescribing the reporting procedures required of the Executive Director and officers of the Board.

In 1938, the second year of its operation, GHA's participant load was only 2,600. By the mid-fiscal year 1967-68, this figure exceeded 70,000.

APPENDIX B

PRENATAL COUNSELING PROJECT NIMH 503-A1

IDENTIFYING SOCIAL DATA

NAME: Address: Case #_____

                                                                          GHA #_____
                                         Telephone: Counselor_____
                         WIFE   HUSBAND   Obstetrician____
                                                                          D.E.D._____
BIRTHDATE   _____   _____   Date of Marriage_____
    Age at Pregnancy   _____   _____   Pregnancy Diagnosed

BIRTHPLACE   _____   _____   _____

                                                                 Accepted_____
RELIGIOUS
    AFFILIATION   _____   _____

HIGHEST SCHOOL
    GRADE   _____   _____

OCCUPATION   _____   _____

RACE   _____   _____

FATHER'S OCCUPATION   _____   _____

MOTHER'S OCCUPATION   _____   _____

SIBLINGS: Age Sex   Residence   Age Sex   Residence
            __ __   _____ __ __   _____
            __ __   _____ __ __   _____
            __ __   _____ __ __   _____
            __ __   _____ __ __   _____

MEDICAL HISTORY
    Asthma
    Cancer   _____   _____
    TB   _____   _____
    Ulcers   _____   _____
    Diabetes   _____   _____
    Other   _____   _____
    Marked physical   _____   _____
        disabilities   _____   _____

ORDINAL POSITION IN
    FAMILY   _____   _____

IF PARENT IS DEAD, YEAR   _____   _____

PREVIOUS MARITAL STATUS   _____   _____

PREVIOUS PREGNANCIES   _____

PSYCHIATRIC CARE, YEAR   _____   _____

OTHER PERSONS LIVING   _____
    IN HOME

1/30/64

4/15/64 REVISED
MH503-A2

GROUP HEALTH ASSOCIATION, INC.
Washington, D. C.

Prenatal Counseling Project

RATING SCHEDULE - PRENATAL

CASE NO._____

PERSON ASSESSING_____
              (Initials)(Date)
CONJOINT ASSESSMENT_____
                 (Date)

I.   SOCIAL BACKGROUND AND LIFE HISTORY

    A.   Extended Family (Check pertinent items)

	H U S B A N D			W I F E		
1. Proximity: In same community	Parents	Siblings	Other Sig- nificant Members	Parents	Sibls.	Other Sig- nificant Members
In another "						
2. Contact: Approx. Weekly						
Approx. Monthly						
Approx. Every Few Months						
Approx. Yearly or less often						

    B.   Religion

                  Husband   Wife

              ___ Plays no role . . . . . (1) ___
              ___ Plays little role . . . .(2) ___
              ___ Moderate influence . . (3) ___
              ___ Considerable influence (4) ___
              ___ Very influential . . . . (5) ___

C. Experiences in Being Mothered - Perception of Mother's Handling of
   Maternal·Role (Circle appropriate number below)

1. ANXIETY

1	2	3	4	5
Intense disruptive anxiety				Little or no anxiety

2. EMPATHY WITH CHILD

1	2	3	4	5
Insensitive even to expressed need		Awareness of child's varying needs and moods		Very sensitive and aware (even when minimally cued)

3. CLOSENESS TO CHILD

1	2	3	4	5
Distant		Close		Very close

4. INTRUSIVENESS

1	2	3	4	5
Intense aggressive involvement				Little or no intrusion on individuality

5. MOTHER'S REACTION TO HER MATERNAL ROLE

1	2	3	4	5
Actively resented demands	Disappointed, frustrated	Ambivalent	Satisfied	Marked gratification in her role

6. MOTHER-DAUGHTER RELATIONSHIP: EXTENT TO WHICH MOTHER SATISFIED EMOTIONAL
   NEEDS - INFANCY TO AGE 12

1	2	3	4	5
Support needs essentially unmet				Support needs essentially met

7. MOTHER-DAUGHTER RELATIONSHIP: EXTENT TO WHICH MOTHER SATISFIED EMOTIONAL
   NEEDS - AFTER AGE 12

1	2	3	4	5
Support needs essentially unmet				Support needs essentially met

CASE NO._____

D. Experiences Related to Development of Identity

8. IDENTIFICATION WITH PARENTS
    Major identification: With father_____ With mother_____;
                           No definite identification with either_____

9. SCHOOL ACHIEVEMENT

1	2	3	4	5
Consistent academic failure	Poor student	Average student	Good student	Consistent academic success

10. SCHOOL ADJUSTMENT

1	2	3	4	5
Behavior poor (in trouble)	Intermittent trouble	Intermittently adaptive	Adaptive behavior	Successful and rewarding

11. WORK PERFORMANCE   None____

1	2	3	4	5
Consistent job failure	Low job performance	Average job performance	Above average	Progressive successful job experience

12. PEER RELATIONSHIPS

1	2	3	4	5
Lonely, isolated		Fairly close		Close and meaningful

13. INTEREST IN YOUNGER CHILDREN

1	2	3	4	5
Resentful	Interested	Mild	Moderate	Eager

14. EXPERIENCE WITH YOUNGER CHILDREN

1	2	3	4	5
Little or none	Some	Moderate	Considerable	Constant responsibility for younger children

CASE NO._____

II. CURRENT PERSONALITY (Check pertinent items)

15. Diagnostic Classification
    15.1____Normal - Normal
    15.2____Normal with tendency towards psychosomatic disorders
    15.3____Normal with tendency towards psychoneurotic disorders
    15.4____Normal with tendency towards character or personality disorders
    15.5____   Borderline psychotic
    15.6____Psychosomatic
    15.7____Psychoneurotic
    15.8____Character and personality disorders
    15.9____Psychotic
    15.0____Others (specify):

16. Predominant Defenses
    16.1____Denial
    16.2____Repression
    16.3____Projection
    16.4____Intellectualization
    16.5____Reaction formation
    16.6____Regression
    16.7____Isolation
    16.8____Acting Out
    16.9____Other (Specify):

17. Predominant Defense System (use if appropriate)
    17.1____Obsessional
    17.2____Hysterical
    17.3____Affective
    17.4____Acting Out
    17.5____Somatization
    17.6____Schizoid
    17.7____Other (Specify):

18. Intellectual Adaptation - Control
    ____Largely emotional
    ____Not excessively one or the other - balanced
    ____Largely governed by logic and reason

19. Intellectual Adaptation - Mode of thinking
    ____Predominantly philosophical and contemplative
    ____Contemplative
    ____Not excessively one or the other
    ____Practical
    ____Picky

20. Emotional Adaptation - Characteristic way of expressing feeling

    20.1____Hostile and explosive (Rate 1 - 5, from high to low)
    20.2____Impulsive (Rate 1 - 5, from high to low)
    20.3____Repressed (Rate 1 - 5, from high to low)
    20.4____Tender and affectionate (Rate 1 - 5, from low to high)
    20.5____Adapted (Rate 1 - 5, from low to high)

II.   CURRENT PERSONALITY (Cont'd.)

21.   ANXIETY (Circle appropriate number)

1	2	3	4	5
Intense dis-ruptive anxiety				Little or no anxiety

22.   EASE OF FANTASY PRODUCTION

1	2	3	4	5
Constricted - Little or no fantasy	Spontaneous but not especially creative	Spontaneous, creative	Tendency towards fantasy living	Excessive fan-tasy living

23.   CONCERN FOR APPEARANCE (Concern with and pleasure in appearance, desire to please)

1	2	3	4	5
Inappropriate neglect				Excessive preoccupa-tion with physical care and appearance

24.   GRATIFICATION IN FEMALE SEXUALITY

1	2	3	4	5
No enjoyment, or actual distaste		Moderate enjoyment		Marked enjoyment

25.   RESPONSIVENESS TO HUSBAND

1	2	3	4	5
Ungiving		Moderately giving		Fully Giving

26.   RESPONSIVENESS TO OTHERS - GIVING AND NURTURANT QUALITY

1	2	3	4	5
Ungiving		Moderately giving		Highly generous; very giving

27.   FLEXIBILITY

1	2	3	4	5
Highly resistant to change or stress		Accommodates after some resistance or delay to change and ordinary stress		Easy accommodation to change (able to "roll with the punches")

28.   SENSE OF HUMOR

1	2	3	4	5
Little or None		Moderately good		Keen

CASE NO._____

II. CURRENT PERSONALITY (Cont'd.)

29. OVERT DEPENDENCY BEHAVIOR

1	2	3	4	5
Clinging to dependency status		Emancipated, adult give-and-take		Marked independence

30. COVERT, UNDERLYING DEPENDENCY PATTERN

1	2	3	4	5
Very strong dependency wishes		Moderate dependency wishes		Little dependency wishes

31. ABILITY TO MEET OWN NEEDS, INCLUDING PLEASURE

1	2	3	4	5
Poor		Average		Marked Ability

32. PASSIVE AGGRESSIVE PATTERN

1	2	3	4	5
Extremely passive				Aggressive

33. SUPEREGO

1	2	3	4	5
Weak superego		Strong superego but can yield		Stringent or rigid unyielding superego demands with guilt if not met

34. INSIGHT INTO SELF

1	2	3	4	5
No insight	Little insight	Fair degree of insight	Considerable insight	Very insightful

35. ACCEPTANCE OF OWN IDENTITY

1	2	3	4	5
Strong rejection of identity		Ambivalence		Positive attitudes - self acceptance

36. SENSE OF SUCCESS AS A WIFE

1	2	3	4	5
Evaluates self as unsuccessful		Evaluates self as fairly adequate		Evaluates self as highly successful

37. SENSE OF SUCCESS AS HOMEMAKER

1	2	3	4	5
Evaluates self as poor		Evaluates self as average		Evaluates self as successful

CASE NO._____

II. CURRENT PERSONALITY (Cont'd.)

38. ACHIEVEMENT OF AN ADULT ROLE

1	2	3	4	5
Childishness		Ambivalence as to adult status		Distinctly mature and clear as to adult status

39. CAPACITY FOR CLOSENESS

1	2	3	4	5
Shallow and distant		Fairly close		Intense meaningful relationships

40. ABILITY TO TAKE HELP

1	2	3	4	5
No acceptance	Tends to defeat or deflect help	Optimal acceptance	Accepts help passively	Extremely dependent

41. ABILITY TO GIVE HELP AND SUPPORT

1	2	3	4	5
Unable to give	Gives grudingly	Gives on own terms	Gives on request	Gives freely on sensing need

42. NEED TO CONTROL

1	2	3	4	5
Rigidly controlling		Neither submissive nor controlling		Submits easily

43. OVERALL EVALUATION OF ADAPTIVE BEHAVIOR

1	2	3	4	5
Defenses basically inadequate to deal with needs				Defenses highly adequate

CASE NO._____

III. CURRENT LIFE SITUATION

    A. Family Adaptation

44. DEPENDENCY BEHAVIOR

1	2	3	4	5
Clings to wife for support	Moderately dependent on wife	Adult give-and-take	Largely independent	Renunciation of any dependency

45. EMPATHY

1	2	3	4	5
Insensitive even to expressed needs		Awareness of varying moods and needs		Very sensitive & aware (even when minimally cued)

46. COMMUNICATION

1	2	3	4	5
Very inhibited about talking to wife	Moderately inhibited	Cautious about initiating talk re feelings	Fairly open	Uninhibited and free

47. AFFECTION

1	2	3	4	5
Minimal				Intense

48. HOSTILITY

1	2	3	4	5
Intense				Minimal

49. SEXUAL ADJUSTMENT

1	2	3	4	5
Restricted & unsatisfying		Generally satisfying (no specific problem)		Highly satisfying

50. DECISION PROCESS

1	2	3	4	5
Resolved only after serious conflict		Resolution achieved without major threat to relationship		Flexibility in arriving at joint decisions, each moving from dominant to passive position without threat to self or the relationship

III. CURRENT LIFE SITUATION (Cont'd.)

51. REACTION TO WIFE IN RE PREGNANCY

1	2	3	4	5.
Dejected	Unresponsive	Contented	Very satisfied	Enthusiastic

52. REACTION TO BABY-TO-BE

1	2	3	4	5
Dejected	Unresponsive	Contented	Very satisfied	Enthusiastic

53. EXTENT TO WHICH HUSBAND ALLOWS DEPENDENCY

1	2	3	4	5.
Impatient, hostile attitude towards wife's dependency		Allows dependency in stress situations		Responds fully to wife's need for support

54. HUSBAND"S FOSTERING OF SELF-CONFIDENCE IN WIFE AS A MOTHER

1	2	3	4	5
Attitudes & actions generally belittling and destructive		Expresses intermittent doubt & questions about wife's capacity to become a mother		Fully sustains wife in belief in her capacity as a mother

55. FEELINGS RE SHARING WIFE

1	2	3	4	5
Clearly impatient & jealous of sharing wife		Normally able to share wife		Eager to share wife with a child

56. CONGRUENCE OF THE PREGNANCY WITH CURRENT WAY OF LIFE

1	2	3	4	5
Disruptive, incongruent	Interruptive but manageable	Generally consonant with aims and resources	Consonant	Highly consonant

57. CONGRUENCE OF THE PREGNANCY WITH LONG-TIME PLANS

1	2	3	4	5
Disruptive, incongruent	Interruptive but manageable	Generally consonant with aims and resources	Consonant	Highly consonant

58. IDENTITY AS COUPLE

1	2	3	4	5
Completely individualistic		Both identity as a married couple & identity as individuals		Little individual differentiation; couple acts as symbiotic unit

III. CURRENT LIFE SITUATION (Cont'd.)

59. HUSBAND-WIFE ADAPTATION

1	2	3	4	5
Very poor adaptation	Poor adaptation	Intermittently good	Good	Excellent

B. Current Stresses (Check pertinent items)

60._____Anxiety about financial security

61._____Food and management problems

62._____ Illness or recent death in extended family

63._____ Illness of husband or wife

64._____ Problems with relatives

65._____ Problems re spouse of previous marriage

66._____ Problems re friends

67._____ Job dissatisfaction for wife

68._____ Job dissatisfaction for husband

69._____ Religious differences

70._____ Other (specify, such as: political differences, etc.)

CASE NO. _____
PERSON ASSESSING _____
                    (initials) (Date)
CONJOINT ASSESSMENT _____ (Date)
TRIMESTER: 1st_____ 3rd_____

IV.   PREGNANCY EXPERIENCE

71.   Problems in conception? Yes____, No_____

72.   Planned pregnancy? Yes_____, No_____

73   PREDOMINANT ATTITUDE OR MOOD (Circle appropriate number)

1	2	3	4	5
Extremely reject-ing of pregnancy	Moderately rejecting	Contented	Very satisfied	Enthusiastic

74.   HOPES OR EXPECTATIONS RE SEX OF CHILD (check)

_____Male, _____Female, _____No specific preference

75.   CLARITY OF IMAGE OF CHILD (circle)

1	2	3	4	5
No visualization or image of child		Wavering or unclear image		Visualizes infant in some detail and clarity

76.   PLANS FOR INFANT FEEDING (Check)

_____Breast, _____Bottle, _____No choice made prior to delivery

Rate the following items from (1) Intense disruptive anxiety to (5)Little or no anxiety, and circle appropriate number

77. ANXIETIES AND FEARS RE: PHYSICAL ASPECTS	1	2	3 4 5
78. ANXIETIES AND FEARS RE: BODY IMAGE	1	2	3 4 5
79. ANXIETIES AND FEARS RE: DELIVERY	1	2	3 4 5
80. ANXIETIES AND FEARS RE: INFANT FEEDING	1	2	3 4 5
81. ANXIETIES AND FEARS RE: UNBORN BABY	1	2	3 4 5
82. ANXIETIES AND FEARS RE: SEXUAL ROLE WITH HUSBAND	1	2	3 4 5
83. ANXIETIES AND FEARS RE: CARE OF INFANT-TO-BE	1	2	3 4 5

84.   DEPENDENCY PATTERN TO HUSBAND (Circle)

1	2	3	4	5
Clings to husband for support in al-most all areas		Mutual give-and-take		Renounces any dependency on husband

85.   DEPENDENCY PATTERN TO OTHERS

Clings to others for support or decision	Emancipated, adult give-and-take	Renunciation of any dependency on other people

CASE NO._____

IV. PREGNANCY EXPERIENCE (Cont'd.)

86. MOTHER-DAUGHTER RELATIONSHIP DURING PREGNANCY

1	2	3	4	5
Support needs essentially unmet				Support needs essentially met

87. CLARITY IN VISUALIZING SELF AS MOTHER

1	2	3	4	5
Unable to picture self as a mother		Can visualize self as mother but not clearly		Visualizes self as mother with great claity

88. CONFIDENCE IN VISUALIZING SELF AS MOTHER

1	2	3	4	5
Visualizes self as very unsure in that role		Visualizes self as handling the mother role sometimes confidently, sometimes uncertainly		Visualizes self handling the role of mother with confidence & assurance

89. ACTIVITY AND INACTIVITY IN PREGNANCY

1	2	3	4	5
Denial (Overactivity)		Constructive use of the passivity in personal gowth		Avoidance of all activity (even that which is well within capacity)

90. PATTERNS OF CARRYING CUSTOMARY RESPONSIBILITIES

1	2	3	4	5
Shifts responsibilities to others (husband, etc.) as completely & quickly as possible,i.e.,she uses pregnancy to evade them.				Shifts responsibilities only as her growing physical limitations demand, i.e., appropriately

91. NARCISSISM

1	2	3	4	5
Little or no concern with self		Appropriately concerned about self, i.e.,not out of perspective		Excessive preoccupation and concern with self

Rev. 8/17/64

CASE NO. _____

IV. PREGNANCY EXPERIENCE (cont'd)   TRIMESTER: 1st_____3rd_____

92. EFFECT OF PREGNANCY ON SEXUAL RELATIONSHIP WITH HUSBAND

1	2	3	4	5
Decreased sat- isfaction		No change		Increased satis- faction

93. EFFECT OF PREGNANCY ON FEELING OF WELL-BEING

1	2	3	4	5
Hypochondriacal	Diminished vitality	Little effect	Good effect	Marked en- hancement of feelings of well-being

94. ADAPTABILITY TO CHANGES OF PREGNANCY

1	2	3	4	5
Resents changes precipitated by the pregnancy		Accepts & adjusts to the changes		Enthusiastically accepts & makes smooth adaptation to changes

95. EVIDENCE OF GROWTH TOWARDS NEW FAMILY IDENTIFICATION

1	2	3	4	5
Little or none		Shows a trend		Marked evidence

Rate the following items from (1) Little significance to (5) Marked significance, and circle appropriate number.

96.	PREGNANCY AS:	CONFIRMATION OF FEMININE IDENTITY	1 2 3 4 5
97.	PREGNANCY AS:	VALIDATION OF SUCCESS AS RELATED TO MOTHER, SIBLS., OTHERS	1 2 3 4 5
98.	PREGNANCY AS:	EXTENSION OF SELF	1 2 3 4 5
99.	PREGNANCY AS:	VALIDATION OF COUPLE IN THEIR IDENTITY	1 2 3 4 5

MH503-A2
REV. 8/11/64

CASE NO. _____
PERSON ASSESSING_____
             (Initials) (Date)
CONJOINT ASSESSMENT_____
               (Date)

Prenatal Rating Schedule: 7th Month

I. Pregnancy Experience

73. PREDOMINANT ATTITUDE OR MOOD (Circle appropriate number)

1	2	3	4	5
Extremely reject-ing of pregnancy	Moderately rejecting	Contented	Very satisfied	Enthusiastic

74. HOPES OR EXPECTATIONS RE SEX OF CHILD (Check)

____Male, ____Female, ____No specific preference

75. CLARITY OF IMAGE OF CHILD (Circle)

1	2	3	4	5
No visualiza-tion or image of child		Wavering or unclear image		Visualizes infant in some detail & clarity

76. PLANS FOR INFANT FEEDING (Check)

____Breast,____Bottle,____No choice made prior to delivery

Rate the following items from (1) Intense disruptive anxiety to (5) Little or no anxiety, and circle appropriate number.

77. ANXIETIES AND FEARS RE: PHYSICAL ASPECTS 1   2   3   4   5
78. ANXIETIES AND FEARS RE: BODY IMAGE 1   2   3   4   5
79. ANXIETIES AND FEARS RE: DELIVERY 1   2   3   4   5
80. ANXIETIES AND FEARS RE: INFANT FEEDING 1   2   3   4   5
81. ANXIETIES AND FEARS RE: UNBORN BABY 1   2   3   4   5
82. ANXIETIES AND FEARS RE: SEXUAL ROLE WITH HUSBAND 1   2   3   4   5
83. ANXIETIES AND FEARS RE: CARE OF INFANT-TO-BE 1   2   3   4   5

84. DEPENDENCY PATTERN TO HUSBAND (Circle)

1	2	3	4	5
Clings to hus-band for support in almost all areas		Mutual give-and-take		Renounces any de-pendency on hus-band

85. DEPENDENCY PATTERN TO OTHERS

1	2	3	4	5
Clings to others for support or decision		Emancipated, adult give-and-take		Renunciation of any dependency on other people

Prenatal Rating Schedule: 7th Month

86.   MOTHER-DAUGHTER RELATIONSHIP DURING PREGNANCY   .

1	2	3	4	5
Support needs essentially unmet				Support needs essentially met

87.   CLARITY IN VISUALIZING SELF AS MOTHER

1	2	3	4	5
Unable to picture self as a mother		Can visualize self as mother but not clearly		Visualizes self as mother with great clarity

88.   CONFIDENCE IN VISUALIZING SELF AS MOTHER

1	2	3	4	5
Visualizes self as very unsure in that role		Visualizes self as handling the mother role sometimes confidently, sometimes uncertainly		Visualizes self handling the role of mother with confidence & assurance

89.   ACTIVITY AND INACTIVITY IN PREGNANCY

1	2	3	4	5
Denial (Overactivity)		Constructive use of the passivity in personal growth		Avoidance of all activity (even that which is well within capacity)

90.   PATTERNS OF CARRYING CUSTOMARY RESPONSIBILITIES

1	2	3	4	5
Shifts responsibilities to others (husband, etc.) as completely & quickly as possible, i.e., she uses pregnancy to evade them.				Shifts responsibilities only as her growing physical limitations demand, i.e.,appropriately

91.   NARCISSISM

1	2	3	4	5
Little or no concern with self		Appropriately concerned about self, i.e., not out of perspective		Excessive preoccupation and concern with self

Prenatal Rating Schedule: 7th Month

92. EFFECT OF PREGNANCY ON SEXUAL RELATIONSHIP WITH HUSBAND

1	2	3	4	5
Decreased sat- isfaction		No change		Increased satisfac- tion

93. EFFECT OF PREGNANCY ON FEELING OF WELL-BEING

1	2	3	4	5
Hypochondriacal	Diminished vitality	Little effect	Good effect	Marked enhancement of feeling of well- being

94. ADAPTABILITY TO CHANGES OF PREGNANCY

1	2	3	4	5
Resents changes precipitated by the pregnancy		Accepts & adjusts to the changes		Enthusiastically accepts and makes smooth adaptation to changes

95. EVIDENCE OF GROWTH TOWARDS NEW FAMILY IDENTIFICATION

1	2	3	4	5
Little or none		Shows a trend		Marked evidence

<u>59.</u> HUSBAND-WIFE ADAPTATION

1	2	3	4	5
Very poor Adaptation	Poor adapta- tion	Intermittently good	Good	Excellent

Rate the following items from (1) Little significance to (5)Marked significance and <u>circle</u> <u>appropriate</u> <u>number.</u>

96. PREGNANCY AS: CONFIRMATION OF FEMININE IDENTITY   1   2   3   4   5
97. PREGNANCY AS: VALIDATION OF SUCCESS AS RELATED
                    TO MOTHER,SIBLS.,OTHERS   1   2   3   4   5
98. PREGNANCY AS: EXTENSION OF SELF   1   2   3   4   5
99. PREGNANCY AS: VALIDATION OF COUPLE IN THEIR IDENTITY   1   2   3   4   5

REV. 3/1/65

MH503-A2
8/7/64

CASE NO. _____

PERSON ASSESSING_____
(Initials) (Date)

CONJOINT ASSESSMENT_____
(Date

Prenatal Rating Schedule: 9th Month

I. Pregnancy Experience

73. PREDOMINANT ATTITUDE OR MOOD (Circle appropriate number)

1	2	3	4	5
Extremely reject-ing of pregnancy	Moderately rejecting	Contented	Very satisfied	Enthusiastic

74. HOPES OR EXPECTATIONS RE SEX OF CHILD (Check)

____Male, ____Female,____No specific preference

75. CLARITY OF IMAGE OF CHILD (Circle)

1	2	3	4	5
No visualization or image of child		Wavering or unclear image		Visualizes infant in some detail and clarity

76. PLANS FOR INFANT FEEDING (Check)

____Breast, ____Bottle, ____No choice made prior to delivery

Rate the following items from (1) Intense disruptive anxiety to (5) Little or no anxiety, and circle appropriate number.

77. ANXIETIES AND FEARS RE: PHYSICAL ASPECTS 1   2   3   4   5
78. ANXIETIES AND FEARS RE: BODY IMAGE 1   2   3   4   5
79. ANXIETIES AND FEARS RE: DELIVERY 1   2   3   4   5
80. ANXIETIES AND FEARS RE: INFANT FEADING 1   2   3   4   5
81. ANXIETIES AND FEARS RE: UNBORN BABY 1   2   3   4   5
82. ANXIETIES AND FEARS RE: SEXUAL ROLE WITH HUSBAND 1   2   3   4   5
83. ANXIETIES AND FEARS RE: CARE OF INFANT-TO-BE 1   2   3   4   5

84. DEPENDENCY PATTERN TO HUSBAND (Circle)

1	2	3	4	5
Clings to hus-band for support in almost all areas		Mutual give-and-take		Renounces any de-pendency on husband

85. DEPENDENCY PATTERN TO OTHERS

1	2	3	4	5
Clings to others for support or decision		Emancipated, adult give-and-take		Renunciation of any dependency on other people

8/7/64

Prenatal Rating Schedule: 9th Month   CASE NO._____

I. Pregnancy Experience (Cont'd.)

86. MOTHER-DAUGHTER RELATIONSHIP DURING PREGNANCY

1	2	3	4	5
Support needs essentially unmet				Support needs essentially met

87. CLARITY IN VISUALIZING SELF AS MOTHER

1	2	3	4	5
Unable to picture self as a mother		Can visualize self as mother but not clearly		Visualizes self as mother with great clarity

88. CONFIDENCE IN VISUALIZING SELF AS MOTHER

1	2	3	4	5
Visualizes self as very unsure in that role		Visualizes self as handling the mother role sometimes confidently, sometimes uncertainly		Visualizes self handling the role of mother with confidence & assurance

89. ACTIVITY AND INACTIVITY IN PREGNANCY

1	2	3	4	5
Denial (Overactivity)		Constructive use of the passivity in personal growth		Avoidance of all activity (even that which is well within capacity)

90. PATTERNS OF CARRYING CUSTOMARY RESPONSIBILITIES

1	2	3	4	5
Shifts responsibilities to others (husband,etc.) as completely & quickly as possible,i.e., she uses pregnancy to evade them				Shifts responsibilities only as her growing physical limitations demand,i.e. appropriately

91. NARCISSISM

1	2	3	4	5
Little or no concern with self		Appropriately concerned about self, i.e., not out of perspective		Excessive preoccupation and concern with self

REVISED 10/5/64

CASE NO._____

Prenatal Rating Schedule: 9th Month

I. Pregnancy Experience (Cont'd.)

92. EFFECT OF PREGNANCY ON SEXUAL RELATIONSHIP WITH HUSBAND

1	2	3	4	5
Decreased satisfaction		No change		Increased satisfaction

93. EFFECT OF PREGNANCY ON FEELING OF WELL-BEING

1	2	3	4	5
Hypochondriacal	Diminished vitality	Little effect	Good effect	Marked enhancement of feeling of well-being

94. ADAPTABILITY TO CHANGES OF PREGNANCY

1	2	3	4	5
Resents changes precipitated by the pregnancy		Accepts & adjusts to the changes		Enthusiastically accepts & makes smooth adaptation to changes

95. EVIDENCE OF GROWTH TOWARDS NEW FAMILY IDENTIFICATION

1	2	3	4	5
Little or none		Shows a trend		Marked evidence

59. HUSBAND-WIFE ADAPTATION

1	2	3	4	5
Very poor adaptation	Poor adaptation	Intermittently good	Good	Excellent

Rate the following items from (1) Little significance to (5) Marked significance, and circle appropriate number.

96. PREGNANCY AS: CONFIRMATION OF FEMININE IDENTITY 1 2 3 4 5
97. PREGNANCY AS: VALIDATION OF SUCCESS AS RELATED
                  TO MOTHER, SIBLS., OTHERS 1 2 3 4 5
98. PREGNANCY AS: EXTENSION OF SELF 1 2 3 4 5
99. PREGNANCY AS: VALIDATION OF COUPLE IN THEIR IDENTITY 1 2 3 4 5

REVISED 10/5/64

Prenatal Rating Schedule: 9th Month

II. Woman's Response to Project

A. Subjective Reaction of Woman in Response to Project

Rate the following items from (1) Not at all to (5) Much
and circle appropriate number:

100. Degree of Helpfulness: SUPPORTIVE (Sustaining)   1   2   3   4   5
101. Degree of Helpfulness: EDUCATIONAL(Informational & Anticipatory)
                                                        1   2   3   4   5
102. Degree of Helpfulness: INSIGHT-STIMULATING (Clarification
      or intensified self-understanding or understanding of
      spouse or infant)   1   2   3   4   5

Rate the following items from (1) No significance to
(5) Marked Significance and circle appropriate number:

103. Areas of Help: HUSBAND-WIFE RELATIONSHIP   1   2   3   4   5
104. Areas of Help: RELATIONSHIP TO HER MOTHER   1   2   3   4   5
105. Areas of Help: DEALING WITH ANXIETIES ABOUT PREGNANCY 1   2   3   4   5
106. Areas of Help: SEEING SELF IN MATERNAL ROLE   1   2   3   4   5
107. Areas of Help: CHANGING FEELINGS ABOUT SELF 1   2   3   4   5

B. Objective Evaluation

108. Degree of Helpfulness: SUPPORTIVE   1   2   3   4   5
109. Degree of Helpfulness: EDUCATIONAL   1   2   3   4   5
110. Degree of Helpfulness: INSIGHT-STIMULATING 1   2   3   4   5
111. Areas of Help: HUSBAND-WIFE RELATIONSHIP   1   2   3   4   5
112. Areas of Help: RELATIONSHIP TO HER MOTHER   1   2   3   4   5
113. Areas of Help: DEALING WITH ANXIETIES ABOUT PREGNANCY 1   2   3   4   5
114. Areas of Help: SEEING SELF IN MATERNAL ROLE   1   2   3   4   5
115. Areas of Help: CHANGING FEELINGS ABOUT SELF 1   2   3   4   5

CASE NO._____
CONJOINT ASSESSMENT_____
(Date)

Prenatal Rating Schedule: 9th Month

116. SUMMARY OF SUBJECTIVE REACTION OF WOMAN IN RESPONSE TO PROJECT

1	2	3	4	5
Not at all useful or negative reaction		Somewhat useful		Clearly useful

117. SUMMARY OF OBJECTIVE EVALUATION RE WOMAN'S RESPONSE TO PROJECT

1	2	3	4	5
Not at all useful or negative reaction		Somewhat useful		Clearly useful

C. Overall Evaluation of Pregnancy Experience

118. SUBJECTIVE REACTION OF WOMAN TO PHYSICAL ASPECTS OF THE PREGNANCY

1	2	3	4	5
Extremely difficult	Difficult	Neither especially difficult or easy	Easy	Very easy

119. MEDICAL EVALUATION OF THE PREGNANCY

1	2	3	4	5
Extremely difficult	Difficult	Neither especially difficult or easy	Easy	Very easy

120. SUBJECTIVE REACTION TO THE EMOTIONAL EXPERIENCE OF THE PREGNANCY

1	2	3	4	5
Sees pregnancy as unsatisfying experience	Matter-of-fact, neutral attitude	Fluctuating feelings	Moderately satisfying	Sees pregnancy as extremely satisfying experience

121. OBJECTIVE EVALUATION OF TOTAL PREGNANCY EXPERIENCE (Physical and Emotional)

1	2	3	4	5
Extremely poor adjustment to pregnancy	Poor adjustment	Fair adjustment	Good adjustment	Excellent adjustment

Rev. 3/1/65

GROUP HEALTH ASSOCIATION, INC.
PRENATAL PROJECT NIMH NO.503-A2

PRENATAL: MEDICAL OBSERVATIONS

NAME OF PATIENT _____
GHA# _____ EDC _____

CHECK BELOW WHERE PERTINENT ON THIS VISIT.

VISIT TO OBSTETRICAL DEPT. (Circle Number)
1 2 3 4 5 6 7 8 9 10 11 12 13 14
Date of Visit _____
Obstetrician _____

A. PHYSICAL SYMPTOMS

| | CURRENT VISIT | | | | | | | | |
| | 1. Degree | | | 2. Treatment Prescribed | | | | 3. Patient's Acceptance of Prescribed Treatment Advised at Prior Visit* | | |
Nature of Complaint	Marked	Moderate	Slight	Reassurance of normalcy or transient aspect	Medication	Diet	Other	Followed	Partially Followed	Not followed
Frequency of Urination										
Breast Enlargement										
Sleepiness & Constant Fatigue										
Nausea										
Vomiting										
Headache										
Abdominal Pain										
Backache										
Leg Cramp										
Edema										
Constipation										
Hemorrhoids										
Faintness or fainting										
Dizziness										
Vaginal Discharge--spotting										
Galactorrhea										
Weight loss or no gain										
Other (specify)										

*Since these ratings require reference to the form for the prior visit, please complete CURRENT ratings on both pages before you consult the prior form.

REV. 3/5/64

REVISED 4/14/65
MH503-03

PRENATAL: MEDICAL OBSERVATIONS

NAME OF PATIENT_____

CHECK BELOW WHERE PERTINENT TO CURRENT VISIT.

B. PATIENT'S APPEARANCE (<u>Circle</u> <u>Appropriate</u> <u>number</u>)

1	2	3	4	5
Poorly groomed		Well groomed		Markedly well groomed

C. THE QUICKENING EXPERIENCE
_____1. Anxious
_____2. Matter-of-fact
_____3. Pleasurable response
_____4. Other (Specify):

COMMENTS, IF ANY: (Include statements re husband's reaction):

D. QUESTIONS RAISED RE:
_____1. Sexual activity during pregnancy
_____2. Nature of delivery - natural childbirth
_____3. Nature of delivery - sedation:
_____a. Desires little
_____b. Desires much
_____4. Labor
_____5. Other (Specify):

E. BREAST FEEDING
_____1. Plans to breast-feed
_____2. Plans to bottle-feed
_____3. Plans combination feeding
_____4. Undecided:
_____a. Because of job plans
_____b. Because of husband's attitude
_____c. Other expressed reactions (Specify):

F. EMOTIONAL STATUS
_____1. Withdrawn or depressed
_____2. Anxious
_____3. Content
_____4. "Fine"
_____5. Other (Specify):

G. RELATIONSHIP TO OBSTETRICIAN
_____1. Resistant
_____2. Demanding
_____3. Unduly dependent
_____4. Cooperative
_____5. Other (Specify):

REV. 4/15/65
MH503-03

MEDICAL STAFF OBSERVATIONS
LABOR AND DELIVERY: PSYCHOLOGICAL ASPECTS

Case No. _____   Date_____
Name of Patient_____   Obstetrician_____

CHECK AND FILL IN BELOW
A. Physical Aspects
    1. Normal Delivery: Yes____, No____
    2. Timing:
        a. On time____; b. Overdue____(over 42 weeks); c. Premature___(Infant
                                                under 5 lbs.)
    3. Labor:
        a. False Labor - how soon before true labor?___How long did it last?____
        b. Was it necessary to stimulate labor? Yes___, No___
        c. On admission:
            1) Stage at which admitted: Early___; Midpoint___; Late____
               (Early = 1 - 3 cm. dilated; Midpoint = 4-6 cm.; Late = 7-10 cm.)
            2) How much dilated in centimeters _____
            3) Character of the contractions:
                  a) Interval _____
                  b) Intensity _____
                  c) Duration _____
        d. Reactions to:
            1) Pain: Over reacted____; Normal reaction____, Little reaction___
            2) Procedures: Over reacted___; Normal reaction___;Little reaction___.
        e. Patient's Cooperation During Labor: (Circle appropriate number)

            1   2   3   4   5
        Poor cooperation   Excellent Cooperation

        f. Duration of Labor:
            Very short (below 6 hrs.)___; Short (6-12 hrs.)___;
            Average (12 - 15 hrs.)____; Moderately long (15 - 18 hrs.)___;
            Prolonged (Over 18 hrs.)____.
        g. Factors Influencing Duration of Labor:
            1) Anxiety 1   2   3   4   5
            Intense disruptive anxiety   Little or no anxiety
            2) Size of baby in relation to pelvis ____
            3) Position of Baby ____
            4) Other (Specify) ____

    4. Complications: YES   NO
        a. While in Hospital: ___   ___
            If "yes" state nature of complication briefly in non-medical
            language if possible.

                                          YES   NO
        b. Postpartum, following hospitalization: ___ ___
            If "yes" state nature of complication.

            Indicate when it occurred (in number of weeks postpartum)_____

REV. 4/15/65
MH503-03

MEDICAL STAFF OBSERVATIONS
LABOR AND DELIVERY: PSYCHOLOGICAL ASPECTS

Case number _____
Name of Patient _____

5. Anesthetics:
    a. Analgesia:
        1) At what stage of labor was it administered? None___; Early___;
                                                        Midpoint___; Late___.
        2) Did patient request it? Yes___, No___
        3) Drug given _____Dosage _____
    b. Sedation:
        1) At what stage of labor was it administered? None___; Early___;
                                                        Midpoint___; Late___.
        2) Did patient request it? Yes___, No_____.
        3) Drug given_____Dosage_____
    c. Anesthesia:
        1) Type requested by patient:
            a) General ____
            b) Regional ___
            c) No anesthesia ____
            d) No choice (left to doctor to decide) ___
        2) Type administered:
            a) None ____
            b) General ___; At what stage? Midpoint ___;Late____.
            c) Regional:
                (1) Caudal___; At what stage administered? Midpoint__;Late__
                (2) Spinal___; At what stage administered? Midpoint__;Late__
                (3) Local ___; At what stage administered? Midpoint__;Late__
6. Complaints During Post-Partum Stay in Hospital:
    a. Nature of Complaint: b. Degree: c. Medical Basis(Check):
        1) Stitches: Slight___; Marked__ No basis__; Slight___;Marked__
        2) Headache: Slight___; Marked__ No basis__; Slight___;Marked__
        3) Breasts: Slight___; Marked__ No basis__; Slight___;Marked__
        4) Aspects of
    Hospital Affecting
    Care or Comfort:
    (State what aspect): Slight___; Marked__ No basis__; Slight___;Marked__

                                    Wife   Husband
B. First Response to Infant: _____1. Welcoming_____
                                _____2. Accepting_____
                                _____3. Ambivalent____
                                _____4. Negative _____
                                _____5. Rejecting_____

C. Mood and Emotional State While in Hospital:
    ____1. Euphoric
    ____2. Contented
    ____3. Anxious or fearful
    ____4. Depressed temporarily (for a day or a few days)
    ____5. Continuously depressed
D. Support Given to Woman by Others - Your Impression:
    Amount: Husband   Mother   Other (Specify)
      Little
      Average   ____   ____   ____
      Marked support ____   ____   ____

3/1/65
Revised

<u>SCHEDULE D</u>

CASE NO. _____
PERSON ASSESSING_____
              (Initials) (Date)
CONJOINT ASSESSMENT _____
                    (Date)

<u>Labor and Delivery Rating Schedule</u>

1. <u>Psychological Aspects</u>

150. SUBJECTIVE REACTION OF WOMAN TO LABOR AND DELIVERY EXPERIENCE

0	1	2	3	4	5
	Extremely diffi-cult (painful, prolonged, or highly disturbing emotionally)	Difficult	Neither diffi-cult nor easy	Rela-tively easy	Very easy

2. <u>Medical Aspects: Summary Evaluation</u>

151. MEDICAL EVALUATION (Overall)

0	1	2	3	4	5
	Extremely dif-ficult (painful, prolonged, or highly disturb-ing emotionally)	Difficult	Neither diffi-cult nor easy	Rela-tively easy	Very easy

MH503-A2
REV. 8/7/64

SCHEDULE EI____ , FI____ , GI____

CASE NO. _____
PERSON ASSESSING _____
(Initials) (Date)

Chronological Age of Infant_____
(In months)

I. Postnatal Rating Schedule: Infant Characteristics

A. INTELLECTUAL FUNCTIONS

(200) 1. Developmental Level (Bayley Infant Scale of Mental Develop.): DIQ:___

(201) 2. Object Responsiveness (Alertness, interest & responsiveness to objects)

0	1	2	3	4	5
C.R.	Very low. Completely unresponsive. Behavior suggests lack of awareness of objects or lack of discrimination between animate and inanimate stimulation.	Low--Tends to be passive in response to objects; rarely shows excitement or positive response.	Midpoint	Moderately high--sustained focus or attention. Moderate interest-- interested much of the time, indicated by sustained focus or attention to object, change in activity level or facial expression.	Very high--very much interested. Consistently shows vigorous response to objects - e.g., marked change in activity level, approach movements, excitement.

B. MOTOR FUNCTIONS

(202) 1. Level of Motor Development (Bayley Scale): DMQ_____

(203) 2. Activity Level - (Self-initiated activity as reflected in energy
level, body motion, arm, leg movements, head movements, crawling
movements.)

0	1	2	3	4	5
	Very high, hyperactive	Moderately high, tends to be hyperactive	Moderate	Low, tends to be hypoactive	Very low, hypoactive

(204) 3. Tension - (Overall impression of how tense or relaxed baby is including arms, legs, body, face, expression, tremors)

0	1	2	3	4	5
	Very tense	Moderately tense	Midpoint	Moderately relaxed	Very relaxed

I. Postnatal Rating Schedule: Infant Characteristics

C. AFFECT

(205)   1. Characteristic Mood (Interview and Observation)

0	1	2	3	4	5
	Actively un-happy much of the time	Passively un-happy much of the time	Passively con-tented	Actively happy	Actively happy most of the time

(206)   2. Mode of Expression of Negative Feelings: Crying

0	1	2	3	4	5
	Rare expression of negative feelings. Almost never cries. Makes no protest in situations which would seem to be highly frustrating ones.	Mild expression of negative feelings; seldom cries vigorously. May occasionally fuss mildly. Is easily soothed.	Moderate exression of negative feelings. Cries vigorously in few situations, under strong provocation; otherwise cries with moderate vigor.	Strong expression of negative feelings. Cries vigorously in many situations, with moderate provocation.	Unusually strong expression of feelings. Cries vigorously much of the time, screams, has "temper tantrums".

(207)   3. Affective Stability

0	1	2	3	4	5
	Highly unstable--much fluctuation in mood from moment to moment	Moderately unstable	Tends to be stable,with some variability in mood	Stable--mood predictable and consistent much of the time	Extremely stable-unusual stability; very rare fluctuation in mood

D. SOCIAL CHARACTERISTICS

(208)   1. Level of Social Responsiveness

0	1	2	3	4	5
	Very low. Completely unresponsive. Behavior suggest lack of awareness of people or lack of discrimination between animate and in-animate stimulation.	Low - tends to be passive in response to people; rarely shows excitement or positive response.	Midpoint	Moderately high--sustained focus or attention to voice. Moderate interest--interested in people much of the time, indicated by sustained focus or attention to voice or face, change in activity level or facial expression.	Very high --very much interested in people. Consistently shows vigorous response to people - e.g., marked change in activity level, approach movements, excitement.

SCHEDULE EI___, FI___, GI___

CASE NO. _____

I. Postnatal Rating Schedule: Infant Characteristics

(209)   2. <u>Appropriateness of Social Responsiveness for Age Level</u> (Based on Bayley Norms)

    ____Above Norm

    ____Appropriate - At Norm

    ____Inappropriate - Somewhat below Norm

    ____Inappropriate - Markedly below Norm

E. COPING CHARACTERISTICS

(210)   1. <u>Adaptability</u> - (Capacity to handle change, based on reactions to changes in scheduling - in expected sequences or daily routines; reactions to new foods, changes in formula; reactions to new situations - change in crib, removal of familiar objects from environment, move to new house; reactions to giving up established patterns of gratification; reactions to new people.)

0	1	2	3	4	5
	Very low adaptability. Usually shows strong and prolonged disturbance.	Low adaptability. Tends to be disturbed by change. Shows moderate degree of disturbance.	Midpoint -- sometimes accepts change without disturbance; more often shows mild disturbance.	Moderate adaptability.	High adaptability -- Accepts all kinds of change well, without overt disturbance. Seems to respond positively.

(211)   2. <u>Irritability</u> - Ease of Being Upset (Fries Test, Interview)

0	1	2	3	4	5
	Very low threshold-- very easily upset by apparently minor annoyances.	Moderately low threshold.	Average	High threshold	Very high threshold -- rarely upset; only upset by very strong stimulus

(212)   3. <u>Vulnerability to Stress</u> (Ease of disintegration of functioning under conditions of fatigue, hunger, excessive stimulation, "psychological stress")

0	1	2	3	4	5
	Extremely vulnerable-- Unusually low threshold for stress. Slight stress results in rapid and complete deterioration in functioning.	Highly vulnerable. Tends to be easily disorganized by mild stress.	Midpoint	Moderately low vulnerability. Tends to maintain integration in response to moderately strong stress stimulation.	Low vulnerability -- very high threshold. Maintains integration, rarely shows deterioration in functioning, even in response to strong stress.

SCHEDULE EI___ , FI___ , GI___

CASE NO._____

I. Postnatal Rating Schedule: Infant Characteristics

(213)   4. Ease of Recovery From Being Upset

0	1	2	3	4	5
	Long delay before re- covery from being upset		Moderate delay before recovery from being upset		Very rapid recovery from being upset

(214)   5. Goal-Directedness (Bayley Scale)

0	1	2	3	4	5
	Very low goal- directedness. No evidence of directed ef- fort to at- tain goals.	Low goal- directedness. Characteris- tically shows brief interest, makes a few attempts at problem solu- tion but not to completion.	Moderate goal- directedness. Tends to be moderately vigorous and persistent	Highly goal- directed	Very highly goal-directed. Extremely vig- orous and per- sistent in at- temps to reach goal or solve problem.

(215) F. OVERALL RATING

0	1	2	3	4	5
	Extremely poor- ly integrated infant. Charac- terized by sig- nificant devia- tions in many areas of func- tioning.	Poorly inte- grated. Tends to have more than average number of prob- lems of moder- ate severity.	Midpoint. On the whole ap- pears to be functioning adequately, but having difficulties in a few areas.	Well-integrated infant	Extremely well- integrated; smoothly functioning infant.

Rev. 11/4/63

V. PEDIATRIC EVALUATION OF INFANT

Name of Patient (infant)_____

Mother's Name_____

Father's Name _____

GHA#_____Birthdate_____

EXAMINATION DATES: (Check which visit)
In Hospital_____
6 weeks _____
12 weeks _____
18 weeks _____
24 weeks _____

Appointment was _____Kept
                 _____Cancelled
                 _____Not kept
If late for appointment, how long?_____
The baby was brought by (check one or more):
_____Mother
_____Father
_____Nurse
_____Babysitter
_____Relative (specify):
_____Friend of family
If mother was not present, specify reason:

A. Physical Status
   1. Birth weight _____lbs, _____oz, _____percentile. (6 week check only)
   2. Weight, this examination _____lbs, _____oz, _____percentile
   3. PKU test result _____ (6 week check only)
   4. Physical condition:
      _____Evidence of neglect (dirty skin, clothing, etc., specify:)

      _____Physical defects not previously noted:

   5. Neurological Status
      a. Moro Reflex present _____Yes, _____No
      b. Deep tendon reflexes; check if:

	Biceps	Knee Jerk	Ankle Jerk
Symmetrical			
Sluggish			
Brisk (Normal)			
Hyperactive			
Clonus			
Absent			

      c. Muscle Tone

	lt Arm	Rt Arm	Lt Leg	Rt Leg
Spasticity				
Increased				
Normal				
Decreased				
Flaccidity				

d. Activity Level
_____1. Hyperactive
_____2. Normal - moderate activity
_____3. Hypoactive

e. Irritability
_____1. Abnormal irritability - hypersensitivity - e.g., crying occurs frequently in response to many mild stimuli. Crying characteristic much of the time.
_____2. Above average irritability - crying in response to mild stimulation; crying frequently does not appear to be related to normal conditions of discomfort,hunger, etc.
_____3. Normal irritability - crying in response to intense stimulation or in response to fatigue, hunger, etc.
_____4. Below normal irritability - hyposensitivity - lack of response to stimulation or to fatigue, hunger, etc.
_____5. Extremely lethargic - marked hyposensitivity - lack of response to intense stimulation.

f. Cry is: _____Normal, _____Abnormal(specify):

6. Sleep, approximate number hours _____
Sleeps through the night_____. Age of onset_____.

B.. Feeding Behavior:
1. Type of feeding: _____Breast, _____Bottle
2. Initial difficulty (if any) with feeding:
_____a. Marked (explain):
_____b. Moderate
_____c. None
3. Complete for breast-fed babies only:
Mother's level of comfort with breast-feeding
_____a. Comfortable
_____b. Uncomfortable (explain):

4. Sucking: _____Weak, _____Strong (Record mother's impression):

5. If breast-feeding has been given up since the last visit, why:

6. Supplemental formula needed (breast-fed only) _____Yes, _____No.
Why started:

7. Spitting-up. Indicate Mother's Reaction:
_____a. Casual, matter-of-fact
_____b. Irritated or uncomfortable
8. Crying Pattern: _____Much, _____Little (Mother's statement):
Can a diagnosis of colic be made? _____Yes, _____No. If Yes,indicate:
a. Age of onset _____
b. Treatment and results:_____

C. Mother's Reaction:
1. Confidence in Coping With Maternal Role:
_____a. Highly confident
_____b. Fairly sure of herself
_____c. Unsure of herself in some ways but fairly sure in others
_____d. Feels great difficulty in coping with the situation
_____e. Extremely helpless and overwhelmed

2. Pediatrician's impression of the mother's reaction to the baby AT THE TIME OF THIS EXAMINATION
   a. Acceptance
   _____1) Relatively rejecting
   _____2) Indifferent
   _____3) Ambivalent
   _____4) Accepting
   _____5) Enthusiastic
   b. Anxiety
   _____1) Intense disruptive anxiety
   _____2) Anxious overconcern
   _____3) Moderate anxiety
   _____4) Mild
   _____5) Little or no anxiety

3. Pediatrician's impression of the mother's reaction to the professional relationship AT THE TIME OF THIS EXAMINATION. The mother is:
   _____a. Overly dependent
   _____b Passively accepting
   _____c. Independent (appropriate behavior)
   _____d. Hostile
   _____e. Belligerent

REV. 9/28/64

PEDIATRIC EVALUATION OF INFANT

D. Pediatrician's Evaluation of Infant's Overall Adaptation as of This
    Examination Period

   1. Overall Evaluation: Feeding (as evidence of mother-child adaptation)

0	1	2	3	4	5
Can't Rate	Erratic and difficult for mother and child		Some minor feeding problems but essentially both are coping with them		Smooth; no feeding problems

   2. Adjustment to Routines (Feeding, sleeping, bathing, toileting and play
       periods)

0	1	2	3	4	5
C.R.	Very poor adjustment to most routines		Fair adjustment to most routines		Very good adjustment to most routines

   3. Developmental Status (Summary Evaluation of Physical and Neurological
       Status, Motor Development and General Impression of Level of
       Responsiveness)

0	1	2	3	4	5
C.R.	Below expectations for age level		At age level expectations		Above age level expectations

   4. Overall Integration of Infant

0	1	2	3	4	5
C.R.	Extremely poorly integrated infant. Characterized by significant deviation in many areas of functioning	Poorly integrated. Tends to have more than average number of problems of moderate severity	Midpoint. On the whole appears to be functioning adequately, but having difficulties in a few areas	Well-integrated infant	Extremely well-integrated smoothly functioning infant

MH503-A2
6/26/64
Revised

Conjoint - Rater _____
                   (Initials) (Date)

III. Postnatal Rating Scale: Maternal Adaptation
      A. MOTHER-INFANT ADAPTATIONS   Outside Help 1st 2 wks.Foll. Delivery:
                                         None___ ½-time help___, Full time___
                                         Outside Help Subsequent to 1st 2 wks:
                                         None___ ½-time help___, Full time___

(300) 1. Coordination of Routines (Degree to which routines of baby
           care and household run smoothly)

0	1	2	3	4	5
	Chaotic, Disorganized	Somewhat dis-organized	Fair coor-dination	Good coor-dination	Excellent coor-dination; in-fant routines & household run smoothly

       2. Accommodation to the Infant

(301)   a. Amount of Physical Contact

0	1	2	3	4	5
	Low--infant often not held for feedings and rarely for play or com-forting		Moderate--infant held for feedings		High--child held during much of waking time; fre-quent play periods during day

(302)   b. Quality of Physical Contact (Ease, awkwardness, tension or
               relaxation, pleasure or distaste, closeness or distance in
               physical contact with baby)

0	1	2	3	4	5
	Low physical involvement		Moderate physi-cal involvement; occassional close-ness but some aloofness evident		Very close physi-cal involvement

(303)   c. Degree of Expression of Affection (Demonstrated feeling
               response of mother judged by the way she talks to and
               about baby, tenderness in handling for feeding, bath,
               etc. Facial expression and emotional tone in presence
               of baby.)

0	1	2	3	4	5
	Not demon-strative; tends to be reserved	Matter-of-fact	Inconsis-tent, am-bivalent; sometimes warm,some-times cool	Usually affec-tionate and expressive	Affectionate, warm, fond-ling, very expressive

MH503-A2
6/26/64 Rev.

III. Postnatal Rating Scale: A. Mother-Infant Adaptations (Cont'd.)

(304)   d. Sensitivity and Responsiveness (Includes awareness and responsiveness to infant's needs, the ability to interpret and
respond accurately to needs and feelings of baby from
simple cues-gestures, grimaces, body movements, cry.)

0	1	2	3	4	5
C.R.	Fails to respond to obvious cues		Moderately able to follow infant's cues		Highly sensitive & responsive to child's cues -- tends to anticipate needs before obvious indications (like crying)

(305)   e. Acceptance-Rejection: Overall Evaluation

0	1	2	3	4	5
	Dissatisfied	Mildly dissatisfied	Generally accepting with some ambivalence	Satisfied	Complete acceptance without reservation

(306)   1) Acceptance-Rejection: Sex

0	1	2	3	4	5
	Dissatisfied	Mildly dissatisfied	Generally accepting with some ambivalence	Satisfied	Complete acceptance without reservation

(307)   2) Acceptance-Rejection: Appearance

0	1	2	3	4	5
	Dissatisfied	Mildly dissatisfied	Generally accepting with some ambivalence	Satisfied	Complete acceptance without reservation

(308)   3) Acceptance-Rejection: Individual Characteristics

0	1	2	3	4	5
	Dissatisfied	Mildly dissatisfied	Generally accepting with some ambivalence	Satisfied	Complete acceptance without reservation

MH503-A2
6/26/64 Rev.

III. Postnatal Rating Scale: A. Mother-Infant Adaptations (Cont'd.)

(309)   f. Emotional Involvement (Depth of mother's feeling towards the
             child; salience of the child in mother's life and the
             degree of investment in the child's future.)

0	1	2	3	4	5
C.R.	Little emotional involvement with child	Moderate emotional involvement characterized by moderate feeling & occasional strong feeling	Strong emotional involvmment in relationship; considerable involvement in child's life but with some objectivity	Strong emotional involvement in relationship & in child's life with little objectivity	Extreme emotional involvement in relationship; overwhelming involvement in child's life with no objectivity.

(310)   g. Individualization (The extent to which mother perceives child
             as an individual and the extent to which her bahavior towards
             the infant is guided by an awareness of his unique charac-
             teristics.)

0	1	2	3	4	5
	Sees infant essentially as an undifferentiated part of self		Sees infant sometimes as part of self, sometimes as separate		Views infant as separate in identity and needs

(311)   h. Amount of Stimulation (Motor, social, visual and auditory,
             play and play materials)

0	1	2	3	4	5
	Little or none	Some	Moderate amount	Much	Very much

B. ADAPTATION TO THE MATERNAL ROLE

     1. Adequacy of Coping with Physical Needs of Infant
(312)   a. Feeding

0	1	2	3	4	5
	Mother very inept in handling feeding		Essentially competent		Handles feeding very well; if problems, copes very effectively

(313)   b. Other Routines (Bathing, diapering and dressing)

0	1	2	3	4	5
	Mother very inept in handling		Essentially competent		Handles very well, copes very effectively

III. Postnatal Rating Scale: B. Adaptation to the Maternal Role (Cont'd.)

2. Psychological Adaptation

(314)   a. Feelings in Regard to Care of Physical Needs of Child
(Expression of resentment, distaste, or pleasure in
performances of most routines in any or all areas
of above aspects of infant care.)

0	1	2	3	4	5
	Highly resentful; finds work distasteful or very onerous	Ambivalent	Accepts in matter-of fact way	Moderate enjoyment of most routines	Marked enjoyment of most routines; in general, finds them gratifying

(315)   b. Reaction to Total Dependency of Infant (Expression of
pleasure and gratification or resentment re infant's
total dependence)

0	1	2	3	4	5
	Highly resentful; feels trapped or burdened	Ambivalent	Accepts in matter-of-fact way	Moderately gratified	Highly gratified at being needed

(316)   c. Reaction to Curtailment of Freedom

0	1	2	3	4	5
	Highly resentful		Mildly resentful	Ambivalent	Accepts in matter-of-fact way	Complete acceptance

(317)   d. Anxiety Re Adequacy in Her Role as Mother (Extent to which
she worries or talks about her ability to be a good mother
or other indicators of anxiety might be self-depreciatory
remarks)

0	1	2	3	4	5
	Intense disruptive anxiety		Moderate Anxiety		Little or no anxiety

(318)   e. Anxiety Re Baby (Extent to which she worries about baby's
health, development, normality, dangers to infant, as
seen by her statements, calls to doctor, questions of
Infant Observer, etc.)

0	1	2	3	4	5
	Intense disruptive anxiety		Moderate anxiety		Little or no anxiety

CASE NO. _____

III. Postnatal Rating Scale: B.   Adaptation to the Maternal Role (Cont'd.)

(319)   f.   Reaction re Real Problems with Baby (Illness, accident, dangers, etc.)

0	1	2	3	4	5
	Consistently shows over-concern with real problems	Sometimes over-reacts	Realistic, appropriate concern	Tends to minimize serious-ness of problems	Lack of appro-priate concern; underestimating seriousness of problem

(320)   g.   Prevailing Mood Since Birth of Baby

0	1	2	3	4	5
	Severely de-pressed	Mildly depressed	Fluctuating moods	Mainly happy mood	Marked happi-ness and enthusiasm

   C.   HUSBAND-WIFE ADAPTATION

(323)   1.   Wife's Reaction to Husband's New Role

0	1	2	3	4	5
	Critical, jealous or hostile		Ambivalent feelings towards hus-band in new role		Highly pleased with and proud of husband as father

(324)   2.   Husband's Reaction to Wife as Mother

0	1	2	3	4	5
	Critical, jealous or hostile	Somewhat negative reaction	Ambivalent	Apprecia-tive, sup-portive	Enthusiastic, highly appre-ciative and supportive

(325)   3.   Husband's Reaction to His Role as Father

0	1	2	3	4	5
	Highly resent-ful; disappoin-ted or de-pressed	Somewhat dis-appointed and dissatisfied	Ambivalent	Satisfied	Marked gratifi-cation

(326)   4.   Husband's Reaction to Baby

0	1	2	3	4	5
	Rejecting	Unresponsive	Accepting	Very well satisfied	Enthusiastic, proud

SCHEDULE EIII, FIII, GIII

CASE NO._____

III. Postnatal Rating Scale: C. Husband-Wife Adaptation (Cont'd.)

(327)   5. Responsiveness of Husband to Wife

0	1	2	3	4	5
	Hostile	Largely unre-sponsive	Ambivalent	Essen-tially responsive	Fully respon-sive

(328)   6. Responsiveness of Wife to Husband

0	1	2	3	4	5
	Hostile	Largely unre-sponsive	Ambivalent	Essen-tially responsive	Fully respon-sive

(329)   7. Overall Husband-Wife Adaptation (based on willingness of each to identify and to respond to the desires of the other; mutuality of emotional investment in infant and home; degree of mutual affection)

0	1	2	3	4	5
	Very poor adaptation	Poor adap-tation	Intermit-tently good	Good	Excellent

(330)   8. Effect of Infant on Family Homeostasis (Subjective reaction to change, experienced as disruptive or not)

0	1	2	3	4	5
	Highly dis-ruptive	Disruptive	Somewhat disruptive but not greatly disturbing	Changes largely anticipated and not ex-perienced as disrup-tive	Family life readily adap-tive to arrival of infant

REV. 3/1/65

MH503-A2
REV. 8/11/64

SCHEDULE GIV

CASE NO._____

PERSON ASSESSING_____
(Initials) (Date)

CONJOINT ASSESSMENT_____
(Date)

Postnatal Rating Schedule, 6 Month Evaluation: Current Personality and Stresses

IV.   Current Personality of Woman

416.   Predominant Defenses Used
416.1___Denial
416.2___Repression
416.3___Intellectualization
416.4___ Reaction formation
416.5___Projection
416.6___Regression
416.7___Isolation
416.8___Acting Out
416.9___Other (Specify):

420.   Emotional Adaptation - Characteristic Way of Expressing Feeling
420.1___Hostile and explosive (Rate 1 - 5, from high to low)
420.2___Impulsive (Rate 1 - 5, from high to low)
420.3___Repressed (Rate 1 - 5, from high to low)
420.4___ Tender and affectionate (Rate 1 - 5, from low to high)
420.5___Adapted (Rate 1 - 5, from low to high)

421.   Anxiety

0	1	2	3	4	5
C.R.	Intense disruptive anxiety				Little or no anxiety

422.   Ease of Fantasy Production

0	1	2	3	4	5
	Constricted - little or no fantasy	Spontaneous but not especially creative	Spontaneous, creative	Tendency towards fantasy living	Excessive fantasy living

423.   Concern for Appearance

0	1	2	3	4	5
	Inappropriate neglect				Excessive preoccupation with physical care and appearance

424.   Gratification in Female Sexuality

0	1	2	3	4	5
	No enjoyment, or actual distaste		Moderate enjoyment		Marked enjoyment

Postnatal Rating Schedule, 6 Month Evaluation: Current Personality and Stresses

426. Responsiveness to Others - Giving and Nurturant Quality

0	1	2	3	4	5
	Ungiving		Moderately giving		Highly generous; very giving

427. Flexibility

0	1	2	3	4	5
	Highly resistant to change or stress		Accommodates after some resistance or delay to change and ordinary stress		Easy accommodation to change (able to "roll with the punches")

428. Sense of Humor

0	1	2	3	4	5
	Little or none		Moderately good		Keen

429. Overt Dependency Behavior

0	1	2	3	4	5
	Clinging to dependency status		Emancipated, adult give-and-take		Marked independence

430. Covert, Underlying Dependency Pattern

0	1	2	3	4	5
	Very strong dependency wishes		Moderate dependency wishes		Little dependency wishes

431. Ability to Meet Own Needs, Including Pleasure

0	1	2	3	4	5
	Poor		Average		Marked ability

432. Passive-Aggressive Pattern

0	1	2	3	4	5
	Extremely passive				Aggressive

433. Superego

0	1	2	3	4	5
	Weak superego		Strong superego but can yield		Stringent or rigid unyielding superego demands with guilt if not met

CASE NO._____

Postnatal Rating Schedule, 6 Month Evaluation: Current Personality and Stresses

434. Insight Into Self

0	1	2	3	4	5
	No insight	Little insight	Fair degree of insight	Considerable insight	Very insightful

435. Acceptance of Own Identity

0	1	2	3	4	5
	Strong rejection of identity		Ambivalence		Positive attitudes -- self-acceptance

436. Sense of Success as a Wife

0	1	2	3	4	5
	Evaluates self as unsuccessful		Evaluates self as fairly adequate		Evaluates self as highly successful

437. Sense of Success as a Homemaker

0	1	2	3	4	5
	Evaluates self as poor		Evaluates self as average		Evaluates self as successful

400. Sense of Success as a Mother

0	1	2	3	4	5
	Evaluates self as inadequate		Evaluates self as fairly adequate		Evaluates self as highly adequate

438. Achievement of an Adult Role

0	1	2	3	4	5
	Childishness		Ambivalence as to adult status		Distinctly mature and clear as to adult status

439. Capacity for Closeness

0	1	2	3	4	5
	Shallow and distant		Fairly close		Intense meaningful relationships

440. Ability to Take Help

0	1	2	3	4	5
	No acceptance	Tends to defeat or deflect help	Optimal acceptance	Accepts help passively	Extremely dependent

CASE NO._____

Postnatal Rating Schedule, 6 Month Evaluation: Current Personality and Stresses

441. Ability to Give Help and Support

0	1	2	3	4	5
	Unable to give	Gives grudg-ingly	Gives on own terms	Gives on request	Gives freely on sensing need

442. Need to Control

0	1	2	3	4	5
	Rigidly con-trolling		Neither sub-missive nor controlling		Submits easily

443. Overall Evaluation of Adaptive Behavior

0	1	2	3	4	5
	Defenses basic-ally inadequate to deal with needs				Defenses highly adequate

491. Narcissism

0	1	2	3	4	5
	Little or no concern with self		Appropriately concerned about self, i.e.,not out of per-spective		Excessive pre-occupation and concern with self

V. Current Stresses (Check pertinent items)

460.__Anxiety about financial security

461.__Food and management problems

462.__Illness or recent death in extended family

463.__Illness of husband or wife

464.__Problems with relatives

465.__Problems re spouse of previous marriage

466.__Problems re friends

467.__Job dissatisfaction for wife

468.__Job dissatisfaction for husband

469.__Religious differences

470.__Other (Specify, such as: political differences, etc.)

REV. 3/1/65

MH503-A2
RÉV. 8/11/64

SCHEDULE H

CASE NO._____

PERSON ASSESSING_____
(Initials) (Date)
CONJOINT ASSESSMENT _____
(Date)

Postnatal Rating Schedule: 6 Month, Summary Evaluation

I. Infant Adjustment

A. DEVELOPMENTAL STATUS (Infant Observer's Findings):

500. D.I.Q._____, Age Equivalent_____.
Chronological Age___.

501. D.M.Q._____, Age Equivalent_____.

B. PHYSICAL DEVELOPMENT AT 6 MONTH:

502. Height Percentile_____

503. Weight Percentile_____

504. Feeding Adjustment

0	1	2	3	4	5
Can't rate	Infant's feeding adjustment erratic & difficult most of the 6 months' period		Some minor feeding problems persisting through much of the 1st 6 months but essentially infant is coping with them		Smooth adjustment; little or no feeding problems throughout 1st 6 months

505. Illness History

0	1	2	3	4	5
0	Many persistent illnesses		Few and intermittent illnesses		No significant illnesses

506. Overall Physical Status

0	1	2	3	4	5
0	Very poor		Fair		Excellent

507. Basic Evaluation of the Functioning of the Infant - Overall Rating

0	1	2	3	4	5
0	Extremely poorly integrated infant. Characterized by significant deviations in many areas of functioning.	Poorly integrated. Tends to have more than average number of problems of moderate severity	Midpoint. On the whole appears to be functioning adequately but having difficulties in a few areas	Well-integrated infant	Extremely well-integrated; smoothly functioning infant

SCHEDULE H

CASE NO._____

Postnatal Rating Schedule: 6 Month, Summary Evaluation

II. Mother-Infant Adaptation

508. Adequacy in Coping with Physical Needs of Infant

0	1	2	3	4	5
	Very inept and inadequate		Average in coping performance		Highly competent and effective

509. Adequacy in Coping with Emotional Needs of Infant

0	1	2	3	4	5
	Very unrespon- sive and in- sensitive		Fairly sensitive, aware and prompt in responsiveness		Highly sensitive, aware, prompt in responsiveness

III. The Woman in Relation to Herself

510. The Pregnancy Experience in Retrospect: Subjective Reaction of Woman

0	1	2	3	4	5
	Pregnancy seen as extremely unsatisfying experience	Moderately unsatisfying	Matter-of-fact, neutral atti- tude	Moderately satisfying	Pregnancy seen as extremely satisfying ex- perience

511. The Delivery Experience in Retrospect: Subjective Reaction of Woman

0	1	2	3	4	5
	Extremely difficult (painful, pro- longed, or highly dis- turbing emo- tionally)	Difficult	Neither diffi- cult nor easy	Relatively easy	Very easy

512. Mother's Predominant Mood

0	1	2	3	4	5
	Depressed	Mildly depressed	Fairly or inter- mittently happy	Essentially happy	Very happy and enthus- iastic

513. Mother's Satisfaction with Current Situation

0	1	2	3	4	5
	Highly dissat- isfied	Moderately dissatisfied	Ambivalent	Moderately satis- fied	Very well satisfied

Postnatal Rating Schedule: 6 Month, Summary Evaluation

514. Change in Level of Personality Integration (Effectiveness of coping; feelings about self, relationships)

0	1	2	3	4	5
	Markedly de- teriorated (including psychotic reaction)		No significant change		Markedly im- proved

IV. The Family

515. New Family Homeostasis

0	1	2	3	4	5
	Unbalanced, "rocky", unsatisfying for any one or more mem- bers of the family		Sometimes in equi- librium and some- times satisfying for all		Well-balanced, satisfying for all most of the time

516. Husband-Wife Adaptation

0	1	2	3	4	5
	Very poor adaptation	Poor	Intermittently good	Good	Excellent

517. The Family as Environment for Infant's Development (Overall rating based on mother's adaptation to infant, maternal role; father's adaptation to his role as father; husband-wife adaptation)

0	1	2	3	4	5
	Poor	Mediocre	Fairly good	Good	Excellent

V. Response to Project

518. Subjective Reaction of Woman in Response to the Project

0	1	2	3	4	5
	Hostile reac- tion	Neutral reaction-- project experience essentially meaning- less to her	Ambivalence	Positive-- project useful	Highly posi- tive - clarify- ing or insight- stimulating to woman

REV. 10/6/64

CASE NO._____

Postnatal Rating Schedule: 6 Month, Summary Evaluation

519. Objective Evaluation

0	1	2	3	4	5
	Hostile reaction	Neutral reaction-- project experience essentially meaningless to her	Ambiva-lent	Positive-- project useful	Highly positive-- clarifying or insight-stimulating to woman

VI. Relation with Own Mother

520. Emulation of Own Mother

0	1	2	3	4	5
	Tendency to be opposite from the familial picture		Tendency to establish a new pattern, appropriate to herself and husband		Tendency to be entirely like the pattern of her own mother

521. Closeness with Own Mother

0	1	2	3	4	5
	Distant		Close		Very Close

APPENDIX C

Compendium
Factor Scales

Scale No.	Name of Factor	Schedule	No. of Items in Factor
1	Perception of Experience Being Mothered	A. I.C.	5

- Item 2, Empathy with Child   <u>Ratings</u>

    Insensitive even to expressed need ------------ (1)
    Awareness of Child's varying
       needs and moods ---------------------------- (3)
    Very sensitive and aware (even when minimally
       cued) ------------------------------------- (5)

- Item 3, Closeness to Child

    Distant ------------------------------------- (1)
    Close --------------------------------------- (3)
    Very Close ---------------------------------- (5)

- Item 5, Mother's Reaction to Her Maternal Role

    Actively resented demands -------------------- (1)
    Disappointed, frustrated --------------------- (2)
    Ambivalent ----------------------------------- (3)
    Satisfied ------------------------------------ (4)
    Marked gratification in her role ------------- (5)

- Item 6, Mother-Daughter Relationship: Extent to Which Mother
  Satisfied Emotional Needs - Infancy to Age 12

    Support needs essentially unmet -------------- (1)
    Support needs essentially met ---------------- (5)

- Item 7, Mother-Daughter Relationship: Extent to Which Mother
  Satisfied Emotional Needs - After Age 12

    Support needs essentially unmet -------------- (1)
    Support needs essentially met ---------------- (5)

Scale No.	Name of Factor	Schedule	No. of Items in Factor
2	Interest in Children	A.I.C.	2

- Item 13, Interest in Younger Children

Ratings

Resentful -------------- (1)
Interested ------------- (2)
Mild ------------------- (3)
Moderate --------------- (4)
Eager------------------- (5)

- Item 14, Experience with Younger Children

Little or none ---------- (1)
Some ------------------- (2)
Moderate --------------- (3)
Considerable ----------- (4)
Constant responsibility
 for younger children --- (5)

Scale No.	Name of Factor	Schedule	No. of Items in Factor
3	School and Peer Relationships	A. I.C.	3

- Item 9, School Achievement   Ratings

        Consistent academic failure -- (1)
        Poor student ---------------- (2)
        Average student ------------- (3)
        Good student ---------------- (4)
        Consistent academic success -- (5)

- Item 10, School Adjustment

        Behavior poor (in trouble)---- (1)
        Intermittent trouble --------- (2)
        Intermittently adaptive------- (3)
        Adaptive behavior ----------- (4)
        Successful and rewarding ----- (5)

- Item 12, Peer Relationships

        Lonely, isolated ------------ (1)
        Fairly close ---------------- (3)
        Close and meaningful --------- (5)

Scale No.	Name of Factor	Schedule	No. of Items in Factor
4	Ego Strength	A.II.	9

- Item 20.5, Emotional Adaptation - Characteristic Way of Expressing Feeling

  Ratings

  Adapted ------------------------------Rate 1-5, from low to high)

- Item 21, Anxiety

  Intense disruptive anxiety --------------------------- (1)
  Little or no anxiety -------------------------------- (5)

- Item 27, Flexibility

  Highly resistant to change or stress ----------------- (1)
  Accommodates after some resistance or delay to change
     and ordinary stress ------------------------------ (3)
  Easy accommodation to change (able to "roll with the
     punches") --- (5)

- Item 28, Sense of Humor

  Little or none --------------------------------------- (1)
  Moderately good -------------------------------------- (3)
  Keen --- (5)

- Item 30, Covert, Underlying Dependency Pattern (Based on Psychological Tests - Psychologist's Rating Only)

  Very strong dependency wishes ------------------------ (1)
  Moderate dependency wishes --------------------------- (3)
  Little dependency wishes ----------------------------- (5)

- Item 31, Ability to Meet Own Needs, Including Pleasure

  Poor --- (1)
  Average -- (3)
  Marked ability --------------------------------------- (5)

- Item 35, Acceptance of Own Identity

  Strong rejection of identity ------------------------- (1)
  Ambivalence -- (3)
  Positive attitudes - self acceptance ----------------- (5)

- Item 38, Achievement of an Adult Role

  Childishness --- (1)
  Ambivalence as to adult status ----------------------- (3)
  Distinctly mature and clear as to adult status -------- (5)

- Item 43, Overall Evaluation of Adaptive Behavior

  Defenses basically inadequate to deal with needs ------ (1)
  Defenses highly adequate ----------------------------- (5)

Scale No.	Name of Factor	Schedule	No. of Items in Factor
5	Nurturance	A. II.	8

- Item 20.4, Emotional Adaptation - Characteristic
  Way of Expressing Feeling   Ratings

  Tender and Affectionate   (Rate 1 - 5, from low to high)

- Item 24, Gratification in Female Sexuality

  No enjoyment, or actual distaste --------------------- (1)
  Moderate enjoyment --------------------------------- (3)
  Marked enjoyment ---------------------------------- (5)

- Item 25, Responsiveness to Husband

  Ungiving --- (1)
  Moderately giving ---------------------------------- (3)
  Fully giving --------------------------------------- (5)

- Item 26, Responsiveness to Others - Giving and Nurturant Quality

  Ungiving --- (1)
  Moderately giving ---------------------------------- (3)
  Highly generous; very giving ---------------------- (5)

- Item 36, Sense of Success as a Wife

  Evaluates self as unsuccessful --------------------- (1)
  Evaluates self as fairly adequate ------------------ (3)
  Evaluates self as highly successful ---------------- (5)

- Item 37, Sense of Success as Homemaker

  Evaluates self as poor ----------------------------- (1)
  Evaluates self as average -------------------------- (3)
  Evaluates self as successful ----------------------- (5)

- Item 41, Ability to Give Help and Support

  Unable to give ------------------------------------- (1)
  Gives grudingly ------------------------------------ (2)
  Gives on own terms --------------------------------- (3)
  Gives on request ----------------------------------- (4)
  Gives freely on sensing need ----------------------- (5)

* - Item 16, Number of Predominant Defenses

       1 - Denial   6 - Regression
       2 - Repression   7 - Isolation
       3 - Intellectualization   8 - Acting Out
       4 - Reaction formation   9 - Other
       5 - Projection

*In all scales but this, the items were added to obtain the total factor scale
score. In this scale, the factor scale score is arrived at by subtracting
from the total score of the first 8 ratings the number of predominant defense

Scale No.	Name of Factor	Schedule	No. of Items in Factor
6	Husband's Responsiveness to Wife	A. III.	9

Ratings

- Item 45, Empathy

Insensitive even to expressed needs ----- (1)
Awareness of varying moods and needs ----- (3)
Very sensitive and aware (even
    when minimally cued) ------------------- (5)

- Item 46, Communication

Very inhibited about talking
    to wife ------------------------------- (1)
Moderately inhibited -------------------- (2)
Cautious about initiating talk re
    feelings ------------------------------ (3)
Fairly open ----------------------------- (4)
Uninhibited and free -------------------- (5)

- Item 47, Affection

Minimal --------------------------------- (1)
Intense --------------------------------- (5)

- Item 48, Hostility

Intense --------------------------------- (1)
Minimal --------------------------------- (5)

- Item 49, Sexual Adjustment

Restricted and unsatisfying ------------- (1)
Generally satisfying (no
    specific problem) --------------------- (3)
Highly satisfying ----------------------- (5)

- Item 50, Decision Process

Resolved only after serious conflict ----- (1)
Resolution achieved without major
    threat to relationship ---------------- (3)
Flexibility in arriving at joint
    decisions, each moving from
    dominant to passive position
    without threat to self or the
    relationship -------------------------- (5)

Scale No.	Name of Factor	Schedule	No. of Items in Factor
6 (cont'd.)	Husband's Responsiveness to Wife	A. III.	9

- Item 53, Extent to Which Husband Allows Dependency

Ratings

Impatient, hostile attitude towards
wife's dependency ------------------------- (1)
Allows dependency in stress situations ---------- (3)
Responds fully to wife's need for
support ------------------------------------- (5)

- Item 54, Husband's Fostering of Self-Confidence in Wife as a Mother

Attitudes and actions generally belittling
and destructive ---------------------------- (1)
Expresses intermittent doubt and questions
about wife's capacity to become a mother------- (3)
Fully sustains wife in belief in her capacity
as a mother---------------------------------- (5)

- Item 59, Husband-Wife Adaptation

Very poor adaptation --------------------------- (1)
Poor adaptation-------------------------------- (2)
Intermittently good --------------------------- (3)
Good -- (4)
Excellent-------------------------------------- (5)

Scale No.	Name of Factor	Schedule	No. of Items in Factor
7	Husband's Responsiveness to Pregnancy	A. III.	5

Ratings

- Item 51, Reaction to Wife in re Pregnancy

Dejected ----------------------------------- (1)
Unresponsive ------------------------------- (2)
Contented -------------------------------- (3)
Very Satisfied----------------------------- (4)
Enthusiastic ----------------------------- (5)

- Item 52, Reaction to Baby-to-be

Dejected ----------------------------------- (1)
Unresponsive ------------------------------- (2)
Contented--------------------------------- (3)
Very satisfied --------------------------- (4)
Enthusiastic ----------------------------- (5)

- Item 55, Feelings re Sharing Wife

Clearly impatient and jealous of sharing
wife ----------------------------------- (1)
Normally able to share wife --------------- (3)
Eager to share wife with a child ---------- (5)

- Item 56, Congruence of the Preg. with Current Way of Life

Disruptive, incongruent ------------------- (1)
Interruptive but manageable --------------- (2)
Generally consonant with aims and
resources ----------------------------- (3)
Consonant -------------------------------- (4)
Highly consonant ------------------------- (5)

- Item 57, Congruence of the Preg. with Long-time Plans

Disruptive, incongruent-------------------- (1)
Interruptive but manageable --------------- (2)
Generally consonant with aims and
resources ----------------------------- (3)
Consonant -------------------------------- (4)
Highly consonant ------------------------- (5)

Scale No.	Name of Factor	Schedule	No. of Items in Factor
8	Adaptation to Pregnancy Experience	A. IV.	4

Ratings

- Item 73, Predominant Attitude or Mood

    Extremely rejecting of pregnancy ------------- (1)
    Moderately rejecting ------------------------ (2)
    Contented ----------------------------------- (3)
    Very satisfied ------------------------------ (4)
    Enthusiastic -------------------------------- (5)

- Item 77, Anxieties and Fears Re: Physical Aspects

    Intense disruptive anxiety ------------------ (1)
    Little or no anxiety------------------------- (5)

- Item 93, Effect of Pregnancy on Feeling of Well-Being

    Hypochondriacal ----------------------------- (1)
    Diminished vitality ------------------------- (2)
    Little effect ------------------------------- (3)
    Good effect --------------------------------- (4)
    Marked enhancement of feelings of
      well-being -------------------------------- (5)

- Item 94, Adaptability to Changes of Pregnancy

    Resents changes precipitated by the pregnancy- (1)
    Accepts and adjusts to the changes ---------- (3)
    Enthusiastically accepts and makes smooth
      adaptation to changes --------------------- (5)

Scale No.	Name of Factor	Schedule	No. of Items in Factor
9	Visualization of Self as Mother	A. IV.	4

- Item 80, Anxieties and Fears Re: Infant Feeding

Intense disruptive anxiety -------------------- (1)
Little or no anxiety ------------------------- (5)

- Item 83, Anxieties and Fears Re: Care of Infant-to-be

Intense disruptive anxiety -------------------- (1)
Little or no anxiety ------------------------- (5)

- Item 87, Clarity in Visualizing Self as Mother

Unable to picture self as a mother ------------ (1)
Can visualize self as mother but not
  clearly ------------------------------------- (3)
Visualizes self as mother with great clarity --- (5)

- Item 88, Confidence in Visualizing Self as Mother

Visualizes self as very unsure in that role ---- (1)
Visualizes self as handling the mother
  role sometimes confidently, sometimes
  uncertainly --------------------------------- (3)
Visualizes self handling the role of
  mother with confidence and assurance --------- (5)

Scale No.	Name of Factor	Schedule	No.of Items in Factor
10	Reaction to Characteristic Fears of Pregnancy	A. IV.	4

Ratings

- Item 77, Anxieties and Fears Re: Physical Aspects

  Intense disruptive anxiety --------------------- (1)
  Little or no anxiety -------------------------- (5)

- Item 79, Anxieties and Fears Re: Delivery

  Intense disruptive anxiety -------------------- (1)
  Little or no anxiety -------------------------- (5)

- Item 81, Anxieties and Fears Re: Unborn Baby

  Intense disruptive anxiety -------------------- (1)
  Little or no anxiety -------------------------- (5)

- Item 82, Anxieties and Fears Re: Sexual Role with Husband

  Intense disruptive anxiety -------------------- (1)
  Little or no anxiety -------------------------- (5)

Scale No.	Name of Factor	Schedule	No. of Items In Factor
11	Adaptation to Pregnancy Experience	B	4

Ratings

- Item 73, Predominant Attitude or Mood

Extremely rejecting of pregnancy ------------------(1)
Moderately rejecting-------------------------------(2)
Contented ---(3)
Very satisfied ------------------------------------(4)
Enthusiastic --------------------------------------(5)

- Item 77, Anxieties and Fears Re: Physical Aspects

Intense disruptive anxiety ------------------------(1)
Little or no anxiety ------------------------------(5)

- Item 93, Effect of Pregnancy on Feeling of Well-Being

Hypochondriacal -----------------------------------(1)
Diminished vitality -------------------------------(2)
Little effect -------------------------------------(3)
Good effect ---------------------------------------(4)
Marked enhancement of feelings of
well-being-------------------------------------(5)

- Item 94, Adaptability to Changes of Pregnancy

Resents changes precipitated by the pregnancy ------(1)
Accepts and adjusts to the changes ----------------(3)
Enthusiastically accepts and makes smooth
adaptation to changes -------------------------(5)

Scale No.	Name of Factor	Schedule	No. of Items in Factor
12	Confirmation of Sexual Identity	B	4

- Item 82, Anxieties and Fears Re: Sexual Role with Husband

    Ratings

    Intense disruptive anxiety --------------(1)
    Little or no anxiety -------------------(5)

- Item 92, Effect of Pregnancy on Sexual Relationship with Huiband

    Decreased satisfaction ------------------(1)
    No change -------------------------------(3)
    Increased satisfaction ------------------(5)

- Item 96, Pregnancy as: Confirmation of Feminine Identity

    Little significance ---------------------(1)
    Marked significance ---------------------(5)

- Item 97, Pregnancy as: Validation of Success as Related to Mother, Siblings, Others

    Little significance ---------------------(1)
    Marked significance---------------------(5)

Scale No.	Name of Factor	Schedule	No. of Items in Factor
13	Reaction to Pregnancy Fears	B	4

Ratings

- Item 77, Anxieties and Fears Re: Physical Aspects

  Intense disruptive anxiety ----------------------- (1)
  Little or no anxiety ---------------------------- (5)

- Item 79, Anxieties and Fears Re: Delivery

  Intense disruptive anxiety ---------------------- (1)
  Little or no anxiety---------------------------- (5)

- Item 81, Anxieties and Fears re: Unborn Baby

  Intense disruptive anxiety------------------------ (1)
  Little or no anxiety ---------------------------- (5)

- Item 86, Mother-Daughter Relationship During Pregnancy

  Support needs essentially unmet ------------------ (1)
  Support needs essentially met -------------------- (5)

Scale No.	Name of Factor	Schedule	No. of Items in Factor
14	Visualization of Self as Mother	B	3

Ratings

- Item 87, Clarity in Visualizing Self as Mother

    Unable to picture self as a mother ------------ (1)
    Can visualize self as mother but not clearly --- (3)
    Visualizes self as mother with great clarity --- (5)

- Item 88, Confidence in Visualizing Self as Mother

    Visualizes self as very unsure in that role ---- (1)
    Visualizes self as handling the mother role
    sometimes confidently, sometimes
    uncertainly ------------------------------- (3)
    Visualizes self handling the role of mother
    with confidence and assurance -------------- (5)

- Item 98, Pregnancy as: Extension of Self

    Little significance --------------------------- (1)
    Marked significance -------------------------- (5)

Scale No.	Name of Factor	Schedule	No. of Items in Factor
15	Response to Project Experience	C. II.	2

Ratings

- Item 116, Summary of Subjective Reaction of Woman in Response to Project

    Not at all useful or negative reaction -------- (1)
    Somewhat useful ------------------------------ (3)
    Clearly useful ------------------------------- (5)

- Item 117, Summary of Objective Evaluation Re Woman's Response to Project

    Not at all useful or negative reaction -------- (1)
    Somewhat useful ------------------------------ (3)
    Clearly useful ------------------------------- (5)

Scale No.	Name of Factor	Schedule	No. of Items in Factor
16	Overall Reaction to Pregnancy Experience	C.II.	4

<u>Ratings</u>

- Item 118, Subjective Reaction of Woman to
  Physical Aspects of the Pregnancy

    Extremely difficult------------------------- (1)
    Difficult ---------------------------------- (2)
    Neither especially difficult or easy -------- (3)
    Easy --------------------------------------- (4)
    Very easy ---------------------------------- (5)

- Item 119, Medical Evaluation of the Pregnancy

    Extremely difficult ------------------------ (1)
    Difficult ---------------------------------- (2)
    Neither especially difficult or easy -------- (3)
    Easy --------------------------------------- (4)
    Very easy ---------------------------------- (5)

- Item 120, Subjective Reaction to the Emotional
  Experience of the Pregnancy

    Sees pregnancy as unsatisfying experience ----(1)
    Matter-of-fact, neutral attitude ----------- (2)
    Fluctuating feelings ----------------------- (3)
    Moderately satisfying ---------------------- (4)
    Sees pregnancy as extremely satisfying
      experience ------------------------------ (5)

- Item 121, Objective Evaluation of Total
  Pregnancy Experience (Physical & Emotional)

    Extremely poor adjustment ------------------ (1)
    Poor adjustment ---------------------------- (2)
    Fair adjustment ---------------------------- (3)
    Good adjustment ---------------------------- (4)
    Excellent adjustment ----------------------- (5)

Scale No.	Name of Factor	Schedule	No. of Items in Factor
17	Infant Adjustment	E-I	8
19	" "	F-I	8
21	" "	G-I	8

- Item 204, Tension (Overall impression of how tense or relaxed baby is, including arms, legs, body, face, expression, tremors)

Ratings

Very tense	(1)
Moderately tense	(2)
Midpoint	(3)
Moderately relaxed	(4)
Very relaxed	(5)

- Item 205, Characteristic Mood (Interview and Observation)

Actively unhappy much of the time	(1)
Passively unhappy much of the time	(2)
Passively contented	(3)
Actively happy	(4)
Actively happy most of the time	(5)

- Item 207, Affective Stability

Highly unstable -- much fluctuation in mood from moment to moment	(1)
Moderately unstable	(2)
Tends to be stable, with some variability in mood	(3)
Stable -- mood predictable and consistent much of the time	(4)
Extremely stable -- unusual stability; very rare fluctuation in mood	(5)

- Item 210, Adaptability (Capacity to handle change, based on reactions to changes in scheduling - in expected sequences or daily routines; reactions to new foods, changes in formula; reactions to new situations - change in crib, removal of familiar objects from environment, move to new house; reactions to giving up established patterns of gratification; reactions to new people)

Very low adaptability. Usually shows strong and prolonged disturbance	(1)
Low adaptability. Tends to be disturbed by change. Shows moderate degree of disturbance	(2)
Midpoint -- sometimes accepts change without disturbance; more often shows mild disturbance	(3)
Moderate adaptability	(4)
High adaptability -- accepts all kinds of change well, without overt disturbance. Seems to respond positively	(5)

Scale No.	Name of Factor	Schedule	No. of Items in Factor
17 (cont'd.)	Infant Adjustment	E-I	8
19 "	" "	F-I	8
21 "	" "	G-I	8

- Item 211, Irritability - Ease of Being Upset
(Fries Test, Interview)

Very low threshold---very easily upset by
apparently minor annoyances ------------------ (1)
Moderately low threshold ----------------------- (2)
Average -- (3)
High threshold --------------------------------- (4)
Very high threshold---rarely upset; only upset
by very strong stimulus ---------------------- (5)

- Item 212, Vulnerability to Stress (Ease of disintegration
of functioning under conditions of fatigue, hunger, excessive stimulation, "psychological stress")

Extremely vulnerable - unusually low threshold
for stress. Slight stress results in rapid
and complete deterioration in functioning ----- (1)
Highly vulnerable. Tends to be easily disorganized
by mild stress -------------------------------- (2)
Midpoint --------------------------------------- (3)
Moderately low vulnerability. Tends to maintain integration in response to moderately
strong stress stimulation -------------------- (4)
Low vulnerability -- very high threshold.
Maintains integration, rarely shows deterioration in functioning, even in response to strong
stress -- (5)

- Item 213, Ease of Recovery from Being Upset

Long delay before recovery from being upset ----- (1)
Moderate delay before recovery from being upset - (3)
Very rapid recovery from being upset ----------- (5)

- Item 215, Overall Rating

Extremely poorly integrated infant. Characterized
by significant deviations in many areas of
functioning ----------------------------------- (1)
Poorly integrated. Tends to have more than
average number of problems of moderate
severity -------------------------------------- (2)
Midpoint. On the whole appears to be functioning
adequately, but having difficulties in a few
areas --- (3)
Well-integrated infant ------------------------- (4)
Extremely well-integrated; smoothly functioning
infant -- (5)

Scale No.	Name of Factor	Schedule	No. of Items in Factor
18	Infant Alertness	E-I	3
20	" "	F-I	3
22	" "	G-I	3

- Item 201, Object Responsiveness (Alertness, interest and responsiveness to objects)

Ratings

Very low. Completely unresponsive. Behavior
suggests lack of awareness of objects
or lack of discrimination between
animate and inanimate stimulation -----------------(1)
Low -- Tends to be passive in response to objects;
rarely shows excitement or positive response -------(2)
Midpoint --(3)
Moderately high -- sustained focus or attention.
Moderate interest -- interested much of the time,
indicated by sustained focus or attention to object,
change in activity level or facial expression ------(4)
Very high -- very much interested. Consistently shows
vigorous response to objects - e.g., marked change
in activity level, approach movements, excitement---(5)

- Item 208, Level of Social Responsiveness

Very low. Completely unresponsive. Behavior suggest
lack of awareness of people or lack of discrimination between animate and inanimate stimulation -----(1)
Low - tends to be passive in response to people;
rarely shows excitement or positive response ------(2)
Midpoint --(3)
Moderately high -- sustained focus or attention to
voice. Moderate interest -- interested in people
much of the time, indicated by sustained focus or
attention to voice or face, change in activity
level or facial expression ----------------------(4)
Very high -- very much interested in people. Consistently shows vigorous response to people - e.g.,
marked change in activity level, approach movements,
excitement.---(5)

- Item 214, Goal-Directedness (Bayley Scale)

Very low goal-directedness. No evidence of directed
effort to attain goals ----------------------------(1)
Low goal-directedness. Characteristically shows brief
interest, makes a few attempts at problem solution
but not to completion ------------------------------(2)
Moderate goal-directedness. Tends to be moderately
vigorous and persistent ---------------------------(3)
Highly goal-directed ------------------------------(4)
Very highly goal-directed. Extremely vigorous and
persistent in attempts to reach goal or solve
problem --(5)

Scale No.	Name of Factor	Schedule	No. of Items in Factor
23	Infant Functioning	E-II	3
24	" "	F-II	3
25	" "	G-II	3

- Item 249, Overall Evaluation: Feeding
  (as evidence of mother-child adaptation)   <u>Ratings</u>

    Erratic and difficult for mother and child -- (1)
    Some minor feeding problems but essentially
      both are coping with them ---------------- (3)
    Smooth; no feeding problems ---------------- (5)

- Item 250, Adjustment to Routines (Feeding,
  sleeping, bathing, toileting and play periods)

    Very poor adjustment to most routines ------- (1)
    Fair adjustment to most routines ----------- (3)
    Very good adjustment to most routines ------- (5)

- Item 252, Overall Integration of Infant

    Extremely poorly integrated infant. Charac-
      terized by significant deviation in many
      areas of functioning -------------------- (1)
    Poorly integrated. Tends to have more than
      average number of problems of moderate
      severity -------------------------------- (2)
    Midpoint. On the whole appears to be
      functioning adequately, but having difficul-
      ties in a few areas --------------------- (3)
    Well-integrated infant --------------------- (4)
    Extremely well-integrated, smoothly function-
      ing infant ------------------------------ (5)

Scale No.	Name of Factor	Schedule	No. of Items in Factor
26	Acceptance of Maternal Role	E-III	4

Ratings

- Item 303, Degree of Expression of Affection
  (Demonstrated feeling response of mother judged
  by the way she talks to and about baby, tenderness in handling for feeding, bath, etc.
  Facial expression and emotional tone in presence of baby)

    Not demonstrative; tends to be reserved -------------- (1)
    Matter-of-fact -- usually non-demonstrative ---------- (2)
    Ambivalent --- (3)
    Usually affectionate and expressive------------------ (4)
    Affectionate, warm, fondling, very expressive -------- (5)

- Item 314, Feelings in Regard to Care of Physical Needs
  of Child (Expression of resentment, distaste, or
  pleasure in performances of most routines in any
  or all areas of above aspects of infant care)

    Highly resentful; finds work distasteful or very
      onerous -- (1)
    Ambivalent --- (2)
    Accepts in matter-of-fact way ----------------------- (3)
    Moderate enjoyment of most routines ----------------- (4)
    Marked enjoyment of most routines; in general,
      finds them gratifying ------------------------------ (5)

- Item 315, Reaction to Total Dependency of Infant
  (Expression of pleasure and gratification or
  resentment re infant's total dependence)

    Highly resentful; feels trapped or burdened ---------- (1)
    Ambivalent --- (2)
    Accepts in matter-of-fact way ----------------------- (3)
    Moderately gratified -------------------------------- (4)
    Highly gratified at being needed -------------------- (5)

- Item 316, Reaction to Curtailment of Freedom

    Highly resentful ------------------------------------- (1)
    Mildly resentful ------------------------------------- (2)
    Ambivalent--- (3)
    Accepts in matter-of-fact way ----------------------- (4)
    Complete acceptance --------------------------------- (5)

Scale No.	Name of Factor	Schedule	No. of Items in Factor
27	Acceptance of Infant	E-III	4

Ratings

- Item 305, Acceptance-Rejection: Overall Evaluation

    Dissatisfied ----------------------------------- (1)
    Mildly dissatisfied ---------------------------- (2)
    Generally accepting with some ambivalence -------- (3)
    Satisfied -------------------------------------- (4)
    Complete acceptance without reservation ---------- (5)

- Item 306, Acceptance-Rejection: Sex

    Dissatisfied ----------------------------------- (1)
    Mildly dissatisfied ---------------------------- (2)
    Generally accepting with some ambivalence -------- (3)
    Satisfied -------------------------------------- (4)
    Complete acceptance without reservation ---------- (5)

- Item 307, Acceptance-Rejection: Appearance

    Dissatisfied ----------------------------------- (1)
    Mildly dissatisfied ---------------------------- (2)
    Generally accepting with some ambivalence -------- (3)
    Satisfied -------------------------------------- (4)
    Complete acceptance without reservation ---------- (5)

- Item 308, Acceptance-Rejection: Individual Characteristics

    Dissatisfied ----------------------------------- (1)
    Mildly dissatisfied ---------------------------- (2)
    Generally accepting with some ambivalence -------- (3)
    Satisfied -------------------------------------- (4)
    Complete acceptance without reservation ---------- (5)

Scale No.	Name of Factor	Schedule	No. of Items in Factor
28	Individualization of Infant	E-III	3

Ratings

- Item 310, Individualization (The extent to which mother perceives child as an individual and the extent to which her behavior towards the infant is guided by an awareness of his unique characteristics)

    Sees infant essentially as an undifferentiated part of self --------------------------------- (1)
    Sees infant sometimes as part of self, sometimes as separate --------------------------- (3)
    Views infant as separate in identity and needs-- (5)

- Item 317, Anxiety re Adequacy in her Role as Mother (Extent to which she worries or talks about her ability to be a good mother or other indicators of anxiety such as self-depreciatory remarks)

    Intense disruptive anxiety -------------------- (1)
    Moderate anxiety ------------------------------ (3)
    Little or no anxiety-------------------------- (5)

- Item 318, Anxiety re Baby (Extent to which she worries about baby's health, development, normality, dangers to infant, as seen by her statements, calls to doctor, questions of Infant Observer, etc.)

    Intense disruptive anxiety -------------------- (1)
    Moderate anxiety ------------------------------ (3)
    Little or no anxiety -------------------------- (5)

Scale No.	Name of Factor	Schedule	No. of Items in Factor
29	Responsiveness to Infant	E-III	4

- Item 301, Amount of Physical Contact

  Low--infant often not held for feedings
  and rarely for play or comforting -------------- (1)
  Moderate--infant held for feedings and
  necessary routines and occasionally for play ---- (3)
  High--child held during much of waking time;
  frequent play periods during day --------------- (5)

- Item 302, Quality of Physical Contact (Ease,
  awkwardness, tension or relaxation, pleasure or
  distaste, closeness or distance in physical
  contact with baby)

  Low physical involvement ------------------------- (1)
  Moderate physical involvement -- occasional
  closeness but some aloofness evident ----------- (3)
  Very close physical involvement ------------------ (5)

- Item 304, Sensitivity and Responsiveness (Includes
  awareness and responsiveness to infant's needs,
  the ability to interpret and respond accurately to
  needs and feelings of baby from simple cues-gestures,
  grimaces, body movement, cry)

  Fails to respond to obvious cues ------------------ (1)
  Moderately able to follow infant's cues ---------- (3)
  Highly sensitive and responsive to child's cues--
  tends to anticipate needs before obvious indications (like crying) --------------------------- (5)

- Item 311, Amount of Stimulation (Motor, social, visual
  and auditory, play and play materials)

  Little or none ----------------------------------- (1)
  Some --- (2)
  Moderate amount ---------------------------------- (3)
  Much --- (4)
  Very much -- (5)

Scale No.	Name of Factor	Schedule	No. of Items in Factor
30	Responsiveness to Infant	F-III	3

Ratings

- Item 301, Amount of Physical Contact

    Low--infant often not held for feedings and
      rarely for play or comforting ------------------- (1)
    Moderate--infant held for feedings and
      necessary routines and occasionally for play ----- (3)
    High--child held during much of waking time;
      frequent play periods during day --------------- (5)

- Item 302, Quality of Physical Contact
(Ease, awkwardness, tension or relaxation, pleasure or
distaste, closeness or distance in physical contact
with baby)

    Low physical involvement -------------------------- (1)
    Moderate physical involvement -- occasional
      closeness but some aloofness evident ------------ (3)
    Very close physical involvement ------------------- (5)

- Item 303, Degree of Expression of Affection
(Demonstrated feeling response of mother judged by the
way she talks to and about baby, tenderness in handling
for feeding, bath, etc. Facial expression and emotional
tone in presence of baby)

    Not demonstrative; tends to be reserved ----------- (1)
    Matter-of-fact -- usually non-demonstrative -------- (2)
    Ambivalent -- (3)
    Usually affectionate and expressive --------------- (4)
    Affectionate, warm, fondling, very expressive ------- (5)

Scale No.	Name of Factor	Schedule	No. of Items in Factor
31	Acceptance of Infant	F-III	3

Ratings

- Item 305, Acceptance-Rejection: Overall Evaluation

    Dissatisfied --- (1)
    Mildly dissatisfied --------------------------------- (2)
    Generally accepting with some ambivalence ------------ (3)
    Satisfied --- (4)
    Complete acceptance without reservation -------------- (5)

- Item 307, Acceptance-Rejection: Appearance

    Dissatisfied --- (1)
    Mildly dissatisfied --------------------------------- (2)
    Generally accepting with some ambivalence ------------ (3)
    Satisfied --- (4)
    Complete acceptance without reservation -------------- (5)

- Item 308, Acceptance-Rejection: Individual Characteristics

    Dissatisfied --- (1)
    Mildly dissatisfied --------------------------------- (2)
    Generally accepting with some ambivalence ------------ (3)
    Satisfied --- (4)
    Complete acceptance without reservation -------------- (5)

Scale No.	Name of Factor	Schedule	No. of Items in Factor
32	Confidence in Maternal Role	F-III	4

Ratings

- Item 304, Sensitivity and Responsiveness
  (Includes awareness and responsiveness to infant's
  needs, the ability to interpret and respond
  accurately to needs and feelings of baby from
  simple cues-gestures, grimaces, body movements, cry)

  Fails to respond to obvious cues -------------------- (1)
  Moderately able to follow infant's cues --------------(3)
  Highly sensitive and responsive to child's cues --
      tends to anticipate needs before obvious indica-
      tion (like crying) ------------------------------ (5)

- Item 314, Feelings in Regard to Care of Physical Needs
  of Child (Expression of resentment, distaste, or
  pleasure in performances of most routines in any or
  all areas of above aspects of infant care)

  Highly resentful; finds work distasteful or
      very onerous ------------------------------------- (1)
  Ambivalent --- (2)
  Accepts in matter-of-fact way ----------------------- (3)
  Moderate enjoyment of most routines ----------------- (4)
  Marked enjoyment of most routines; in general,
      finds them gratifying --------------------------- (5)

- Item 317, Anxiety re Adequacy in Her Role as Mother
  (Extent to which she worries or talks about her ability
  to be a good mother or other indicators of anxiety such
  as self-depreciatory remarks)

  Intense disruptive anxiety -------------------------- (1)
  Moderate anxiety ------------------------------------ (3)
  Little or no anxiety -------------------------------- (5)

- Item 318, Anxiety re Baby (Extent to which she worries
  about baby's health, development, normality, dangers to
  infant, as seen by her statements, calls to doctor,
  questions of Infant Observer, etc.)

  Intense disruptive anxiety -------------------------- (1)
  Moderate anxiety ------------------------------------ (3)
  Little or no anxiety -------------------------------- (5)

Scale No.	Name of Factor	Schedule	No. of Items in Factor
33	Acceptance of Maternal Role	F-III	3

Ratings

- Item 315, Reaction to Total Dependency of Infant
  (Expression of pleasure and gratification or
  resentment re infant's total dependence)

    Highly resentful; feels trapped or burdened ------- (1)
    Ambivalent --------------------------------------- (2)
    Accepts in matter-of-fact way -------------------- (3)
    Moderately gratified ----------------------------- (4)
    Highly gratified at being needed ----------------- (5)

- Item 316, Reaction to Curtailment of Freedom

    Highly resentful --------------------------------- (1)
    Mildly resentful --------------------------------- (2)
    Ambivalent --------------------------------------- (3)
    Accepts in matter-of-fact way -------------------- (4)
    Complete acceptance ------------------------------ (5)

- Item 320, Prevailing Mood Since Birth of Baby

    Severely depressed ------------------------------- (1)
    Mildly depressed --------------------------------- (2)
    Fluctuating moods -------------------------------- (3)
    Mainly happy mood -------------------------------- (4)
    Marked happiness and enthusiasm ------------------ (5)

Scale No.	Name of Factor	Schedule	No. of Items in Factor
34	Responsiveness to Infant	G-III	5

- Item 301, Amount of Physical Contact .... Ratings

    Low-- infant often not held for feedings and rarely
      for play or comforting ------------------------------- (1)
    Moderate--infant held for feedings and necessary
      routines and occasionally for play ------------------ (3)
    High--child held during much of waking time; frequent
      play periods during day ---------------------------- (5)

- Item 302, Quality of Physical Contact (ease, awkwardness,
    tension or relaxation, pleasure or distaste, closeness
    or distance in physical contact with baby)

    Low physical involvement ---------------------------- (1)
    Moderate physical involvement - occasional closeness
      but some aloofness evident ------------------------- (3)
    Very close physical involvement --------------------- (5)

- Item 303, Degree of Expression of Affection (Demonstrated
    feeling response of mother judged by the way she talks
    to and about baby, tenderness in handling for feeding,
    bath, etc. Facial expression and emotional tone in
    presence of baby)

    Not demonstrative; tends to be reserved ------------- (1)
    Matter-of-fact; usually non-demonstrative ----------- (2)
    Ambivalent -- (3)
    Usually affectionate and expressive ----------------- (4)
    Affectionate, warm, fondling, very expressive ------- (5)

- Item 314, Feelings in Regard to Care of Physical Needs
    of Child (Expression of resentment, distaste, or
    pleasure in performance of most routines in any or
    or all areas of above aspects of infant care)

    Highly resentful; finds work distasteful or very
      onerous --- (1)
    Ambivalent --- (2)
    Accepts in matter-of-fact way ----------------------- (3)
    Moderate enjoyment of most routines ----------------- (4)
    Marked enjoyment of most routines; in general, finds
      them gratifying ------------------------------------- (5)

- Item 315, Reaction to Total Dependency of Infant (Expression
    of pleasure and gratification or resentment re infant's
    total dependence)

    Highly resentful; feels trapped or burdened --------- (1)
    Ambivalent --- (2)
    Accepts in matter-of-fact way ----------------------- (3)
    Moderately gratified -------------------------------- (4)
    Highly gratified at being needed -------------------- (5)

Scale No.	Name of Factor	Schedule	No. of Items in Factor
35	Acceptance of Infant and Maternal Role	G-III	6

-Item 305, Acceptance-Rejection: Overall Evaluation

```
Dissatisfied ------------------------------------------- (1)
Mildly dissatisfied ----------------------------------- (2)
Generally accepting with some ambivalence ------------- (3)
Satisfied --------------------------------------------- (4)
Complete acceptance without reservation --------------- (5)
```

-Item 307, Acceptance-Rejection: Appearance

```
Dissatisfied ------------------------------------------- (1)
Mildly dissatisfied ----------------------------------- (2)
Generally accepting with some ambivalence ------------- (3)
Satisfied --------------------------------------------- (4)
Complete acceptance without reservation --------------- (5)
```

-Item 308, Acceptance-Rejection: Individual Characteristics

```
Dissatisfied ------------------------------------------- (1)
Mildly dissatisfied ----------------------------------- (2)
Generally accepting with some ambivalence ------------- (3)
Satisfied --------------------------------------------- (4)
Complete acceptance without reservation --------------- (5)
```

-Item 315, Reaction to Total Dependency of Infant
(Expression of pleasure and gratification or resentment re
infant's total dependence)

```
Highly resentful; feels trapped or burdened ----------- (1)
Ambivalent -------------------------------------------- (2)
Accepts in matter-of-fact way ------------------------- (3)
Moderately gratified ---------------------------------- (4)
Highly gratified at being needed ---------------------- (5)
```

-Item 316, Reaction to Curtailment of Freedom

```
Highly resentful -------------------------------------- (1)
Mildly resentful -------------------------------------- (2)
Ambivalent -------------------------------------------- (3)
Accepts in matter-of-fact way ------------------------- (4)
Complete acceptance ----------------------------------- (5)
```

-Item 320, Prevailing Mood Since Birth of Baby

```
Severely depressed ------------------------------------ (1)
Mildly depressed -------------------------------------- (2)
Fluctuating moods ------------------------------------- (3)
Mainly happy mood ------------------------------------- (4)
Marked happiness and enthusiasm ----------------------- (5)
```

Scale No.	Name of Factor	Schedule	No. of Items in Factor
36	Individualization	G-III	3

-Item 310, Individualization (The extent to which mother perceives child as an individual and the extent to which her behavior towards the infant is guided by an awareness of his unique characteristics)

Rating

                            an

Sees infant essentially as/undifferentiated part of self -- (1)

Sees infant sometimes as part of self, sometimes as separate -- (3)

Views infant as separate in identity and needs ------- (5)

-Item 317, Anxiety re Adequacy in Her Role as Mother (Extent to which she worries or talks about her ability to be a good mother or other indicators of anxiety such as self-depreciatory remarks)

Intense disruptive anxiety ------------------------- (1)

Moderate anxiety ----------------------------------- (3)

Little or no anxiety ------------------------------- (5)

-Item 318, Anxiety re Baby (Extent to which she worries about baby's health, development, normality, dangers to infant, as seen by her statements, calls to doctor, questions of Infant Observer, etc.)

Intense disruptive anxiety ------------------------- (1)

Moderate anxiety ----------------------------------- (3)

Little or no anxiety ------------------------------- (5)

Scale No.	Name of Factor	Schedule	No. of Items in Factor
37	Husband-Wife Adaptation	E-III	6
39	" "	F-III	6
41	" "	G-III	6

- Item 323, Wife's Reaction to Husband's New Role   Ratings

    Critical, jealous or hostile ----------------------- (1)
    Ambivalent feelings towards husband in new role ----- (3)
    Highly pleased with and proud of husband as father -- (5)

- Item 324, Husband's Reaction to Wife as Mother

    Critical, jealous or hostile ----------------------- (1)
    Somewhat negative reaction ------------------------- (2)
    Ambivalent --- (3)
    Appreciative, supportive --------------------------- (4)
    Enthusiastic, highly appreciative and supportive ---- (5)

- Item 327, Responsiveness of Husband to Wife

    Hostile -- (1)
    Laregly unresponsive ------------------------------- (2)
    Ambivalent --- (3)
    Essentially responsive ----------------------------- (4)
    Fully responsive ----------------------------------- (5)

- Item 328, Responsiveness of Wife to Husband

    Hostile -- (1)
    Largely unresponsive ------------------------------- (2)
    Ambivalent --- (3)
    Essentially responsive ----------------------------- (4)
    Fully responsive ----------------------------------- (5)

- Item 329, Overall Husband-Wife Adaptation (Based on
willingness of each to identify and to respond to the
desires of the other; mutuality of emotional investment
in infant and home; degree of mutual affection)

    Very poor adaptation ------------------------------- (1)
    Poor adaptation ------------------------------------ (2)
    Intermittently good -------------------------------- (3)
    Good --- (4)
    Excellent -- (5)

- Item 330, Effect of Infant on Family Homeostasis (Subjective
reaction to the change, experienced as disruptive or not)

    Highly disruptive ---------------------------------- (1)
    Disruptive --- (2)
    Somewhat disruptive but not greatly disturbing ------ (3)
    Changes largely anticipated and not experienced as
      disruptive -------------------------------------- (4)
    Family life readily adaptive to arrival of infant --- (5)

Scale No.	Name of Factor	Schedule	No. of Items in Factor
38	Reaction to Paternal Role	E-III	2
40	" " " "	F-III	2
42	" " " "	G-III	2

Ratings

- Item 325, Husband's Reaction to His Role as Father

 Highly resentful; disappointed or depressed ---------- (1)
 Somewhat disappointed and dissatisfied -------------- (2)
 Ambivalent --- (3)
 Satisfied -- (4)
 Marked gratification --------------------------------- (5)

- Item 326, Husband's Reaction to Baby

 Rejecting -- (1)
 Unresponsive --- (2)
 Accepting -- (3)
 Very well satisfied --------------------------------- (4)
 Enthusiastic, proud --------------------------------- (5)

Scale No.	Name of Factor	Schedule	No of Items in Factor
43	Ego Strength (Postnatal)	G-IV	9

- Item 420.5, Emotional Adaptation - Characteristic
Way of Expressing Feeling   Ratings

      Adapted ------------------------------(Rate 1-5, from low to high

- Item 421, Anxiety

      Intense disruptive anxiety---------------------------- (1)
      Little or no anxiety --------------------------------- (5)

- Item 427, Flexibility

      Highly resistant to change or stress ----------------- (1)
      Accommodates after some resistance or delay to change
        and ordinary stress ------------------------------- (3)
      Easy accommodation to change (able to "roll with the
        punches") --- (5)

- Item 428, Sense of Humor

      Little or none --------------------------------------- (1)
      Moderately good -------------------------------------- (3)
      Keen --- (5)

- Item 430, Covert, Underlying Dependency Pattern (Based on
Psychological Tests - Psychologist's Rating Only)

      Very strong dependency wishes ----------------------- (1)
      Moderate dependency wishes -------------------------- (3)
      Little dependency wishes ---------------------------- (5)

- Item 431, Ability to Meet Own Needs, Including Pleasure

      Poor --- (1)
      Average -- (3)
      Marked ability --------------------------------------- (5)

- Item 435, Acceptance of Own Identity

      Strong rejection of identity ------------------------ (1)
      Ambivalence -- (3)
      Positive attitudes - self acceptance ---------------- (5)

- Item 438, Achievement of an Adult Role

      Childishness --- (1)
      Ambivalence as to adult status ---------------------- (3)
      Distinctly mature and clear as to adult status ------- (5)

- Item 443, Overall Evaluation of Adaptive Behavior

      Defenses basically inadequate to deal with needs ----- (1)
      Defenses highly adequate ---------------------------- (5)

Scale No.	Name of Factor	Schedule	No. of Items in Factor
44	Nurturance	G-IV, G-III	8

- Item 420.4, Emotional Adaptation - Characteristic
Way of Expressing Feeling   Ratings

    Tender and affectionate   (Rate from 1-5, from low to high)

- Item 424, Gratification in Female Sexuality

    No enjoyment, or actual distaste -------------------- (1)
    Moderate enjoyment ---------------------------------- (3)
    Marked enjoyment ------------------------------------ (5)

- Item 328, Responsiveness of Wife to Husband

    Hostile --- (1)
    Largely unresponsive ------------------------------ (2)
    Ambivalent -- (3)
    Essentially responsive ---------------------------- (4)
    Fully responsive ---------------------------------- (5)

- Item 426, Responsiveness to Others - Giving and Nurturant Quality

    Ungiving -- (1)
    Moderately giving --------------------------------- (3)
    Highly generous; very giving ---------------------- (5)

- Item 436, Sense of Success as a Wife

    Evaluates self as unsuccessful -------------------- (1)
    Evaluates self as fairly adequate ----------------- (3)
    Evaluates self as highly successful --------------- (5)

- Item 437, Sense of Success as a Homemaker

    Evaluates self as poor ---------------------------- (1)
    Evaluates self as average ------------------------- (3)
    Evaluates self as successful ---------------------- (5)

- Item 441, Ability to Give Help and Support

    Unable to give ------------------------------------ (1)
    Gives grudgingly ---------------------------------- (2)
    Gives on own terms -------------------------------- (3)
    Gives on request ---------------------------------- (4)
    Gives freely on sensing need ---------------------- (5)

*- Item 416. Number of Predominant Defenses Used

    1 - Denial   6 - Regression
    2 - Repression   7 - Isolation
    3 - Intellectualization   8 - Acting Out
    4 - Reaction formation   9 - Other
    5 - Projection

*In all scales but this, the items were added to obtain the total factor scale score. In this scale, the factor scale score is arrived at by subtracting high the total score of the first 8 ratings the number of predominant defenses.

Scale No.	Name of Factor	Schedule	No. of Items in Factor
45	Family Adaptation	H	5

-Item 512, Mother's Predominant Mood　　　　　　　　　　　Ratings

```
Depressed ----------------------------------------------------- (1)
Mildly depressed --------------------------------------------- (2)
Fairly or intermittently happy ----------------------------- (3)
Essentially happy -------------------------------------------- (4)
Very happy and enthusiastic -------------------------------- (5)
```

-Item 513, Mother's Satisfaction with Current Situation

```
Highly dissatisfied ------------------------------------------ (1)
Moderately dissatisfied -------------------------------------- (2)
Ambivalent --------------------------------------------------- (3)
Moderately satisfied ----------------------------------------- (4)
Very well satisfied ------------------------------------------ (5)
```

-Item 515, New Family Homeostasis

```
Unbalanced, "rocky", unsatisfying for any one or more mem-
  bers of the family ---------------------------------------- (1)
Sometimes in equilibrium and sometimes satisfying for all -- (3)
Well-balanced, satisfying for all most of the time --------- (5)
```

-Item 516, Husband-Wife Adaptation

```
Very poor adaptation ----------------------------------------- (1)
Poor --------------------------------------------------------- (2)
Intermittently good ------------------------------------------ (3)
Good --------------------------------------------------------- (4)
Excellent ---------------------------------------------------- (5)
```

-Item 517, The Family as Environment for Infant's Development
(Overall rating based on mother's adaptation to infant, maternal
role; father's adaptation to his role as father; husband-wife
adaptation)

```
Poor --------------------------------------------------------- (1)
Mediocre ----------------------------------------------------- (2)
Fairly good -------------------------------------------------- (3)
Good --------------------------------------------------------- (4)
Excellent ---------------------------------------------------- (5)
```

340

Scale No.	Name of Factor	Schedule	No. of Items in Factor
46	Mother-Infant Adaptation	H	4

Ratings

- Item 504, Feeding Adjustment

Infant's feeding adjustment erratic and difficult
most of the 6 months' period --------------------- (1)
Some minor feeding problems persisting through much
of the 1st 6 months but essentially infant is
coping with them ------------------------------- (3)
Smooth adjustment; little or no feeding problems
throughout 1st 6 months ------------------------ (5)

- Item 507, Basic Evaluation of the Functioning of the
Infant - Overall Rating

Extremely poorly integrated infant. Characterized
by significant deviations in many areas of
functioning ------------------------------------ (1)
Poorly integrated. Tends to have more than average
number of problems of moderate severity ---------- (2)
Midpoint. On the whole appears to be functioning
adequately but having difficulties in a few areas - (3)
Well-integrated infant ---------------------------- (4)
Extremely well-integrated; smoothly functioning
infant -- (5)

- Item 508, Adequacy in Coping with Physical Needs of Infant

Very inept and inadequate ------------------------- (1)
Average in coping performance --------------------- (3)
Highly competent and effective -------------------- (5)

- Item 509, Adequacy in Coping with Emotional Needs of Infant

Very unresponsive and insensitive ----------------- (1)
Fairly sensitive, aware and prompt in responsiveness- (3)
Highly sensitive, aware, prompt in responsiveness --- (5)

APPENDIX D. INITIAL FACTOR ANALYSES

SCHEDULE A-I. Experiences in Being Mothered and Ego Development

Item	Loadings				h^2*	N	Mean	S.D.
	I	II	III	IV				
Wife's Experiences Being Mothered:								
1 Her Mother's Anxiety	.36	-.40	-.46		.52	62	3.49	1.03
2 Her Mother's Empathy	.79				.68	62	2.84	1.09
3 Her Mother's Closeness	.83				.74	62	3.26	1.24
4 Her Mother's Intrusiveness			-.80		.68	62	3.31	1.20
5 Her Mother's Reaction to Maternal Role	.85				.76	62	3.69	1.02
6 Mother-Daughter Relationship: to Age 12	.82				.73	62	3.21	1.12
7 Mother-Daughter Relationship: After Age 12	.83				.72	62	3.00	1.17
Wife's Ego Development:								
9 School Achievement				.54	.36	62	3.71	0.86
10 School Adjustment				.67	.46	62	3.92	0.73
11 Work Performance			.66		.60	62	3.23	1.09
12 Peer Relationships				.66	.55	62	3.00	0.91
13 Interest in Younger Children		.84			.73	62	3.48	1.04
14 Experience with Younger Children		.71			.55	61	2.90	1.42
Proportion of common variance	.45	.20	.18	.17	1.00			
Factor Scale	1	2	--	3				

*Sum of h^2 = 8.08

SCHEDULE A-II.   Prenatal Current Personality

Item	Loadings I	Loadings II	Loadings III	h²*	N	Mean	S.D.
No. of Defenses			-.46	.28	62	2.81	0.97
20.1 Hostility				.29	62	3.56	0.93
20.2 Impulsive		.76		.62	62	3.23	1.21
20.3 Repressed		-.57		.41	62	2.76	1.14
20.4 Tender and Affectionate	.66	-.49	.56	.61	62	3.32	0.91
20.5 Adapted	.73		.42	.63	62	3.08	0.89
21 Anxiety			.52	.57	61	2.73	0.96
24 Gratification Female Sexuality	.42			.36	62	2.93	0.83
25 Responsiveness to Husband			.76	.78	62	3.13	0.93
26 Responsiveness to Others			.51	.43	62	2.98	0.82
27 Flexibility	.73			.58	62	3.03	1.04
28 Sense of Humor	.70			.61	62	2.37	0.96
30 Covert Dependency	.63			.45	60	1.80	0.76
31 Ability to Meet Own Needs	.60			.40	59	3.13	0.86
34 Insight into Self	.44			.31	62	2.44	0.80
35 Acceptance of Own Identity	.72			.59	62	3.39	0.80
36 Sense of Success as Wife			.73	.64	62	3.65	0.77
37 Sense of Success as Homemaker	.71		.57	.41	62	3.44	1.03
38 Achievement of Adult Role		-.44		.66	62	2.87	0.86
39 Capacity for Closeness			.47	.43	62	3.34	0.87
41 Ability to Give Help				.30	62	3.39	0.82
43 Overall Evaluation of Adaptive Behavior	.79			.78	62	2.97	0.99
Proportion of common variance	.50	.16	.34	1.00			
Factor Scale	4	--	5				

*Sum of h² = 11.24

SCHEDULE A-III. Prenatal – Husband's Impact

Item	Loadings I	Loadings II	h^2*	N	Mean	S.D.
45 Empathy	.83		.68	62	3.03	0.99
46 Communication	.57		.34	62	3.60	0.98
47 Affection	.80		.67	62	3.61	0.88
48 Hostility	.64		.43	62	3.48	1.17
49 Sexual Adjustment	.53		.31	62	2.97	0.87
50 Decision Process	.74		.60	62	3.19	1.11
51 Reaction to Wife in re Pregnancy		.75	.57	62	3.65	0.87
52 Reaction to Baby-to-be		.74	.60	62	3.71	0.78
53 Extent Husband Allows Dependency	.59	.46	.56	61	3.38	1.13
54 Husband's Fostering Self-Conf. Wife as Mother	.56	.46	.53	61	4.08	0.97
55 Feelings re Sharing Wife		.69	.50	62	3.53	1.21
56 Congruence Pregnancy w/Current Life		.62	.39	62	3.52	1.04
57 Congruence Pregnancy w/Long-time Plans		.70	.52	62	4.42	0.76
59 Husband-Wife Adaptation	.79		.71	62	3.52	1.04
Proportion of common variance	.58	.42	1.00			
Factor Scale	6	7				

*Sum of h^2 = 7.41

SCHEDULE A-IV. First Trimester Pregnancy Experience

Item		Loadings			h^2*	N	Mean	S.D.
	I	II	III	IV				
73 Predominant Mood	.76				.68	62	3.52	0.86
75 Clarity of Image	.50	.48			.33	57	2.74	1.16
77 Anxieties & Fears re Phys. Aspects			.61		.67	62	3.47	1.22
78 Anxieties & Fears re Body Image					.26	62	3.65	1.09
79 Anxieties & Fears re Delivery			.79		.70	62	3.11	1.17
80 Anxieties & Fears re Infant Feeding		.65			.43	61	4.03	0.93
81 Anxieties & Fears re Unborn Baby			.55		.39	61	3.30	1.24
82 Anxieties & Fears re Sex Role w/ Husb.			.54		.35	59	4.12	1.02
83 Anxieties & Fears re Care of Infant		.68			.59	62	3.58	1.14
86 Mother-Daught. Relat. during Preg.				.50	.28	60	3.07	1.22
87 Clarity Visualization Self as Mother		.60			.46	62	2.82	1.00
88 Confidence " Self as Mother		.64			.63	61	3.05	1.07
90 Responsibility Patterns					.20	62	4.26	0.99
92 Pregnancy Effect on Sex					.19	60	2.45	0.95
93 Pregnancy Effect Feeling of Well-Being	.67				.56	62	2.61	0.95
94 Adaptability to Pregnancy Changes	.78				.66	62	3.06	0.87
95 Evidence of Growth New Family Identif.				.58	.42	62	2.90	0.99
96 Preg. as Confirm. Feminine Identity					.25	61	3.51	1.07
97 Preg. as Validation of Success				.56	.38	62	3.92	1.08
98 Preg. as Extension of Self					.16	60	3.65	0.97
99 Preg. as Validation of Couple		.47		.46	.45	62	3.39	1.45
Proportion of common variance	.30	.29	.24	.17	1.00			
Factor Scale	8	9	10	--				

*Sum of h^2 = 9.04

SCHEDULE B. Second Trimester Pregnancy Experience

Item	I	II	III	IV	V	h^{2}*	N	Mean	S.D.
73 Predominant Mood	.71					.80	60	3.68	0.98
75 Clarity of Image	.77				.42	.46	57	2.84	1.24
77 Anxieties & Fears re Phys. Aspects				.40		.78	60	3.72	1.09
78 Anxieties & Fears re Body Image				.59		.39	60	3.85	1.12
79 Anxieties & Fears re Delivery		.63				.47	60	3.07	0.99
80 Anxieties & Fears re Infant Feed.				.57		.46	60	4.10	0.95
81 Anxieties & Fears re Unborn Baby						.35	60	3.22	0.96
82 Anxieties & Fears re Sex Role w/Husband			.40			.34	60	4.13	0.98
83 Anxieties & Fears re Care of Infant		.60				.43	60	3.85	0.86
86 Mother-Daught.Relationship during Pregnancy				.44		.24	58	3.24	1.27
87 Clarity Visualiz. Self as Mother					.87	.85	59	3.31	1.00
88 Confidence " Self as Mother	.48				.47	.63	60	3.38	0.90
90 Responsibility Pattern	.50					.27	60	4.15	0.95
92 Pregnancy Effect on Sex			.42			.29	59	2.46	1.10
93 Pregnancy Effect Feeling Well-Being	.70					.57	60	3.13	1.11
94 Adaptability to Preg. Changes	.78					.74	60	3.43	1.16
95 Evid. of Growth New Fam. Identif.		.83				.83	60	3.42	1.00
96 Preg. as Confirm. Femin. Identity			.55			.39	59	3.22	1.08
97 Preg. as Validat. of Success			.66			.45	60	4.03	1.16
98 Preg. as Extension of Self					.53	.37	58	3.52	1.05
99 Preg. as Validation of Couple		.75				.67	60	3.72	1.10
59 Husband-Wife Adaptation						.31	60	3.77	0.81
Proportion of common variance	.29	.22	.16	.16	.17	1.00			
Factor Scale	11	--	12	13	14				

*Sum of h^{2} = 11.09

SCHEDULE C-II. Summary and Overall Evaluation of Pregnancy Experience

Item	Loadings		h^{2*}	N	Mean	S.D.
	I	II				
116 Subjective Reaction - Response to Project		.92	.85	62	3.71	1.01
117 Objective Eval. - Response to Project		.92	.85	62	3.63	1.00
118 Subjective Reaction - Phys. Aspects Preg.	.90		.83	62	3.65	1.09
119 Medical Evaluation of Pregnancy	.70		.50	62	3.95	1.08
120 Subjective Reaction to Emo. Exper. of Preg.	.84		.72	62	3.68	1.25
121 Objective Eval. Total Pregnancy Exper.	.90		.82	62	3.69	1.03
Proportion of common variance	.63	.37	1.00			
Factor Scale	16	15				

*Sum of h^2 = 4.57

SCHEDULE E-I. Infant Characteristics

Item	Loadings		h²*	N	Mean	S.D.
	I	II				
Chronological Age			.06	59	10.14	0.92
200 DIQ		.73	.54	57	101.70	10.58
201 Object Responsiveness		.60	.37	55	2.15	0.73
202 DMQ		.53	.29	56	118.02	11.63
204 Tension	.39		.17	56	3.02	0.70
205 Characteristic Mood	.45		.23	56	2.77	0.54
207 Affective Stability	.63		.40	55	2.96	0.67
208 Level of Social Responsiveness		.57	.34	56	2.00	0.69
209 Appropriate Social Responsiveness		.46	.22	55	3.13	0.47
210 Adaptability	.50		.26	53	4.17	0.75
211 Irritability	.58		.43	53	3.19	0.98
212 Vulnerability to Stress	.79		.62	55	3.09	0.78
213 Ease of Recovery from Upset	.69		.47	56	3.84	0.93
214 Goal Directedness		.62	.40	56	1.70	0.63
215 Overall Rating	.65		.45	56	3.57	0.74
Proportion of common variance	.55	.45	1.00			
Factor Scale	17	18				

*Sum of h² = 5.29

SCHEDULE F-I. Infant Characteristics

Item	I	II	III	h²*	N	Mean	S.D.
Chronological Age			.60	.53	58	30.22	1.43
200 DIQ		.68		.49	57	101.25	10.34
201 Object Responsiveness		.83		.69	57	2.75	0.76
202 DMQ			-.58	.45	57	116.79	9.54
204 Tension	.60			.39	58	3.10	0.85
205 Characteristic Mood	.53		-.42	.54	58	2.95	0.80
207 Affective Stability	.89			.81	58	2.98	0.87
208 Level of Social Responsiveness		.63		.42	58	3.16	0.59
209 Appropriate Social Responsiveness			-.58	.34	55	3.22	0.50
210 Adaptability	.63			.43	58	3.66	0.81
211 Irritability	.70			.49	56	2.91	0.79
212 Vulnerability to Stress	.76			.62	57	2.93	0.73
213 Ease of Recovery from Upset	.76			.58	58	3.78	0.88
214 Goal Directedness		.60		.38	57	2.12	0.63
215 Overall Rating	.80			.66	58	3.48	0.80
Proportion of common variance	.55	.28	.17	1.00			
Factor Scale	19	20	--				

*Sum of h² = 7.82

SCHEDULE G-I. Infant Characteristics

Item	Loadings I	Loadings II	Loadings III	h²*	N	Mean	S.D.
Chronological Age				.30	58	60.17	1.60
200 DIQ		.40		.43	57	106.65	7.55
201 Object Responsiveness		.51	.78	.62	58	3.62	0.64
202 DMQ		.46		.36	57	107.39	12.11
204 Tension	.69			.49	58	3.40	0.86
205 Characteristic Mood	.60			.61	58	3.57	0.94
207 Affective Stability	.82			.67	57	3.37	0.86
208 Level of Social Responsiveness				.57	58	3.84	0.62
209 Appropriate Social Responsiveness		.65	.72	.48	56	3.16	0.50
210 Adaptability	.62			.39	57	3.93	0.73
211 Irritability	.74			.59	57	3.21	0.86
212 Vulnerability to Stress	.73			.57	57	3.32	0.66
213 Ease of Recovery from Upset	.57		.78	.36	56	4.02	0.82
214 Goal Directedness				.61	58	3.19	0.63
215 Overall Rating	.78			.76	58	3.78	0.73
Proportion of common variance	.52	.25	.23	1.00			
Factor Scale	21	--	22				

*Sum of h² = 7.81

SCHEDULE E-II. Pediatric Evaluation of Infant

Item	Loadings I	Loadings II	h^2*	N	Mean	S.D.
232 Cry		-.57	.33	56	1.04	0.42
233 Sleeps through Night			.33	55	14.33	2.08
235 Sleeps through Night - Age Onset	.53		.07	41	4.83	1.34
237 Initial Feeding Difficulty			.27	57	2.44	0.76
242 Cry Pattern	.52	.71	.52	56	1.75	0.48
243 Colic		.80	.66	57		
245 Mother's Confidence Coping w/Maternal Role	.66		.48	55	4.13	0.98
246 Mother's React. to Infant re Acceptance	.61		.48	54	5.57	0.77
249 Overall Evaluation: Feeding	.90		.81	41	3.88	1.23
250 Infant's Adjustment to Routines	.80		.64	36	4.28	0.78
251 Developmental Status			.02	41	3.07	0.41
252 Overall Integration of Infant	.51		.33	40	3.78	0.80
Proportion of common variance	.64	.36	1.00			
Factor Scale	23	--	--			

*Sum of h^2 = 4.94

SCHEDULE **F-II.** Pediatric Evaluation of Infant

	Item	Loadings		h^{2*}	N	Mean	S.D.
		I	II				
232	Cry		.82	.71	56	0.89	0.53
233	Sleeps through Night			.09	53	13.58	1.98
242	Cry Pattern		.73	.53	55	1.91	0.29
245	Mother's Confid. Coping w/Maternal Role	.43	.57	.51	54	4.33	0.82
246	Mother's React. to Infant re Acceptance	.68	.42	.64	55	4.35	0.84
249	Overall Evaluation: Feeding Behavior	.78		.62	38	4.13	1.28
250	Infant's Adjustment to Routines	.79		.68	36	4.53	0.81
251	Developmental Status	.61		.38	38	3.21	0.47
252	Overall Integration of Infant	.80		.65	38	3.95	0.80
	Proportion of common variance	.61	.39	1.00			
	Factor Scale	24	--				

*Sum of h^2 = 4.81

SCHEDULE G-II. Pediatric Evaluation of Infant

Item		Loadings			h^{2*}	N	Mean	S.D.
		I	II	III				
232	Cry		-.74		.62	58	0.76	0.51
233	Sleeps through Night		-.61		.39	58	13.40	1.36
242	Cry Pattern		.75		.60	58	1.95	0.22
245	Mother's Confidence Coping w/Maternal Role	.68			.63	57	4.51	0.68
246	Mother's Reaction to Infant re Acceptance	.36		.44	.32	58	4.55	0.65
249	Overall Evaluation: Feeding Behavior	.77			.60	57	4.40	0.94
250	Infant's Adjustment to Routines	.76			.59	51	4.73	0.60
251	Developmental Status			.80	.69	56	3.36	0.59
252	Overall Integration of Infant	.36		.53	.48	57	4.02	0.79
Proportion of common variance		.40	.32	.28	1.00			
Factor Scale		25	--	--				

*Sum of h^2 = 4.92

SCHEDULE E-III. Mother-Infant Adaptation

Item	I	II	III	IV	h^2*	N	Mean	S.D.
			Loadings					
300 Coordination of Routines	.49				.27	59	4.10	0.96
301 Amount of Physical Contact				.67	.50	59	3.83	0.77
302 Quality of Physical Contact	.40	.37		.44	.50	59	3.95	0.88
303 Degree of Expression of Affection	.62			.41	.55	59	4.02	0.84
304 Sensitivity and Responsiveness	.46			.58	.67	59	3.27	0.81
305 Accept.-Reject.: Overall Evaluation		.87			.85	59	4.54	0.73
306 Accept.-Reject. re Sex		.68			.63	59	4.75	0.66
307 Accept.-Reject. re Appearance		.58			.48	59	4.71	0.53
308 Accept.-Reject. re Indiv. Char.		.73			.69	54	4.37	0.89
310 Individualization			.78		.62	56	3.13	1.12
311 Amount of Stimulation	.47				.35	59	3.07	0.89
312 Coping w/ Phys. Needs Infant: Feeding	.40				.25	58	3.81	0.96
313 Coping w/ Phys. Needs Infant: Routines					.27	59	4.10	0.89
314 Feelings re Physical Care	.72				.58	59	3.68	0.97
315 React. Total Dependency of Infant	.74	.35			.72	59	3.81	1.25
316 React. Curtailment of Freedom	.68	.35			.59	59	3.71	1.20
317 Anxiety re Adequacy in Role as Mother			.52		.48	59	3.88	1.07
318 Anxiety re Baby			.54		.41	59	4.24	0.93
320 Prevailing Mood	.49				.35	59	3.56	0.90
Proportion of common variance	.36	.28	.16	.20	1.00			
Factor Scale	26	27	28	29				

*Sum of h^2 = 9.76

SCHEDULE F-III. Mother-Infant Adaptation

Item		Loadings				h2*	N	Mean	S.D.
		I	II	III	IV				
300	Coordination of Routines			.45		.29	59	4.10	0.94
301	Amount of Physical Contact	.75				.59	59	3.64	0.83
302	Quality of Physical Contact	.77				.63	59	3.88	0.81
303	Degree of Expression of Affection	.66			.40	.70	59	3.98	0.75
304	Sensitivity & Responsiveness		.42	.50		.54	58	3.26	0.89
305	Accept.-Reject.: Overall Evaluation		.77			.60	59	4.49	0.70
306	Accept.-Reject. re Sex		.55			.31	59	4.81	0.43
307	Accept.-Reject. re Appearance					.36	59	4.76	0.54
308	Accept.-Reject. re Indiv. Char.		.89			.81	59	4.31	0.88
310	Individualization					.22	58	3.33	1.08
311	Amount of Stimulation	.44		.40		.28	59	3.47	0.94
312	Coping w/ Phys. Needs Infant: Feeding		.47	.41		.41	59	3.85	1.10
313	Coping w/ Phys. Needs Infant: Routines	.48		.53		.41	59	4.44	0.65
314	Feelings re Physical Care					.54	59	3.41	1.05
315	React. Total Dependency of Infant				.54	.44	59	3.81	1.21
316	React. Curtailment of Freedom				.85	.76	59	3.78	1.04
317	Anxiety re Adequacy in Role as Mother			.64		.46	59	4.12	0.95
318	Anxiety re Baby			.65		.44	59	4.49	0.82
320	Prevailing Mood			.48	.62	.62	59	3.53	0.84
	Proportion of common variance	.27	.27	.25	.21	1.00			
	Factor Scale	30	31	32	33				

*Sum of h2 = 9.41

SCHEDULE G-III. Mother-Infant Adaptation

Item		Loadings I	Loadings II	Loadings III	h^2*	N	Mean	S.D.
300	Coordination of Routines		.73		.64	57	4.26	0.88
301	Amount of Physical Contact	.59			.36	57	3.28	0.88
302	Quality of Physical Contact	.84			.75	57	3.88	0.91
303	Degree of Expression of Affection	.78			.70	57	4.11	0.70
304	Sensitivity & Responsiveness	.45			.41	57	3.44	0.89
305	Accept.-Reject.: Overall Evaluation		.69	.38	.70	57	4.41	0.75
306	Accept.-Reject. re Sex		.42		.28	57	4.82	0.50
307	Accept.-Reject. re Appearance		.55		.43	57	4.77	0.46
308	Accept.-Reject. re Individual Characteristics	.40	.60		.61	57	4.37	0.79
310	Individualization			.48	.31	55	3.22	0.92
311	Amount of Stimulation	.49			.24	57	3.56	0.95
312	Coping w/ Physical Needs Infant: Feeding	.45			.27	57	4.35	0.69
313	Coping w/ Physical Needs Infant: Routines	.39			.20	56	4.55	0.66
314	Feelings re Physical Care	.57			.48	57	3.65	0.92
315	Reaction Total Depend. of Infant	.54	.61		.72	57	3.93	1.08
316	React. Curtailment of Freedom		.53		.42	57	3.86	1.11
317	Anxiety re Adequacy in Role as Mother			.53	.37	57	4.37	0.82
318	Anxiety re Baby			.51	.26	57	4.49	0.76
320	Prevailing Mood	.36	.58		.48	57	3.53	0.76
	Proportion of common variance	.45	.38	.17	1.00			
	Factor Scale	34	35	36				

*Sum of h^2 = 8.63

SCHEDULE E-III. Husband-Wife Adaptation

	Item	Loadings		h^{2*}	N	Mean	S.D.
		I	II				
323	Wife's Reaction to Husband's New Role	.81		.70	59	4.29	0.79
324	Husband's Reaction to Wife's New Role	.81		.66	58	3.97	0.95
325	Husband's Reaction fo Role as Father		.84	.75	57	4.44	0.76
326	Husband's Reaction to Baby		.91	.84	59	4.44	0.82
327	Response of Husband to Wife	.82		.73	58	4.00	0.82
328	Response of Wife to Husband	.84		.71	59	4.02	0.78
329	Overall Husband-Wife Adaptation	.88		.79	59	3.90	0.90
330	Infant Effect on Family Homeostasis	.56		.42	59	3.64	1.17
	Proportion of common variance	.68	.32	1.00			
	Factor Scale	37	38				

*Sum of h^2 = 5.60

SCHEDULE F-III. Husband-Wife Adaptation

Item	Loading I	Loading II	h^2*	N	Mean	S.D.
323 Wife's Reaction to Husband's New Role	.76		.64	59	4.19	0.88
324 Husband's Reaction to Wife's New Role	.63	.47	.62	59	4.03	0.96
325 Husband's Reaction to Role as Father		.78	.71	59	4.37	0.67
326 Husband's Reaction to Baby		.86	.75	59	4.39	0.72
327 Response of Husband to Wife	.87		.81	59	3.85	0.94
328 Response of Wife to Husband	.74		.59	59	3.92	0.88
329 Overall Husband-Wife Adaptation	.98		.98	59	3.78	1.02
330 Infant Effect on Family Homeostasis	.56	.48	.55	59	3.73	1.26
Proportion of common variance	.65	.35	1.00			
Factor Scale	39	40				

*Sum of h^2 = 5.65

SCHEDULE G-III. Husband-Wife Adaptation

Item	Loadings		h^{2*}	N	Mean	S.D.
	I	II				
323 Wife's Reaction to Husband's New Role	.72	.41	.69	57	4.25	0.76
324 Husband's Reaction to Wife's New Role	.70		.51	57	4.05	0.85
325 Husband's Reaction to Role as Father	.48	.69	.71	57	4.46	0.68
326 Husband's Reaction to Baby		.92	.84	57	4.63	0.70
327 Response of Husband to Wife	.88		.81	57	3.68	0.98
328 Response of Wife to Husband	.75		.56	57	3.98	0.83
329 Overall Husband-Wife Adaptation	.92		.89	56	3.79	0.95
330 Infant Effect on Family Homeostasis	.71		.64	57	3.86	1.09
Proportion of common variance	.70	.30	1.00			
Factor Scale	41	42				

*Sum of h^2 = 5.65

SCHEDULE G-IV. Six Month Evaluation: Current Peronality

Item	Loadings				h²*	N	Mean	S.D.
	I	II	III	IV				
Number of Defenses	.44			.51	.31	56	2.57	0.87
420.1 Emotional Adapt. - Hostile & Explosive		.60			.58	56	3.57	0.91
420.2 Emotional Adapt. - Impulsive		.62		.58	.73	56	3.86	0.96
420.3 Emotional Adapt. - Repressed				-.67	.50	56	2.84	1.04
420.4 Emotional Adapt. - Tender & Affect.	.71	.69			.54	56	3.30	0.68
420.5 Emotional Adapt. - Adapted	.48	.64			.72	56	2.96	0.76
421 Anxiety					.47	56	3.02	0.90
424 Gratification in Female Sexuality	.59		.46		.63	57	2.89	0.90
426 Responsiveness to Others	.78				.70	57	3.07	0.84
427 Flexibility	.52			-.48	.62	57	2.77	0.98
428 Humor		.51		-.60	.69	57	2.12	0.96
430 Covert Depend. (Psychologist's Rating)		.63			.44	57	1.86	0.91
431 Ability to Meet Own Needs		.40	.43		.64	57	3.10	0.94
434 Insight into Self	.46				.31	57	2.30	0.80
435 Acceptance of Own Identity	.41		.56		.66	57	3.35	0.74
436 Sense of Success as a Wife			.70		.62	57	3.79	0.94
437 Sense of Success as Homemaker			.62		.40	57	3.91	1.07
438 Achievement of Adult Role		.73			.63	57	2.96	0.63
439 Capacity for Closeness	.56				.60	57	2.89	0.90
440 Ability to Take Help					.39	57	3.07	1.10
441 Ability to Give Help	.70				.66	57	3.37	0.75
443 Overall Eval. of Adapt. Behavior	.47	.57			.80	57	2.76	0.93
400 Sense of Success as Mother		.36			.22	56	4.34	0.61
Proportion of common variance	.31	.32	.17	.20	1.00			
Factor Scale	43	44	--	--				

*Sum of h² = 12.86

SCHEDULE H. Six Month, Summary Evaluation

Item	Loadings I	II	III	h²*	N	Mean	S.D.
504 Infant Adjustment : Feeding		.78		.61	58	3.72	0.85
505 Infant Adjustment : Illness History				.12	57	4.33	0.91
506 Infant Adjustment : Overall Physical Status			-.44	.25	58	4.67	0.51
507 Infant Adjustment : Overall Rating		.57		.39	58	3.64	0.69
508 Mother's Adequacy – Coping w/Phys. Needs Infant		.83		.70	58	3.98	0.76
509 Mother's Adequacy – Coping w/Emo. Needs Infant		.45		.44	58	3.05	0.87
510 Pregnancy Experience – Subjective Reaction	.42			.22	57	3.84	1.01
511 Delivery Experience – Subjective Reaction			-.50	.25	57	3.89	1.31
512 Mother's Predominant Mood	.78			.64	58	3.17	0.82
513 Mother's Satisfaction w/ Cur. Situation	.75			.62	58	3.64	0.97
514 Personality Integration		.41	.48	.45	58	3.34	0.61
515 New Family Homeostasis	.87			.82	58	3.45	1.05
516 Husband-Wife Adaptation	.85			.77	58	3.43	0.88
517 Family as Environ. Infant Development	.74			.68	58	2.95	0.85
518 Responsiveness to Project – Subjective			.56	.36	58	3.55	0.92
519 Responsiveness to Project – Objective			.67	.56	58	3.21	0.95
521 Closeness to Own Mother				.13	56	3.18	1.10
Proportion of common variance	.48	.30	.22	1.00			
Factor Scale	45	46	--				

*Sum of h² = 8.02

APPENDIX E: TABLE 1. *Formulas for Calculating Super Factor Scale Scores*

Super Factor	Name	Multiple Correlation		Factor Score Formula	Factor Scales Involved
		R	R²		
I	Feminine Identification	.84	.71	2(F.S. 9) + 3(F.S. 45)	9: Visualization of Self as Mother (4) A-IV 45: Family Adaptation (5) II
II	Infant Adjustment	.85	.73	1(F.S. 19) + 2(F.S. 31) + 2(F.S. 46)	19: Infant Adjustment (S) F-I 31: Acceptance of Infant (3) F-III 46: Mother-Infant Adaptation (4) H
III	Woman's Intelligence	.95	.90	WAIS-FSIQ Score	None
IV	Infant Alertness (at 1 month of age)	.83	.69	9(F.S. 18) + 1(DMQ at 1 mo.)	18: Infant Alertness (3) E-I DMQ E-I
VI	Maternal Responsiveness	.84	.71	2(F.S. 26) + 7(F.S. 29)	26: Acceptance of Maternal Role (4) E-III 29: Responsiveness to Infant (4) E-III
IX	Husband-Wife Adaptation (Prenatal)	.70	.50	1(F.S. 6) + 1(F.S. 7)	6: Husband's Responsiveness to Wife (9) A-III 7: Husband's Responsiveness to Pregnancy (5) A-III
XI	Husband's Responsiveness to Paternal Role	.84	.70	3(F.S. 40) + 1(F.S. 42)	40: Reaction to Paternal Role (2) F-III 42: Reaction to Paternal Role (2) G-III
VIII	Woman's Self-Confidence	.73	.53	1(F.S. 1) + 1(F.S. 13) + 2(F.S. 32)	1: Perception of Being Mothered (5) A-I 13: Reaction to Pregnancy Fears (4) B 32: Confidence in Maternal Role (4) F-III

Those Containing Both Pre- and Postnatal Variables:

I. FEMININE IDENTIFICATION

	Prenatal	L*		Postnatal	L
A. IV.	Visualizing Self as Mother	.64	H.	Family Adaptation	.78
A. II.	Nurturance	.60	G. IV.	Nurturance	.73
A. II.	Ego Strength	.57	G. III.	Acceptance of Maternal Role	.71
A. IV.	Adaptation to Pregnancy Experience	.52	F. III.	Acceptance of Maternal Role	.63
C. II.	Overall Reaction to Pregnancy Experience	.52	E. III.	Acceptance of Maternal Role	.50
			G. III.	Husband-Wife Adaptation	.67
			F. III.	Husband-Wife Adaptation	.56
			E. III.	Husband-Wife Adaptation	.56
			G. IV.	Ego Strength	.64
			G. III.	Responsiveness to Infant	.59

VIII. WOMAN'S SELF-CONFIDENCE

	Prenatal	L		Postnatal	L
A. I.	Perception of Experience in Being Mothered	.64	F. III.	Confidence in Maternal Role	.49
B.	Reaction to Fears of Pregnancy	.53			

IX. HUSBAND-WIFE ADAPTATION

	Prenatal	L		Postnatal	L
A. III.	Husband's Response to Wife	.67	E. III.	Husband-Wife Adaptation	.45
A. III.	Husband's Response to Pregnancy	.52	F. III.	Husband-Wife Adaptation	.40
			E. I.	DIQ	-.49

Those Containing Postnatal Variables Only:

II. INFANT ADJUSTMENT

	Postnatal	L
F. I.	Infant Adjustment	.71
G. I.	Infant Adjustment	.67
E. I.	Infant Adjustment	.55
H.	Mother-Infant Adaptation	.66
F. III.	Acceptance of Infant	.62
F. II.	Infant Functioning	.51
F. III.	Confidence in Maternal Role	.47

IV. INFANT ALERTNESS (1 month)

	Postnatal	L
E. I.	Infant Alertness	.75
E. I.	DMQ	.69
E. III.	Individualization of Infant	.50

VI. MATERNAL RESPONSIVENESS

	Postnatal	L
E. III.	Responsiveness to Infant	.81
F. III.	Responsiveness to Infant	.43
G. III.	Responsiveness to Infant	.41
E. III.	Acceptance of Maternal Role	.65
F. III.	Confidence in Maternal Role	.45
E. II.	Infant Functioning	.43

XI. HUSBAND'S RESPONSIVENESS TO PATERNAL ROLE

	Postnatal	L
F. III.	Reaction to Paternal Role	.82
G. III.	Reaction to Paternal Role	.55
E. III.	Reaction to Paternal Role	.44
F. III.	Acceptance of Infant	.52

That Containing Prenatal Variables Only:

IV. WOMAN'S INTELLIGENCE

	Prenatal	L
FSIQ		.95
VIQ		.87
PIQ		.66
A. I.	School & Peer Relationships	.62
A. II.	Ego Strength	.56
A. IV.	Reaction to Characteristic Fears of Pregnancy	.47

*L is factor loading of variable on super factor.

APPENDIX E: TABLE 3. Means, Standard Deviations, and Significant Differences between Counseled and Control Groups

Scale No.	Name	Schedule	Counseled			Control			F or t	p Level
			Mean	S.D.	S.D.²	Mean	S.D.	S.D.²		
1	Perception of Experience Being Mothered	A-I	15.38	5.37	28.89	17.25	4.19	17.53		
2	Interest in Children	A-I	6.24	2.21	4.90	6.36	2.30	5.28		
3	School and Peer Relationships	A-I	10.52	1.55	2.40	10.79	2.17	4.69		
4	Ego Strength	A-II	25.69	5.68	32.29	25.54	6.91	47.81		
5	Nurturance	A-II	20.17	4.67	21.79	20.39	4.79	22.91		
6	Husband's Responsiveness to Wife	A-III	29.41	6.70	44.82	32.79	6.08	36.92	$t = 2.05$	.05
7	Husband's Responsiveness to Pregnancy	A-III	19.03	3.32	11.03	19.04	3.47	12.04		
8	Adaptation to Pregnancy Experience	A-IV	13.41	2.65	7.04	12.43	3.13	9.81		
9	Visualization of Self as Mother	A-IV	13.48	3.00	9.04	13.54	3.53	12.48		
10	Reaction to Characteristic Fears of Pregnancy	A-IV	14.03	3.72	13.82	14.25	2.86	8.19		
11	Adaptation to Pregnancy Experience	B	13.62	3.40	11.53	14.75	3.77	14.19		
12	Confirmation of Sexual Identity	B	13.59	3.38	11.39	13.96	2.65	7.00		
13	Reaction to Pregnancy Fears	B	12.93	2.45	6.00	14.25	2.95	8.71		
14	Visualization of Self as Mother	B	10.48	2.20	4.83	10.25	2.15	4.64		
15	Response to Project Experience	C-II	8.21	1.54	2.38	6.54	1.55	2.41	$t = 3.98$	.001
16	Overall Reaction to Pregnancy Experience	C-II	15.62	3.68	13.53	14.92	3.41	11.62		
17	Infant Adjustment	E-I	26.59	3.03	9.18	26.39	4.26	18.17		
18	Infant Alertness	E-I	5.76	1.55	2.40	6.11	1.73	2.99		

Scale No.	Name	Schedule	Counseled			Control			F or t	p Level
			Mean	S.D.	S.D.²	Mean	S.D.	S.D.²		
19	Infant Adjustment	F-I	25.27	4.59	21.06	26.36	5.22	27.20		
20	Infant Alertness	F-I	8.13	1.68	2.84	8.04	1.43	2.04		
21	Infant Adjustment	G-I	27.90	4.64	21.52	29.25	4.65	21.60		
22	Infant Alertness	G-I	10.83	1.28	1.65	10.54	1.45	2.11		
23	Infant Functioning	E-II	12.17	1.95	3.79	11.68	1.94	3.78		
24	Infant Functioning	F-II	11.93	2.22	4.92	13.21	1.69	2.84	$t = 2.72$	.05
25	Infant Functioning	G-II	13.10	2.09	4.38	13.25	1.46	2.12	$F = 206$	.02
26	Acceptance of Maternal Role	E-III	15.10	3.82	14.60	15.57	3.28	10.77		
27	Acceptance of Infant	E-III	18.31	2.35	5.51	18.39	2.33	5.43		
28	Individualization of Infant	E-III	11.00	2.14	4.57	11.46	2.49	6.18		
29	Responsiveness to Infant	E-III	14.28	2.34	5.49	13.96	2.70	7.30		
30	Responsiveness to Infant	F-III	11.52	2.13	4.54	11.54	1.97	3.89		
31	Acceptance of Infant	F-III	13.34	1.76	3.09	13.71	1.82	3.32		
32	Confidence in Maternal Role	F-III	15.00	2.96	8.79	15.79	2.17	4.69		
33	Acceptance of Maternal Role	FIII	11.31	2.19	4.79	11.36	2.45	6.02		
34	Responsiveness to Infant	G-III	18.34	3.54	12.52	19.36	3.40	11.57		
35	Acceptance of Infant and Maternal Role	G-III	24.07	3.95	15.64	25.50	3.63	13.15		
36	Individualization	G-III	12.31	1.51	2.29	11.75	1.80	3.23		
37	Husband-Wife Adaptation	E-III	23.86	4.96	24.62	24.18	3.45	11.93	$F = 2.06$	.02
38	Reaction to Paternal Role	E-III	9.21	0.98	0.96	8.68	1.83	3.34	$F = 3.47$	.002
39	Husband-Wife Adaptation	F-III	22.76	4.81	23.12	24.57	5.01	25.07		
40	Reaction to Paternal Role	F-III	9.24	1.90	3.62	8.75	1.27	1.60	$F = 2.26$	.02
41	Husband-Wife Adaptation	G-III	22.93	4.91	24.06	24.36	4.10	16.83		
42	Reaction to Paternal Role	G-III	9.14	1.13	1.21	9.00	1.44	2.07		
43	Ego Strength	G-IV	25.34	5.23	27.31	25.29	5.75	33.10		
44	Nurturance	G-IV	21.86	4.65	21.62	21.96	3.56	12.70		
45	Family Adaptation	H	16.48	3.82	14.76	16.89	4.00	16.03		
46	Mother-Infant Adaptation	H	14.14	2.55	6.48	14.82	2.31	5.34		
	Birthweight (oz.)	—	112.41	14.84	220.18	110.82	15.47	239.41		
	DIQ	E-I	102.34	10.09	101.81	102.14	11.10	123.31		
	DMQ	E-I	118.34	10.53	110.88	117.29	12.60	158.73		

Scale No.	Name	Schedule	Counseled			Control			F or t	p Level
			Mean	S.D.	S.D.²	Mean	S.D.	S.D.²		
	DIQ	F-I	100.86	9.73	94.69	101.93	10.40	108.14		
	DMQ	F-I	116.83	8.30	68.93	116.36	11.16	124.53		
	DIQ	G-I	105.86	6.22	38.69	107.93	8.52	72.59		
	DMQ	G-I	103.45	21.58	465.90	109.36	11.86	140.68	F = 3.30	.002
	Psychological Aspects of Delivery (Item 150)	D	4.07	1.00	1.00	-3.57	1.17	1.37		
	Medical Aspects of Delivery (Item 151)	D	4.24	1.12	1.26	3.96	0.88	0.78		
	VIQ	—	114.17	12.74	162.29	116.96	15.16	229.96		
	PIQ	—	110.72	11.08	122.71	110.50	12.17	148.04		
	FSIQ	—	113.45	11.54	133.18	114.96	12.74	162.41		

APPENDIX E: TABLE 4. Intercorrelations of Super Factor Scores, Stresses, and Medical Symptoms

	I	II	III	IV	VI	VIII	IX	XI	Total Stresses	Med. Sym.	Name of Super Factor
I	—	.12	.32	-.07	.27	.38	.30	.31	-.43	-.19	Feminine Identification
II		—	-.04	-.04	.21	.33	.06	.28	.06	.00	Infant Adjustment
III			—	-.07	.19	.17	.16	.04	-.13	-.36	Woman's Intelligence
IV				—	.14	.07	-.04	-.12	.14	.06	Infant Alertness (1 mo.)
VI					—	.41	.18	.42	.04	-.04	Maternal Responsiveness
VIII						—	.20	.38	-.11	-.17	Woman's Self-Confidence
IX							—	.28	-.45	.09	Husband-Wife Adaptation (3 mos. prenatal)
XI								—	-.04	.05	Husband's Response to Paternal Role
Total Number of Stresses									—	.21	
Number of Medical Symptoms										—	

Intercorrelations

INDEX